W9-APW-394

Manchester Medieval Sources Series

series advisers Rosemary Horrox and Janet L. Nelson

This series aims to meet a growing need amongst students and teachers of medieval history for translations of key sources that are directly usable in students' own work. It provides texts central to medieval studies courses and focuses upon the diverse cultural and social as well as political conditions that affected the functioning of all levels of medieval society. The basic premise of the series is that translations must be accompanied by sufficient introductory and explanatory material, and each volume, therefore, includes a comprehensive guide to the sources' interpretation, including discussion of critical linguistic problems and an assessment of the most recent research on the topics being covered.

already published in the series

Simon Barton and Richard Fletcher *The world of El Cid: Chronicles of the Spanish Reconquest*

J. A. Boyle *Genghis Khan: history of the world conquerer*

Trevor Dean *The towns of Italy in the later Middle Ages*

John Edwards *The Jews in Western Europe, 1400–1600*

Paul Fouracre and Richard A. Gerberding *Late Merovingian France*

Chris Given-Wilson *Chronicles of the Revolution, 1397–1400: the reign of Richard II*

P. J. P. Goldberg *Women in England, c. 1275–1525*

Janet Hamilton and Bernard Hamilton *Christian dualist heresies in the Byzantine world c. 650–c. 1450*

Rosemary Horrox *The Black Death*

Graham A. Loud and Thomas Wiedemann *The history of the tyrants of Sicily by 'Hugo Falcandus', 1153–69*

Michael Staunton *The lives of Thomas Becket*

R. N. Swanson *Catholic England: faith, religion and observance before the Reformation*

Elizabeth van Houts *The Normans in Europe*

Jennifer Ward *Women of the English nobility and gentry, 1066–1500*

David Warner *Ottonian Germany*

THE BLACK DEATH

Medieval Sources*online*

Complementing the printed editions of the Medieval Sources series, Manchester University Press has developed a web-based learning resource which is now available on a yearly subscription basis.

Medieval Sources*online* brings quality history source material to the desktops of students and teachers and allows them open and unrestricted access throughout the entire college or university campus. Designed to be fully integrated with academic courses, this is a one-stop answer for many medieval history students, academics and researchers keeping thousands of pages of source material 'in print' over the Internet for research and teaching.

titles available now at Medieval Sources*online include*

John Edwards *The Jews in Western Europe 1400–1600*

Paul Fouracre and Richard A. Gerberding *Late Merovingian France: History and hagiography 640–720*

Chris Given-Wilson *Chronicles of the Revolution 1397–1400: The reign of Richard II*

P. J. P. Goldberg *Women in England c. 1275–1525*

Janet Hamilton and Bernard Hamilton *Christian dualist heresies in the Byzantine world c. 650–c. 1450*

Rosemary Horrox *The Black Death*

Graham A. Loud and Thomas Wiedemann *The history of the tyrants of Sicily by 'Hugo Falcandus' 1153–69*

Janet L. Nelson *The Annals of St-Bertin: Ninth-century histories, volume I*

Timothy Reuter *The Annals of Fulda: Ninth-century histories, volume II*

R. N. Swanson *Catholic England: faith, religion and observance before the Reformation*

Jennifer Ward *Women of the English nobility and gentry 1066–1500*

visit the site at *www.medievalsources.co.uk*
for further information and subscription prices

THE BLACK DEATH

translated and edited by Rosemary Horrox

Manchester University Press

Copyright © Rosemary Horrox 1994

The right of Rosemary Horrox to be identified as the author of this work has been asserted by her in accordance with the Copyright, Designs and Patents Act 1988.

Published by Manchester University Press
Altrincham Street, Manchester M1 7JA, UK
www.manchesteruniversitypress.co.uk

British Library Cataloguing-in-Publication Data is available

ISBN 978 0 7190 3497 8 hardback

ISBN 978 0 7190 3498 5 paperback

First published by Manchester University Press in hardback 1994

The publisher has no responsibility for the persistence or accuracy of URLs for any external or third-party internet websites referred to in this book, and does not guarantee that any content on such websites is, or will remain, accurate or appropriate.

Typeset by Servis Filmsetting Ltd, Stockport, Cheshire
Printed by TJ Books Ltd, Padstow, Cornwall

FOR MY MOTHER
IN MEMORY OF MY FATHER

Contents

Foreword   *page* xi
Preface and acknowledgements   xii

PART ONE: NARRATIVE ACCOUNTS   1

I: The plague in continental Europe   14

  1. The arrival of the plague   14
  2. The plague in Florence   26
  3. The plague in Padua   34
  4. The plague in Sicily   35
  5. The plague in Avignon   41
  6. The plague seen from Tournai   45
  7. The plague in France according to Jean de Venette   54
  8. The plague in France according to the Great Chronicle   58
  9. The plague in central Europe   59

II: The plague in the British Isles   62

  10. The arrival of the plague at Bristol   62
  11. The arrival of the plague near Bristol   62
  12. The arrival of the plague in Dorset   63
  13. The plague spreads   63
  14. The plague spreads to London   64
  15. The plague in York   65
  16. The plague according to Thomas Walsingham   65
  17. The plague seen from Lincolnshire   66
  18. The plague at Meaux Abbey   67
  19. The plague seen from Rochester   70
  20. The plague according to John of Reading   74
  21. The plague according to Henry Knighton   75
  22. The plague according to Geoffrey le Baker   80
  23. The plague in Ireland   82
  24. The plague in Scotland   84
  25. The second pestilence, 1361   85
  26. The third pestilence, 1369   88

27. The fourth pestilence, 1374-79   88
28. The fifth pestilence, 1390-93   91

PART TWO: EXPLANATIONS AND RESPONSES   93

III: The religious response   111

29. Intercessionary processions (1)   111
30. Intercessionary processions (2)   112
31. The importance of prayer   113
32. The response in Exeter   115
33. A Voice in Rama   115
34. Edward III to the bishops, 5 September 1349   117
35. Causes for gratitude   118
36. Processions against the plague in 1361   119
37. A call for prayers in 1375   120
38. Masses to be said in time of plague   120
39. A prayer against pestilence to the Virgin Mary   124

40. A prayer made to St Sebastian against the mortality   125
41. The sins of the times   126
42. The failings of the clergy   127
43. Divine disapproval of tournaments   130
44. Indecent clothing as a cause of the 1348-49 epidemic   131
45. Indecent clothing as a cause of later outbreaks   131
46. The disobedience of children   134
47. The Sermon of Reason   135
48. The sins of the English   137
49. Be watchful   143
50. Pilgrimage to Merevale, 1361   148
51. A wholesome medicine against the plague   149
52. The flagellants   150
53. The flagellants in England   153
54. Rumours of Antichrist   154
55. Millenarianism in Germany   155

IV: Scientific explanations   158

56. The report of the Paris medical faculty, October 1348   158
57. Simon de Covino, *De Judicio Solis*   163

58. The astrological causes of the plague, Geoffrey de Meaux 167
59. The dangers of corrupted air 173
60. Earthquakes as the cause of plague 177
61. The transmission of plague 182
62. The treatise of John of Burgundy, 1365 184
63. A fifteenth-century treatise on the pestilence 193
64. Ordinances against the spread of plague, Pistoia, 1348 194
65. Plague regulations of Bernabò Visconti, Lord of Milan 203
66. London butchery regulations, 1371 203
67. Parliamentary statute of 1388 205

V: Human agency 207

68. Well-poisoning 207
69. The persecution of the Jews 208
70. Measures taken against the Jews in Lausanne 210
71. Examination of Jews captured in Savoy 211
72. Letter from Cologne to Strassburg 219
73. Mandate of Clement VI concerning the Jews 221
74. Accusations of well-poisoning against the poor 222
75. An accusation of well-poisoning 223

PART THREE: CONSEQUENCES 227

VI: The impact of the plague 248

76. Petrarch on the death of friends 248
77. The death of Princess Joan 250
78. The Wakebridge family 250
79. The death of Abbot Michael of St Albans 252
80. Deaths among the nuns of Malling 253
81. Deaths in Walsham le Willows 256
82. The plague in Lancashire 262
83. A new burial ground in London 266
84. Burial problems in Worcester 268
85. A new burial ground in Newark 269
86. Consecration of new burial grounds in Yorkshire 269
87. A shortage of priests to hear confession 271
88. A papal licence for extra ordinations 273
89. The shortage of secular clergy 273
90. A failed chantry endowment 274

91. The deaths of officials   275
92. A wrong redressed   276
93. An immediate fall in revenue   277
94. Decayed rents   280
95. Unwillingness to take on vacant properties   283
96. The renegotiation of labour services   285
97. A reduction in labour services   286
98. The ordinance of labourers, 18 June 1349   287
99. An episcopal response to the ordinance   290

VII: Repercussions   292

100. Land values before and after the plague   292
101. An increase in value   295
102. Diminished vills   296
103. An early enclosure   299
104. Appropriations of parishes   300
105. An amalgamation of parishes   302
106. Amendments to a chantry foundation, 1351   304
107. Amendment of statutes governing a chantry, 1365   304
108. *Effrenata*   306
109. Unwillingness to take on parochial responsibilities   310
110. William Langland on gadding clergy   310
111. Simon Sudbury increases priests' wages   311
112. The statute of labourers, 1351   312
113. A case under the ordinance of labourers   317
114. Cases brought under the statute of labourers   318
115. A selection of cases from Lincolnshire   319
116. Cases before the justices in Kesteven, 1371   321
117. Additions to the statute of labourers, 1388   323
118. Difficulties in finding tenants   326
119. Rebellious serfs at Wawne   331
120. The sin of pride   339
121. Sumptuary legislation, 1363   340
122. The unprepared death   342
123. The prepared death   344
124. 'It is good to think on death'   347
125. The fate of the sinful   347

Suggestions for further reading   353
Index   357

Foreword

Reversing the trends of a generation ago, current scholarship on the Black Death underlines its huge impact on later medieval Europe. In the present volume, Rosemary Horrox draws on up-to-date research, at the same time making a substantial contribution to it. She brings together a mass of hitherto untranslated, and in many cases unpublished, documents: on this basis readers will form their own assessment. From narrative accounts, often of heart-rending immediacy, the book proceeds to a variety of contemporary responses, drawn from many parts of Christian Europe. Students of intellectual history will find a wealth of pseudo-scientific explanations of the plague ranging from astrological conjunctions, through earthquakes releasing toxic vapours, to well poisoning by Jews – there is, tragically, plentiful documentation here of medieval anti-semitism. Commonest of all were moralising attempts to explain and justify unprecedented disaster in terms of Christian cosmology. Focusing on England, an exceptionally well documented region, Rosemary Horrox offers a wide range of evidence for the plague's variegated repercussions on the economy and, no less complex, on social and religious conduct. Contemporaries reported anomie and amorality, but also intensified piety. The evidence speaks for itself up to a point: Rosemary Horrox's commentary captures survivors' sense of mingled vulnerability and guilt. In this remarkable book, a uniquely difficult subject is presented with the requisite detachment, sensitivity and psychological insight. A distinguished political historian breaks new ground. The later Middle Ages will be studied more fruitfully as a result.

Janet L. Nelson, King's College London

Preface and acknowledgements

This book has grown remorselessly in the making. As the sources piled up I even found myself wildly contemplating the possibility of a second volume. Fortunately my long-suffering editor Jane Thorniley-Walker nipped that particular notion in the bud with her usual tact and good humour – which counts as not the least of her kindnesses during the book's long gestation. But to bring the Black Death within the limits of a single volume has called for some ruthless restrictions and omissions. The sources printed here are predominantly concerned with the British experience of plague in the fourteenth century; and that, sadly, because of the imbalance in the available evidence, very largely means the *English* experience. I have included a chapter of chronicle accounts from elsewhere in Europe, and have drawn some other material from European sources, particularly for Sections IV and V. But Europe remains under-represented here, with nothing from Scandinavia, the Iberian peninsula or eastern Europe. I have also made no attempt to document the movement of the plague across Asia and the Middle and Near East, although the extant sources would have added a valuable extra dimension to the western perspective.

Even within these geographical and chronological limits some aspects of the plague have proved easier to illustrate than others. Much (one might even say most) of the recent scholarly work on the Black Death has been on its demographic and economic impact – areas which demand the comparative study of a mass of manorial and other non-chronicle material from before and after 1348-49. In a volume like this, where a single manorial court roll would occupy many pages, the raw material of such analysis can only be sampled. This raises a related problem. Pride of place must be given to sources which show the plague having an effect. It would be hard to justify the inclusion of very much material which does not mention it at all. The result may be to exaggerate the seriousness and universality of the plague's impact. For historians, as for journalists, the headline, 'Small plague, not many dead' is not news.

In preparing the translations I have used the modern local spelling of place names except where an English version is so well-established that an alternative would seem odd to English-speaking readers. Thus I have referred to Florence and Cologne, rather than to Firenze and Köln. Personal names represent an even greater dilemma for the translator – should the Aragonese ruler of Sicily be John, Juan or Giovanni? And should the Hungarian ruler of Naples, described by a Flemish cleric based in Avignon be Andrew, András, Andrea or André? Any solution is likely to produce some inconsistencies. I have adopted the English spelling for saints, emperors and kings, where to do otherwise might read oddly, but have used the prevalent local spelling for lesser figures. Thus I refer to King John of France, but the Bishop of Tournai appears in his local spelling as Jean des Prés. Similarly, the Virgin Mary appears as such throughout, but place names incorporating her name use the local form, as in Santa Maria la Nuova. Names which have defied identification altogether have been printed in italics.

The English coinage mentioned in the sources is, of course, pre-decimal and I have made no attempt to 'translate' it, either in the text or footnotes. Medieval England shared the pound (£) with the post-decimal currency. The medieval pound was made up of 20 shillings (s), each of which was made up of 12 pence (d). Thus 1s is represented by 5p in the post-decimal coinage, although this means very little given the price inflation of the intervening centuries. The sources also include frequent references to the mark: a unit of account which represented two thirds of a pound, or 13s 4d. I have also made no attempt to give imperial measurements of length and volume in their metric equivalents, not least because there was considerable local variation in some measurements and any such 'translation' would imply an entirely spurious precision.

Medieval writers used the Vulgate text of the Bible, which includes some books not generally part of 'Protestant' Bibles, among them 1 & 2 Maccabees, the Book of Wisdom and Ecclesiasticus. Readers familiar with other translations of the Bible should also note that the Vulgate has different names for some of the books of the Bible, for example the books which appear in most modern translations as 1 & 2 Samuel and 1 & 2 Kings appear in the Vulgate as 1-4 Kings respectively, and the Book of Revelation appears as the Apocalypse. There are also some differences in the numbering of the Psalms and I have used the Vulgate numbering throughout. I have followed the Reims/Douai translation of the Vulgate text except where the author is merely paraphrasing a biblical passage, where I have produced my own translation in order to avoid too abrupt a stylistic break.

All but three of the translations are my own. Dr Susan Tilby generously translated the extract from the *Grandes Chroniques* [8]. The extract from Boccaccio's *Decameron* [2] is from the translation by G. H. McWilliam and is reproduced by permission of the copyright holders, Penguin Books Ltd. The passage from the *Book of the Servant* [75] is from the translation published by the late Professor Clarke of Glasgow University in 1952. In making my translations from the Latin I have benefited greatly from the advice of Lesley Wynne-Davies. In fairness to her I should add that I only consulted her about the passages which had defeated me – not about the ones I thought I understood – and she is not responsible for any remaining errors. I have rendered Latin poetry into prose throughout, in order to secure a fairly close translation without the constraints imposed by trying to write verse. Sources in Middle English have been modernised to a varying degree, from complete translation in the case of Langland to modernisation of the spelling only in the case of Lydgate. The headnote to each text explains the extent of the modernisation.

I am enormously grateful to the friends and colleagues who rallied round and gave me the benefit of their expertise, among them Debbie Banham, John Hatcher, Philip Jones, Rosamond McKitterick, Nigel Morgan, Ted Powell, David Sherlock, Margie Tolstoy and Patrick Zutshi. David Dymond and Janet Gyford helped me in my hunt for the unreferenced local sources cited by Dr Augustus Jessopp in his nineteenth-century essay on the Black Death. Mark Bailey, Barbara English and John Henderson drew my attention to possible sources for inclusion. Richard Britnell spontaneously placed his transcript of the Durham hallmote material at my disposal, and Ray Locke allowed me to use his work on Walsham le Willows. Richard Butterwick generously obtained a microfilm of the manuscript text of Gabriele de' Mussis from the University of Wroclaw so that I could check the accuracy of some readings in the printed edition.

Crown copyright material in the Public Record Office is reproduced by permission of Her Majesty's Stationery Office. Documents 19, 46, 63, 78 and 124 are printed by kind permission of the British Library. Material from the episcopal registers of the archbishops of York is reproduced by permission of the Borthwick Institute of Historical Research. I am also grateful to the following for allowing me to print translations of manuscripts in their care: the Director of the University Library of Wroclaw [1]; the Keeper of the Ely Diocesan Records, Cambridge University Library [106]; the Syndics of Cambridge University Library [120]; the Bodleian Library, Oxford [58]; the Wellcome Institute Library [51]. 33 is printed by permission of Hampshire Record Office, and 50, 104c and 107 by permission of the County Archivist of Staffordshire. 97 is printed by permission of the Suffolk Record Office and Miss D. E. Ridley. The County Archivist of Somerset kindly checked an entry in an episcopal register of the bishop of Bath and Wells to clarify a dubious reading in the published version.

The extract from Knuttson's *A Little Book for the Pestilence* [59] is reproduced by courtesy of the Director and University Librarian, the John Rylands University Library of Manchester. I am grateful to the following editors and publishers for allowing me to publish translations of material published by them: Boydell and Brewer Ltd for 48 and 49; the editors of the English Historical Review for 82, and to them and Dr Antonia Gransden for 12 and 25f; Dr Robert Lerner for 54; the Council of the Early English Text Society for 39b; the Council of the Canterbury and York Society for 34, 80, 99, 105 and 108. Document 73 is translated from S. Simonsohn, *The Apostolic See and the Jews, Documents 492–1404* by permission of the publisher; © 1988 by the Pontifical Institute of Mediaeval Studies, Toronto. To anyone whose permission I have inadvertently failed to obtain, I offer my apologies; full acknowledgement will be made in any future edition if the omission is drawn to my attention.

PART ONE:
NARRATIVE ACCOUNTS

The disease which swept across Europe in the late 1340s seemed to contemporaries to herald the end of the world. To the chroniclers of Padua the plague was a devastation more final than Noah's Flood – when God had left *some* people alive to continue the human race [3]. On the other side of Europe, in Kilkenny, John Clynn left blank pages at the end of his chronicle 'in case anyone should still be alive in the future' [23]. The very enormity of the disaster drove chroniclers to take refuge in clichés: there were not enough living to bury the dead; whole families died together; the priest was buried with the penitent he had confessed a few hours earlier. The same comments appear in chronicle after chronicle, and the result can seem curiously perfunctory, with only the occasional vivid detail bringing the reality of the situation before the reader, such as William Dene's remark that the stench from the mass graves was so appalling that people could hardly bear to go past a churchyard [19].

Alongside these verbal clichés are the numerical ones. The most common claim was that scarcely a tenth of the population survived the plague. Other writers opted for one in five. A few, more modestly, suggested that barely half or a third of mankind was left alive. It is easy to dismiss such claims as meaningless exaggeration: one more example of the notorious medieval tendency to inflate numbers. The mortality rate was clearly nothing like 90% (one in 10 surviving) or even 80% (one in five surviving). But if the figures are exaggerated, they are not meaningless. The chroniclers' resort to them is a measure of their horror and disbelief at the number of deaths they saw around them. The best modern estimates of the death rate in England during the first outbreak of plague cluster between 40% and 55% – which give a probable average mortality of around 47% or 48%. In other words nearly half the population of England died in something like 18 months. Not all of Europe was so badly affected, and even within the worst-affected areas there must have been communities which, for whatever reason, managed to escape relatively lightly, but the Black Death was a human disaster of appalling magnitude.

The name 'Black Death' is a later coinage. Contemporaries do not seem to have put a name to the illness, referring to it in non-specific ways as a mortality or epidemic.¹ Even the words plague or pestilence, which became the standard terms for the disease, were originally non-specific, and have remained so: not all plagues are *the* plague. This is not to say that contemporaries had failed to recognise that they were dealing with a specific disease, or that they were hazy about its manifestations. On the contrary, writers across Europe not only present a consistent picture of the symptoms of the disease, but had realised that the same disease was taking two distinct forms. One, the most common, manifested itself by painful swellings in the groin or armpit, less commonly on the neck, often accompanied or followed by little blisters elsewhere on the body or by a blotchy discolouration of the skin. The first sign of illness was a sudden coldness, and a prickling sensation like pins and needles, accompanied by extreme tiredness and depression. By the time the swellings had formed the patient would be in a high fever, with severe headaches. The victim might well fall into a stupor, or be unable to articulate when conscious.² Several writers note that the matter contained in the swellings and the bodily effluvia were particularly noisome. The other form of the disease attacked the lungs, causing chest pains and breathing difficulties, followed by the coughing up of blood and sputum. This was invariably fatal and killed more quickly than the first form, whose victims lingered for several days, and might even recover.

Not all contemporary writers distinguished explicitly between the two forms of the disease, although the distinction was clearly common knowledge within the papal court at Avignon, where it was familiar to men with no medical training, such as Louis Heyligen [5]. But even writers who conflated all the plague symptoms into a single list were often making the same distinction implicitly. Most believed that the appearance of the swellings was a sign that the body was trying to expel the poisonous matter to its surface, and that if swellings did not form the poison would work inwards, affecting first the lungs and then the brain. They had recognised, in other words, that the swellings and the coughing up of blood from the lungs did not generally occur together.³

1 The claim, repeated by several writers, that in Vienna the plague was characterised as Frau Peste almost certainly refers to post-medieval outbreaks. I have been unable to trace the story back beyond R. Krafft-Ebing, *Geschichte der Pest in Wien*, Leipzig & Wien, 1899.

2 A symptom noted by the Byzantine emperor John VI Cantacuzene in 1347: C. S. Bartsocas, 'Two fourteenth century Greek descriptions of the Black Death', *Journal of the History of Medicine and Allied Sciences* XXI, 1966, p. 396.

3 Medieval explanations of the plague are discussed in more detail in the introduction to Part Two.

What such writers were describing were quite clearly cases of bubonic and pneumonic plague. Plague is primarily a disease of wild rodents, caused by the bacillus *Yersinia pestis*.[4] Once the disease has become well-established in the human population person to person transmission can occur, but in the first instance plague can be transmitted to humans only by the agency of fleas from infected rodents. Bacilli multiply rapidly in the blood of an infected rodent and are ingested by fleas feeding on the animal. Several types of flea can carry the disease, but much the most effective vector is the rat flea: *Xenopsylla cheopis*. This will not, for choice, seek non-rodent hosts if rodents are available, but may be driven to find new hosts as rodent communities are thinned by the plague.

Under normal conditions the plague makes the transition from rodents to humans relatively rarely, in part because the wild rodents in which the disease is endemic are unlikely to come into sufficiently close contact with people for their fleas to move across onto a human host. Thus although plague exists today among the rodent population in parts of the United States, there have been only a handful of cases of people contracting the disease. What seems to have happened in the mid fourteenth century is that ecological changes in central Asia (where wild rodents formed a reservoir of the disease) drove the infected animals out of their existing habitats and into closer proximity to human settlement, allowing the disease to become endemic among the local rat population and facilitating the movement of fleas to human hosts. This is not an entirely speculative scenario. Islamic authors believed that the plague in the east was preceded by famine, floods and earthquakes, and the highly coloured stories of natural prodigies which appear in a number of European sources [5, 9], are garbled versions of the same belief.

A flea carrying the plague bacilli can transmit the disease to a human victim in one of two ways. When an infected flea bites its host it regurgitates bacilli into the blood stream before beginning to feed. Alternatively, the bacilli in the faeces of an infected flea can contaminate abrasions in the host's skin. In either case the result is bubonic plague, which derives its name from the characteristic buboes, or swellings. When the bacilli have entered the human body they are carried by the lymphatic system to the regional lymph node nearest

4 For modern medical views of the plague I have relied largely on *The Pest Anatomized: five centuries of the plague in Western Europe*, Wellcome Institute for the History of Medicine, London, 1985.

the site of infection, where the bacilli multiply, forming large colonies. This generally takes three to eight days, and the resulting swelling can be very large. The most usual site of the swelling is in the groin (presumably because flea bites are most likely to be on the legs), but it can also be in the armpit or under the ear. Blistering may occur around the site of the original bite or contamination, and in severe cases there is likely to be subcutaneous bleeding, causing discolour- ation of the skin. Three or four days after the formation of the bubo, the bacilli reach the blood stream, carrying the infection to other organs, notably the spleen and lungs – and, in very rare cases, the brain. In such cases haemorrhages may occur throughout the body, and the physician Raymond Chalin de Vinario noted bloody urine and bleeding from the bowels in some plague victims.[5]

In pneumonic plague the lungs are the primary, rather than a secondary, seat of infection. This form of the disease is caused by the inhalation of plague bacilli. The most likely source of such airborne bacilli is the droplets of moisture sprayed out by the coughing of someone whose lungs are already infected, but bacilli might also be inhaled in flea faeces from bedding or clothing. The onset of this form of plague is far more rapid than bubonic plague, and is accompanied by coughing and difficulty in breathing. The victim is soon coughing up abundant, blood stained sputum, and death occurs within two days from anoxia (shortage of oxygen) and cardiac failure. The victim's sputum contains large numbers of bacilli and, unlike bubonic plague, this form of the disease is infectious and can be transmitted directly from person to person.

It has been generally assumed that the prevalence of pneumonic plague in the medieval epidemics explains the otherwise rather sur- prising continuance of the disease throughout winter and spring, when rats and their fleas might be expected to be relatively dormant. Contemporary accounts make it clear that pneumonic plague was indeed present on a significant scale – at least in southern and western Europe[6] – but none of them makes a seasonal connection between this form of plague and cold weather, which suggests that pneumonic plague was not the only explanation of the plague's persistence. Another factor is likely to have been a run of mild, damp winters,

---

5 Cited by G. Twigg, *The Black Death: a biological reappraisal*, London, 1984, p. 207.

6 It has recently been argued that this was not the case in northern Europe: O. Benedictow, *Plague in the late medieval Nordic Countries*, Oslo, 1992.

allowing the fleas and their hosts to remain fairly active. Gilles li Muisis specifically comments on the mildness of the winter of 1349-50, when the expected frosts never materialised [6b], and the Paris medical faculty made the same point about 1347-48 [56]. The ratflea, X. cheopis, is happiest at between 20°-25°C, with high humidity – conditions which may well be found in rat burrows during a mild winter, even if the outside temperature drops below the optimum.

The continuing high mortality over the winter months is not the only aspect of the epidemic which has left some historians unhappy with its usual identification with bubonic plague. The medieval disease travelled extremely fast across large areas; faster than can reasonably be explained by the spread of the disease within the rat population. It also seems to have been as active in thinly-populated rural areas as in towns, which are usually assumed to provide the best conditions for the transfer of rat fleas to humans. These apparent difficulties have, in the past, produced two totally different solutions. In his work on bubonic plague, J. F. D. Shrewsbury asserted that the epidemic was indeed plague, and that the fourteenth-century mortality levels could not therefore have been anything like as high as historians had hitherto claimed. The other solution, floated by Graham Twigg, was that a different disease must have been involved – with anthrax his preferred candidate.[7]

In fact the problem is more apparent than real, and both these 'solutions' may be discounted. Part of the answer is that plague does not, strictly, need rats for its transmission; it needs fleas. An infective flea can remain alive for at least eighty days away from its rodent host – long enough to travel considerable distances in traded goods. De' Mussis' account of soldiers contracting the plague from looted bedding (although involving a very much shorter time scale) is obviously explicable in these terms [1]. In addition, plague bacilli can persist in flea faeces for up to five weeks.

More important, however, is the fact that modern assumptions about how plague spreads, and how rapidly this can occur, are based on the observation of epidemics from the nineteenth century onwards, where the spread among humans has been slow and often highly localised. But the modern experience of plague may be misleading. Bacilli, like other organisms, can mutate, and it is now known that a single

7 J. F. D. Shrewsbury, *A History of Bubonic Plague in the British Isles*, Cambridge, 1970; Twigg, *Black Death*.

8 NARRATIVES

mutation in the plague bacillus can produce a massive increase in its virulence.[8] If medieval plague was simply more virulent than its nineteenth-century counterpart several of the apparent anomalies mentioned above would disappear. It evidently did differ from modern plague in a number of ways, notably in its ease of transmission from rodents to humans, something which is now relatively rare even when people come into contact with infected rodents. Similarly, dogs and cats are now considered highly resistant to infection, but medieval observers were in no doubt that household pets were dying with their owners. The librarian at Constantinople, Andronikos Palaeologus, also noticed that birds were dying in large numbers.[9] Medieval Islamic writers observed the same phenomenon and took it to mean that the disease was being carried by birds; something which, if true, could have made a radical difference to the configuration of the epidemic.

The posited virulence of the medieval plague bacillus, compared with its modern equivalent, has the additional advantage of removing the need to appeal to a third form of plague – septicaemic plague – as an explanation of the plague's rapid spread among humans.[10] As its name implies, septicaemic plague is characterised by the extremely rapid proliferation of plague bacilli in the human blood stream, bringing death within a matter of hours, before any of the characteristic plague symptoms have had time to appear. During that period the blood of the victim becomes so super-charged with plague bacilli that a human flea which bites the patient and then moves on to bite another host can spread the infection. The advantage of this explanation to historians troubled by the rapid spread of plague was that it supplied another method of person-to-person transmission by allowing a significant role to the human flea (*Pulex irritans*), which otherwise seems not to be a very efficient plague vector. Cases may have occurred during the epidemic: a number of chroniclers mention examples of men who died suddenly without the formation of buboes or the appearance of any other of the classic plague symptoms. But this form of plague seems to be extremely rare and most recent writers have been wary of giving it a major role in the spread of the 1348-49 epidemic.

However it was being spread, the geographical movement of the plague has now been charted in some detail. It almost certainly began

8 R. E. Lenski, 'Evolution of plague virulence', *Nature*, 11 August 1988, pp. 473-4. I owe this reference to Dr John Hatcher.

9 Bartsocas, 'Two fourteenth century Greek descriptions' p. 395.

10 P. Ziegler, *The Black Death*, Harmondsworth, 1970, p. 29.

in the Asiatic steppe when, as described above, the wild rodents which formed a reservoir of disease migrated into areas of human settlement. The plague was probably active in central Asia in 1331-32. Thence it spread south, to China and India, and west through Transoxiana and Persia. It had reached southern Russia by 1345-46, when it attacked the cities of the Golden Horde, including Astrakhan. By this time it was moving fast down the main trading arteries and, as far as Europe is concerned, the crucial line of transmission seems to have been overland to the Crimea and then by sea from the Genoese trading centres in the Black Sea to Italy. This is the route described by de' Mussis [1], whose version can be supported by eastern accounts. In 1343 Italian merchants were expelled from their trading depot of Tana and took refuge in Caffa. In 1345-46 they were besieged there by Kipchak Khan Janibeg, and in the course of the siege the Khan's army was struck by plague. The besiegers spread the disease to the Genoese within the city by lobbing infected corpses over the walls: an early and apparently highly effective form of germ warfare.

The fleeing Genoese brought the plague to Constantinople in 1347, and in the same year it reached Italy. From there it spread almost literally in all directions. It seems to have been Italian merchants who carried the disease to the eastern Mediterranean and the near East.[11] The plague had crossed the Alpine passes into the Holy Roman Empire within a year. By June 1348 it had reached Bavaria and was in southern Austria by November [9]. Vienna was affected the following year, as was northern Germany. Italian vessels also carried the plague into the western Mediterranean. Contemporary accounts convey an image of a single fleet carrying death from port to port along the French littoral and the western seaboard of the Iberian peninsula; anchoring just long enough to spread the disease before being driven away to infect a new port. This cannot have been literally true, but the picture of plague-bearing ships roaming the sea gives a vivid sense of contemporary paranoia, as does Louis Heyligen's comment that people at Avignon would not eat the new season's spices in case they had come from one of the infected ships [5].

From the Mediterranean coast the plague spread north through France. It was raging in Avignon in the spring of 1348 and had reached Paris by June. At the same time it was moving westwards, through Toulouse to Bordeaux, and it was probably from Gascony

11 M. W. Dols, *The Black Death in the Middle East*, Princeton, 1977, p. 56. For fuller details of the plague's movement in Europe, see Ziegler, *Black Death.*

that it crossed to England in the summer of 1348. Chroniclers disagreed in their identification of its first port of call: Bristol was a favoured, and plausible, candidate; Melcombe (now part of Weymouth) was another; Henry Knighton preferred Southampton [21]. The difference hardly matters. By this date the plague was spreading on several fronts and these ports may well have been affected more or less simultaneously. The plague raged in their hinterland throughout the autumn and winter. By autumn it had reached London. Geoffrey le Baker [22] implies that it had spread eastwards from Gloucester and Oxford, but it is more likely that the capital had been infected independently, from sea-borne trade. Such trade certainly continued throughout the epidemic, and Bergen was infected from London in May 1349.[12]

The plague continued in London thoughout winter and the following spring. By then it had also begun to spread north. If one tries to chart its movements in detail it becomes obvious, as indeed one would expect, that it did not advance evenly in a broad swathe across the country. In spite of the plague's early arrival in Bristol and Dorset, rural Devon seems not to have been affected until the following year [91]. St Albans abbey, a mere day's journey from London, held the disease at bay until early April 1349 [79]. The plague had reached York by late May, but the Lincolnshire Wolds were not affected until July [17]; and Meaux abbey in the East Riding of Yorkshire seems to have escaped until August [18].

One of the most terrifying things about the plague must have been that people could see it coming. The northern Italian cities may, as de' Mussis implies, have been caught entirely by surprise, but most other centres were alerted in advance. Louis Heyligen was able to warn his colleagues in Bruges a year before the plague reached Flanders [5]. Travellers and pilgrims carried home stories of deserted landscapes and uncomfortable personal brushes with death [6a]. In England, the Archbishop of York was already ordering prophylactic processions at the end of July 1348 [29]. By August several of his fellow bishops were taking action – in each case because they thought plague was due to arrive rather than because it already had. Of course, not everyone took these warnings very seriously, and the bishops' descriptions of the horrors in store [33] evidently did not send shivers down every spine. Gilles li Muisis, the Abbot of Tournai, complained that although there were great rumours of the mortality, people did not take much notice until the blow actually fell [6b]. But many people must have suffered the intense anxiety of watching the plague advancing on their homes. William Dene gives a glimpse of such pressures in his not entirely sympathetic description of the elderly Bishop of Rochester, who spent the winter of 1348–49 worrying himself sick about the plague, which was then raging in London but was not to affect Kent seriously until the following spring [19]. The obverse of this reaction was the frenzied rejoicing noted by the chronicler of Saint-Denis in a community which had hitherto escaped the plague, although the neighbouring villages had been affected [8]. In proper moralising fashion the merry-making villagers were promptly struck down by a violent hailstorm.

By the end of 1349 informed opinion in England was beginning to hope that the worst was over. On 28 December the Archbishop of Canterbury ordered people to offer prayers of thanksgiving for their survival [35]. It is difficult to gauge from the chronicles whether people thought that the plague had gone for good – not least because many of the chroniclers were writing after the plague's return in 1361. John of Reading (writing probably in the mid 1360s) clearly had the advantage of hindsight when he noted that, in spite of the lesson of the 1348 plague, people returned to their sinful ways: 'Their greed, scorn and malice were asking to be punished' [20].

When the plague did return to England the chroniclers' treatment of it was fairly cursory. Although a Scottish writer thought this outbreak as bad as the first epidemic [25i] most English sources seem to have thought it less destructive. Almost all of them comment that the second pestilence particularly attacked children and adolescents – a characteristic which explains its relatively low profile in non-chronicle sources such as rentals and court rolls. Perhaps contemporaries found it less disruptive for the same reason, although this is not to belittle the grief it caused. Thomas Brinton, in a sermon preached against the backdrop of the third pestilence, suggested that the death of the innocent is designed by God to jolt their families and friends into good behaviour – oblique testimony to the distress caused by the deaths of children [49].

Later outbreaks of plague generally receive no more than a bare mention in the chronicles, unless, as in Walsingham's account of the fourth pestilence [28] they provided the occasion for an improving *exemplum*. This does not mean that the plague was a spent force.

Although mortality rates never approached the levels experienced in 1348-49 it is clear that national outbreaks of plague continued throughout the fifteenth and sixteenth centuries, that of 1545-46 being particularly severe. Such 'national' outbreaks are, in any case, far from being the whole story. Work is accumulating to show that many manors and religious houses experienced abnormal mortality levels about once every decade in the two centuries after the plague's arrival – although plague may not have been the culprit in every case.[13]

In demographic terms these continuing, modest recurrences of plague have assumed considerable importance in the eyes of recent historians.[14] Although they did not reduce the population as dramatically as the first two national epidemics, they played a major role in preventing its recovery – particularly when, as in the second and third pestilences, the main victims were apparently children and adolescents who had not yet started their own families. Studies of the demographic impact of the major famine in the second decade of the fourteenth century have shown that the population, left to itself, could recover rapidly from such disasters.[15] Some contemporaries, at least, believed that such a recovery was under way after the plague of 1347-49. In France, Jean de Venette thought that woman were conceiving more readily than usual and that 'there were pregnant women wherever you looked' [7], although the English author of the *Eulogium* took the contrary view [13].

If demographic recovery did begin in the 1350s, it was not sustained. Most historians now agree that the English population did not begin to recover until well into the fifteenth century, and that the consequences of a rising population did not really begin to be felt until the sixteenth century. Demographic change is never likely to be mono-causal – personal preference and fertility, as well as mortality, have roles to play in dictating family size – but there seems little reason to doubt that the continuing outbreaks of plague were a significant factor in delaying population recovery.

---

13 There is a good series of figures in C. Dyer, *Lords and Peasants in a Changing Society: the estates of the bishopric of Worcester, 680-1540*, Cambridge, 1980, chapter 9.

14 The best statement of this view is J. Hatcher, *Plague, Population and the English Economy 1348-1530*, London and Basingstoke, 1977.

15 Z. Razi, *Life, Marriage & Death in a Medieval Parish: economy, society and demography in Halesowen 1270-1400*, Cambridge, 1980, chapter 2. But for a warning of the problems inherent in charting population movement in this period see Richard M. Smith, 'Demographic developments in rural England, 1300-48: a survey', in B. M. S. Campbell (ed), *Before the Black Death: studies in the 'crisis' of the early fourteenth century*, Manchester, 1991, pp. 25-78.

What is less clear is whether the regularity of subsequent outbreaks allowed familiarity to breed contempt, or whether (as most modern writers seem to assume) plague remained uniquely terrifying, even after Europe had experienced large-scale outbreaks of other new diseases, such as the sweat or syphilis. Certainly the plague's literary supremacy was unassailable well into the seventeenth century. When writers wished to evoke the transience of human life, or the vulnerability of human plans, they turned to the plague to provide their context, confident that this would arouse all the right responses in their audience. Chaucer's Pardoner sets his sermon on greed as the root of all evil in a countryside terrorised by plague [122], and in the fifteenth-century debate poem, 'A disputation betwixt the body and worms' [124] the pilgrim overhears the macabre argument in a country where the pestilence was 'heavily reigning'. It was an outbreak of plague which prevented the schemes of Shakespeare's 'star-crossed lovers', Romeo and Juliet, from coming to a successful conclusion.

By contrast, historical sources offer a more ambiguous picture. The brevity of chronicle entries after the first outbreak may well say more about the fading attraction of that form of historical writing than about any contemporary lack of interest in the subject. But non-chronicle sources are usually at least as undemonstrative, suggesting, at the very least, that their writers no longer felt that there was anything new to say about the plague and its effects. For them, as for poets and playwrights, the plague had become a familiar explanation, not something which needed explanation itself. People in general, as far as one can judge, no longer reacted to the plague with the passionate terror and urge to repentance which the first outbreak had evoked. The plague continued to cast long shadows.[16] But the survival of mankind in 1347-50 (and the relative mildness of later outbreaks by comparison) had brought the plague into some sort of perspective. It might engender deep insecurity and could bring appalling personal tragedy, but no one any longer expected the world to end.

16 For further discussion of the plague's impact see the introduction to Part Three.

I: The plague in continental Europe

1. The arrival of the plague

Gabriele de' Mussis was a lawyer of Piacenza who died in 1356. His *Historia de Morbo* is the main source for the arrival of the plague in Europe, although it is not true, as his first editor believed, that de' Mussis was actually a passenger on the ship which brought the plague to Genoa – he is now known to have remained in Piacenza throughout the epidemic. The factual details which de' Mussis provides have often been quoted, but this complete translation restores them to their moral framework: an extended meditation on the plague as an expression of divine anger.

A. W. Henschel, 'Document zur Geschichte des schwarzen Todes', in *Archiv für die gesammte Medicin* ed. Heinrich Haeser, II, Jena, 1841, pp. 45-57. I have checked Henschel's printed version against a microfilm of the manuscript (University of Wrocław Library, Ms R 262, fos 74-77v) and made a few emendations.

In the name of God, amen. Here begins an account of the disease or mortality which occured in 1348, put together by Gabriele de' Mussis of Piacenza.

May this stand as a perpetual reminder to everyone, now living and yet to be born, how almighty God, king of heaven, lord of the living and of the dead, who holds all things in his hand, looked down from heaven and saw the entire human race wallowing in the mire of manifold wickedness, enmeshed in wrongdoing, pursuing numberless vices, drowning in a sea of depravity because of a limitless capacity for evil, bereft of all goodness, not fearing the judgements of God, and chasing after everything evil, regardless of how hateful and loathsome it was. Seeing such things he called out to the earth: 'What are you doing, held captive by gangs of worthless men, soiled with the filth of sinners? Are you totally helpless? What are you doing? Why do you not demand human blood in vengeance for this wrongdoing? Why do you tolerate my enemies and adversaries? When confronted by such wantonness you should have swallowed my opponents. Make yourself ready to exercise the vengeance which lies within your power.'

And the earth replied, 'I, established by your power, shall open and swallow up the countless criminals as soon as you give the word. When the enraged Judge gives the signal, with violent thunder from

God vs. sin

heaven, and leads the elements, the planets, the stars and the orders of
angels against the human race in an unspeakable judgement, enlisting
all forms of life to wipe out the sinners at one savage stroke, I shall
refuse the usual harvest, I shall not yield grain, wine and oil.'
God said, 'The exercise of justice belongs to me. I am the life of the
living. I bear the keys of death. I bring retribution, giving each
individual his due. My hands shaped the heavens. I formed light,
created the world and adorned it. Oh you sinner, wretched and yet
more wretched, why have you chosen to resist me and to scorn all my
commands, laws and judgements? Where is the faith of baptism and
the price of my redemption? When I fashioned my creation I never
imagined that you would fall into these snares and come to this end.
I had prepared heaven for you, not hell, and look where you have
brought yourself. When you compelled me, who upheld the spheres, to
descend into the womb of a virgin I endured hunger, thirst, toil,
crucifixion and death – and your deeds, you ingrate, condemn me still
to the cross. I ought to have punished you with eternal death, but pity
conquered me. Behold, I have been merciful towards you, and you have
barely acknowledged the salvation you have gained through me. You
are unworthy of eternal bliss, showing yourself instead to be worthy
of the torments of hell. Leave my earth, I abandon you to be torn into
pieces by dragons. You shall go into the shadows, where there will be
perpetual wailing and gnashing of teeth. Now disaster is at hand; your
strength must have an end. The sight of the vanities and lecheries to
which you have abandoned yourself has provoked me to fury. May evil
spirits arise with the power to devour you. May you have no escape
from this time forward.

'I pronounce these judgements: may your joys be turned to mourning,
your prosperity be shaken by adversity, the course of your life be
passed in never-ending terror. Behold the image of death. Behold I
open the infernal floodgates. Let hunger strike down those it seizes; let
peace be driven from the ends of the earth; let dissensions arise; let
kingdoms be consumed in detestable war; let mercy perish throughout
the world; let disasters, plagues, violence, robberies, strife and all kinds
of wickedness arise. Next, at my command, let the planets poison the
air and corrupt the whole earth; let there be universal grief and
lamentation. Let the sharp arrows of sudden death have dominion
throughout the world. Let no one be spared, either for their sex or
their age; let the innocent perish with the guilty and no one escape.

'Because those I appointed to be shepherds of the world have behaved *lack of religion —o religious authority*

towards their flocks like ravening wolves, and do not preach the word
of God, but neglect all the Lord's business and have barely even urged
repentance, I shall take a savage vengeance on them. I shall wipe them
from the face of the earth. The enemy and adversary will seize their
hidden treasure. They, along with all other wrongdoers, will bear the
heavy burden of their offences. Their office – acquired through deceit
– will not avail them, and because they feared men rather than God,
and valued their grace more highly, they will be branded as hypocrites.
Religion, turned out of doors, will grieve. The treacherous and
maleficent fellowship of priests and clergy, imperilled by their own
failings, will be destroyed. No one will be given rest, poisoned arrows
will strike everyone, fevers will throw down the proud, and incurable
disease will strike like lightning.'

After this warning had been given to mortals, disease was sent forth;
the quivering spear of the Almighty was aimed everywhere and
infected the whole human race with its pitiless wounds. Orion, that
cruel star, and the tail of the dragon and the angel hurling vials of
poison into the sea, and the appalling weather of Saturn were given
leave to harm land and sea, men and trees; advancing from east to west
with plague-bearing steps they poured out the poisoned vessels
throughout the countries of the world, leaving fiery tokens on the
sick.[1] And so the terrible violence of death, running through the world
threatening ruin, devoured mortals by a sudden blow, as I shall
describe below. Mourn, mourn, you peoples, and call upon the mercy
of God.

In 1346, in the countries of the East, countless numbers of Tartars and
Saracens were struck down by a mysterious illness which brought

---

1 This rather clumsy passage mixes apocalyptic and astrological imagery. The angel
   pouring out the vial of poison evokes the seven angels with the seven vials full of
   the wrath of God in Apocalypse 15-16. De' Mussis emphasises the identification
   with his comment that they were permitted to harm land and sea, men and trees –
   a reference to Apocalypse 7.2-3 where an angel ascending from the east forbids the
   four angels to harm the earth, the sea and the trees until the chosen of God have
   been sealed.

   The head and tail of the dragon are the points in the heavens where the course of
   the moon crosses the ecliptic (the circle which defines the path along which the sun
   seems to travel) – the head of the dragon in the moon's northward journey, the tail
   when it is travelling south. They intensify (for good and ill respectively) the power
   of any planet situated in the same house of the zodiac. De' Mussis is not referring
   to a specific astrological conjunction here but is simply using the term, along with
   Saturn (the most harmful of the planets) and Orion (a constellation and not, as de'
   Mussis has it, a star) as examples of malevolent astrological forces. For more on
   medieval astrology see the introduction to Part Two.

sudden death. Within these countries broad regions, far-spreading provinces, magnificent kingdoms, cities, towns and settlements, ground down by illness and devoured by dreadful death, were soon stripped of their inhabitants.

An eastern settlement under the rule of the Tartars called Tana, which lay to the north of Constantinople and was much frequented by Italian merchants, was totally abandoned after an incident there which led to its being besieged and attacked by hordes of Tartars who gathered in a short space of time. The Christian merchants, who had been driven out by force, were so terrified of the power of the Tartars that, to save themselves and their belongings, they fled in an armed ship to Caffa, a settlement in the same part of the world which had been founded long ago by the Genoese.[2]

Oh God! See how the heathen Tartar races, pouring together from all sides, suddenly invested the city of Caffa and besieged the trapped Christians there for almost three years. There, hemmed in by an immense army, they could hardly draw breath, although food could be shipped in, which offered them some hope. But behold, the whole army was affected by a disease which overran the Tartars and killed thousands upon thousands every day. It was as though arrows were raining down from heaven to strike and crush the Tartars' arrogance. All medical advice and attention was useless; the Tartars died as soon as the signs of disease appeared on their bodies: swellings in the armpit or groin caused by coagulating humours, followed by a putrid fever.

The dying Tartars, stunned and stupefied by the immensity of the disaster brought about by the disease, and realising that they had no hope of escape, lost interest in the siege. But they ordered corpses to be placed in catapults and lobbed into the city in the hope that the intolerable stench would kill everyone inside. What seemed like mountains of dead were thrown into the city, and the Christians could not hide or flee or escape from them, although they dumped as many of the bodies as they could in the sea. And soon the rotting corpses tainted the air and poisoned the water supply, and the stench was so overwhelming that hardly one in several thousand was in a position to flee the remains of the Tartar army. Moreover one infected man could carry the poison to others, and infect people and places with the disease by look alone. No one knew, or could discover, a means of defence.

2 Tana (now Azov), lay at the northern end of the Sea of Azov; it was abandoned in 1343 but subsequently recolonised. Caffa (now Feodosiya), on the Crimean peninsula, was one of the chief Black Sea ports.

Thus almost everyone who had been in the East, or in the regions to
the south and north, fell victim to sudden death after contracting this
pestilential disease, as if struck by a lethal arrow which raised a
tumour on their bodies. The scale of the mortality and the form which
it took persuaded those who lived, weeping and lamenting, through
the bitter events of 1346 to 1348 – the Chinese, Indians, Persians,
Medes, Kurds, Armenians, Cilicians, Georgians, Mesopotamians,
Nubians, Ethiopians, Turks, Egyptians, Arabs, Saracens and Greeks
(for almost all the East has been affected) – that the last judgement had
come.

Now it is time that we passed from east to west, to discuss all the
things which we ourselves have seen, or known, or consider likely on
the basis of the evidence, and, by so doing, to show forth the terrifying
judgements of God. Listen everybody, and it will set tears pouring
from your eyes. For the Almighty has said: 'I shall wipe man, whom
I created, off the face of the earth. Because he is flesh and blood, let him
be turned to dust and ashes. My spirit shall not remain among man.'
– 'What are you thinking of, merciful God, thus to destroy your
creation and the human race; to order and command its sudden
annihilation in this way? What has become of your mercy; the faith of
our fathers; the blessed virgin, who holds sinners in her lap; the
precious blood of the martyrs; the worthy army of confessors and
virgins; the whole host of paradise, who pray ceaselessly for sinners;
the most precious death of Christ on the cross and our wonderful
redemption? Kind God, I beg that your anger may cease, that you do
not destroy sinners in this way, and, because you desire mercy rather
than sacrifice, that you turn away all evil from the penitent, and do not
allow the just to be condemned with the unjust.'

– 'I hear you, sinner, dropping words into my ears. I bid you weep.[3]
The time for mercy has passed. I, God, am called to vengeance. It is my
pleasure to take revenge on sin and wickedness. I shall give my signs
to the dying, let them take steps to provide for the health of their souls.'

As it happened, among those who escaped from Caffa by boat were a
few sailors who had been infected with the poisonous disease. Some
boats were bound for Genoa, others went to Venice and to other

---

3 This passage incorporates a slightly strained pun. The sinner is dropping [*instill-
antem*] words into God's ear. God orders him instead to weep [*stille* – an error for
stilla], an echo of Job 16.21: *ad Deum stillat oculus meus* – my eye pours out [tears]
to God.

Christian areas. When the sailors reached *scared, sick people flee, thereby spreading the plague* these places and mixed with the people there, it was as if they had brought evil spirits with them: every city, every settlement, every place was poisoned by the contagious pestilence, and their inhabitants, both men and women, died suddenly. And when one person had contracted the illness, he poisoned his whole family even as he fell and died, so that those preparing to bury his body were seized by death in the same way. Thus death entered through the windows, and as cities and towns were depopulated their inhabitants mourned their dead neighbours.

– Speak, Genoa, of what you have done. Describe, Sicily and Isole Pelagie, the judgements of God.[4] Recount, Venice, Tuscany and the whole of Italy, what you have done.

– We Genoese and Venetians bear the responsibility for revealing the judgements of God. Alas, once our ships had brought us to port we went to our homes. And because we had been delayed by tragic events, and because among us there were scarcely ten survivors from a thousand sailors, relations, kinsmen and neighbours flocked to us from all sides. But, to our anguish, we were carrying the darts of death. While they hugged and kissed us we were spreading poison from our lips even as we spoke.

When they returned to their own folk, these people speedily poisoned the whole family, and within three days the afflicted family would succumb to the dart of death. Mass funerals had to be held and there was not enough room to bury the growing numbers of dead. Priests and doctors, upon whom most of the care of the sick devolved, had their hands full in visiting the sick and, alas, by the time they left they too had been infected and followed the dead immediately to the grave. Oh fathers! Oh mothers! Oh children and wives! For a long time prosperity preserved you from harm, but one grave now covers you and the unfortunate alike. You who enjoyed the world and upon whom pleasure and prosperity smiled, who mingled joys with follies, the same tomb receives you and you are handed over as food for worms. Oh hard death, impious death, bitter death, cruel death, who divides parents, divorces spouses, parts children, separates brothers and sisters. We bewail our wretched plight. The past has devoured us, the present is gnawing our entrails, the future threatens yet greater

---

4 Isole Pelagie: strictly, the islands lying between Sicily and Tunis but the phrase literally means Islands of the Sea and de' Mussis may be referring to all the Mediterranean islands.

dangers. What we laboured to amass with feverish activity, we have
lost in one hour.

Where are the fine clothes of gilded youth? Where is nobility and the
courage of fighters, where the mature wisdom of elders and the regal
throng of great ladies, where the piles of treasure and precious stones?
Alas! All have been destroyed; thrust aside by death. To whom shall
we turn, who can help us? To flee is impossible, to hide futile. Cities,
fortresses, fields, woods, highways and rivers are ringed by thieves –
which is to say by evil spirits, the executioners of the supreme Judge,
preparing endless punishments for us all.

We can unfold a terrifying event which happened when an army was
camped near Genoa. Four of the soldiers left the force in search of
plunder and made their way to Rivarolo on the coast, where the
disease had killed all the inhabitants. Finding the houses shut up, and
no one about, they broke into one of the houses and stole a fleece which
they found on a bed. They then rejoined the army and on the following
night the four of them bedded down under the fleece. When morning
comes it finds them dead. As a result everyone panicked, and thereafter
nobody would use the goods and clothes of the dead, or even handle
them, but rejected them outright.

Scarcely one in seven of the Genoese survived. In Venice, where an
inquiry was held into the mortality, it was found that more than 70%
of the people had died, and that within a short period 20 out of 24
excellent physicians had died. The rest of Italy, Sicily and Apulia and
the neighbouring regions maintain that they have been virtually
emptied of inhabitants. The people of Florence, Pisa and Lucca, finding
themselves bereft of their fellow residents, emphasise their losses. The
Roman Curia at Avignon, the provinces on both sides of the Rhône,
Spain, France, and the Empire cry up their griefs and disasters – all of
which makes it extraordinarily difficult for me to give an accurate
picture.

By contrast, what befell the Saracens can be established from trust-
worthy accounts. In the city of Babylon alone (the heart of the Sultan's
power), 480,000 of his subjects are said to have been carried off by
disease in less than three months in 1348 – and this is known from the
Sultan's register which records the names of the dead, because he
receives a gold bezant for each person buried. I am silent about
Damascus and his other cities, where the number of dead was infinite.
In the other countries of the East, which are so vast that it takes three
years to ride across them and which have a population of 10,000 for

[handwritten annotation at top: plague = punishment for Christian sin = starts in non-Christian lands]

every one inhabitant of the west, it is credibly reported that countless people have died. *[handwritten annotation: not academic, but a personal account]* Everyone has a responsibility to keep some record of the disease and the deaths, and because I am myself from Piacenza I have been urged to write more about what happened there in 1348. Some Genoese, whom the disease had forced to flee, crossed the Alps in search of a safe place to live and so came to Lombardy. Some had merchandise with them and sold it while they were staying in Bobbio, whereupon the purchaser, their host, and his whole household, together with several neighbours, were infected and died suddenly of the disease. One man there, wanting to make his will, died along with the notary, the priest who heard his confession, and the people summoned to witness the will, and they were all buried together on the following day. The scale of the disaster was such that virtually all the inhabitants were subsequently struck down by sudden death and only a tiny handful remained alive.

Another of the Genoese, who was already suffering from the illness, managed to reach Piacenza. Finding himself unwell, he sought out his close friend Fulco della Croce, who gave him shelter. He immediately took to his bed and died, and then straightaway Fulco, with his whole household and many of the neighbours, died too. And that, briefly, is how this disease (spreading rapidly throughout the world) arrived in Piacenza. I don't know where to begin. Cries and laments arise on all sides. Day after day one sees the Cross and the Host[5] being carried about the city, and countless dead being buried. The ensuing mortality was so great that people could scarcely snatch breath. The living made preparations for their burial, and because there was not enough room for individual graves, pits had to be dug in colonnades and piazzas, where nobody had ever been buried before. It often happened that man and wife, father and son, mother and daughter, and soon the whole household and many neighbours, were buried together in one place. The same thing happened in Castell' Arquato and Viguzzolo and in the other towns, villages, cities and settlements, and last of all in the Val Tidone, where they had hitherto escaped the plague.

Very many people died. One Oberto de Sasso, who had come from the infected neighbourhood around the church of the Franciscans, wished to make his will and accordingly summoned a notary and his neighbours as witnesses, all of whom, more than sixty of them, died

---

5 The consecrated Eucharistic wafer. The reference is to priests taking the last sacrament to the dying.

soon after. At this time the Dominican friar Syfredo de Bardis, a man
of prudence and great learning who had visited the Holy Sepulchre,
also died, along with 23 brothers of the same house. There also died
within a short time the Franciscan friar Bertolino Coxadocha of
Piacenza, renowned for his learning and many virtues, along with 24
brothers of the same house, nine of them on one day; seven of the
Augustinians; the Carmelite friar Francesco Todischi with six of his
brethren; four of the order of Mary; more than sixty prelates and
parish priests from the city and district of Piacenza; many nobles;
countless young people; numberless women, particularly those who
were pregnant. It is too distressing to recite any more, or to lay bare
the wounds inflicted by so great a disaster.

Let all creation tremble with fear before the judgement of God. Let
human frailty submit to its creator. May a greater grief be kindled in
all hearts, and tears well up in all eyes as future ages hear what
happened in this disaster. When one person lay sick in a house no one
would come near. Even dear friends would hide themselves away,
weeping. The physician would not visit. The priest, panic-stricken,
administered the sacraments with fear and trembling.

Listen to the tearful voices of the sick: 'Have pity, have pity, my
friends. At least say something, now that the hand of God has touched
me.'

'Oh father, why have you abandoned me? Do you forget that I am your
child?'

'Mother, where have you gone? Why are you now so cruel to me when
only yesterday you were so kind? You fed me at your breast and
carried me within your womb for nine months.'

'My children, whom I brought up with toil and sweat, why have you
run away?'

Man and wife reached out to each other, 'Alas, once we slept happily
together but now are separated and wretched.'

And when the sick were in the throes of death, they still called out
piteously to their family and neighbours, 'Come here. I'm thirsty, bring
me a drink of water. I'm still alive. Don't be frightened. Perhaps I
won't die. Please hold me tight, hug my wasted body. You ought to be
holding me in your arms.'

At this, as everyone else kept their distance, somebody might take pity
and leave a candle burning by the bed head as he fled. And when the

victim had breathed his last, it was often the mother who shrouded her son and placed him in the coffin, or the husband who did the same for his wife, for everybody else refused to touch the dead body. No prayer, trumpet or bell summoned friends and neighbours to the funeral, nor was mass performed. Degraded and poverty-striken wretches were paid to carry the great and noble to burial, for the social equals of the dead person dared not attend the funeral for fear of being struck down themselves. Men were borne to burial by day and night, since needs must, and with only a short service. In many cases the houses of the dead had to be shut up, for no one dared enter them or touch the belongings of the dead. No one knew what to do. Everyone, one by one, fell in turn to death's dart.   *social implications, disease progression*

What a tragic and wretched sight! Who would not shed sympathetic tears? Who would not be shaken by the disastrous plague and the terrors of death? But our hearts have grown hard now that we have no future to look forward to. Alas. Our inheritance has been diverted to strangers, our homes to outsiders. It is only the survivors who can enjoy the relief of tears.

I am overwhelmed, I can't go on. Everywhere one turns there is death and bitterness to be described. The hand of the Almighty strikes repeatedly, to greater and greater effect. The terrible judgement gains in power as time goes by.

– What shall we do? Kind Jesus, receive the souls of the dead, avert your gaze from our sins and blot out all our iniquities.

We know that whatever we suffer is the just reward of our sins. Now, therefore, when the Lord is enraged, embrace acts of penance, so that you do not stray from the right path and perish. Let the proud be humbled. Let misers, who withheld alms from the poor, blush for shame. Let the envious become zealous in almsgiving. Let lechers put aside their filthy habits and distinguish themselves in honest living. Let the raging and wrathful restrain themselves from violence. Let gluttons temper their appetites by fasting. Let the slaves of sloth arise and dress themselves in good works. Let adolescents and youths abandon their present delight in following fashion. Let there be good faith and equity among judges, and respect for the law among merchants. Let pettifogging lawyers study and grow wise before they put pen to paper. Let members of religious orders abandon hypocrisy. Let the dignity of prelates be put to better use. Let all of you hurry to set your feet on the way of salvation. And let the overweening vanity of great ladies, which so easily turns into voluptuousness, be bridled. It was against their arrogance that Isaiah inveighed: 'Because the daughters of Sion are haughty, and have walked with stretched out necks and wanton glances of their eyes, and made a noise as they walked with their feet, and moved in a set pace: the Lord will make bald the crown of the head of the daughters of Sion: and the Lord will discover their hair. In that day, the Lord will take away the ornaments of shoes, and little moons: and chains, and necklaces, and bracelets, and bonnets and bodkins, and ornaments of the legs, and tablets, and sweet balls, and earrings: and rings, and jewels hanging on the forehead: and changes of apparel, and short cloaks, and fine linen, and crisping pins: and looking glasses, and lawns and headbands, and fine veils. And instead of a sweet smell, there shall be a stench: and instead of a girdle, a cord. And instead of curled hair, baldness: and instead of a stomacher, haircloth. Thy fairest men also shall fall by the sword: and thy valiant ones in battle. And her gates shall lament and mourn: and she shall sit desolate on the ground' [Isaiah 3.16-26]. This was directed against the pride of ladies and young people.

For the rest, so that the conditions, causes and symptoms of this pestilential disease should be made plain to all, I have decided to set them out in writing. Those of both sexes who were in health, and in no fear of death, were struck by four savage blows to the flesh. First, out of the blue, a kind of chilly stiffness troubled their bodies. They felt a tingling sensation, as if they were being pricked by the points of arrows. The next stage was a fearsome attack which took the form of an extremely hard, solid boil. In some people this developed under the armpit and in others in the groin between the scrotum and the body. As it grew more solid, its burning heat caused the patients to fall into an acute and putrid fever, with severe headaches. As it intensified its extreme bitterness could have various effects. In some cases it gave rise to an intolerable stench. In others it brought vomiting of blood, or swellings near the place from which the corrupt humour arose: on the back, across the chest, near the thigh. Some people lay as if in a drunken stupor and could not be roused. Behold the swellings, the warning signs sent by the Lord.[6] All these people were in danger of dying. Some died on the very day the illness took possession of them,

---

6 Another pun: *bulla* is a swelling, but it is also the word for the papal seal, and hence for a papal document (or bull). De' Mussis is playing on the idea of the swelling characteristic of the plague being God's seal, notifying the victim of his imminent fate.

others on the next day, others – the majority – between the third and fifth day. There was no known remedy for the vomiting of blood. Those who fell into a coma, or suffered a swelling or the stink of corruption very rarely escaped. But from the fever it was sometimes possible to make a recovery.

I have, however, known a case where, although there was a stench arising from the patient, the use of the best theriac expelled the poison and prevented it proving fatal.[7] If the tumid humour revealed itself in numbness, but not by any external growths, it was a sign of death, because then the poison, passing into the veins of the heart, smothered the patient. But if swellings appeared externally, on the upper or lower body, the patient might be rescued. He could be cured by immediately letting blood from the appropriate part of his body: from his arm if the upper part of the body was affected; from the tendon of the foot if it was the lower part which was affected. When this was followed up with medicinal means, using mallow or a plaster of marsh mallow to ripen the boil and draw the humours from the seat of the illness, and then cutting out the boil, the patients received the blessing of health. But if the bitter fever persisted it stole the life of its victims. It can be asserted, on the clear evidence of experience, that the illness was more dangerous during an eclipse, because then its effect was enhanced, and it was at such times that people died in the greatest numbers.

In the East, in Cathay, which is the greatest country in the world, horrible and terrifying signs appeared. Serpents and toads fell in a thick rain, entered dwellings and devoured numberless people, injecting them with poison and gnawing them with their teeth. In the South, in the Indies, earthquakes cast down whole towns and cities were consumed by fire from heaven. The hot fumes of the fire burnt up infinite numbers of people, and in some places it rained blood, and stones fell from the sky.

Truly, then was a time of bitterness and grief, which served to turn men to the Lord. I shall recount what happened. A warning was given by a certain holy person, who received it in a vision, that in cities, towns and other settlements, everyone, male and female alike, should gather in their parish church on three consecutive days and, each with a lighted candle in their hand, hear with great devotion the mass of the

---

7 Theriac was an ointment, made from snake flesh and other ingredients, which was believed to draw poison from the body. De' Mussis' discussion of the medical treatment of plague is rather obscure and I have drawn on contemporary medical treatises in making sense of it.

Blessed Anastasia, which is normally performed at dawn on Christmas day, and they should humbly beg for mercy, so that they might be delivered from the disease through the merits of the holy mass. Other people sought deliverance through the mediation of a blessed martyr; and others humbly turned to other saints, so that they might escape the abomination of disease. For among the aforesaid martyrs, some, as stories relate, are said to have died from repeated blows, and it was therefore the general opinion that they would be able to protect people against the arrows of death. Finally, in 1350, the most holy Pope Clement ordained a general indulgence, to be valid for a year, which remitted penance and guilt to all who were truly penitent and confessed. And as a result a numberless multitude of people made the pilgrimage to Rome, to visit with great reverence and devotion the basilicas of the blessed apostles Peter and Paul and St John.

Oh, most dearly beloved, let us therefore not be like vipers, growing ever more wicked, but let us rather hold up our hands to heaven to beg for mercy on us all, for who but God shall have mercy on us?[8] With this, I make an end. May the heavenly physician heal our wounds – our spiritual rather than our bodily wounds. To whom be the blessing and the praise and the glory for ever and ever, Amen.

2. The plague in Florence

The introduction to the *Decameron* of Giovanni Boccaccio (1313-75) is the most famous literary treatment of the Black Death. As Boccaccio himself emphasises, however, the description is based on his own experiences in Florence and the picture he gives can be paralleled in chronicle accounts of the period.

This translation by G. H. McWilliam is taken from the Penguin Classics edition of the *Decameron*, Harmondsworth, 1972, pp. 50-58.

I say, then, that the sum of thirteen hundred and forty-eight years had elapsed since the fruitful Incarnation of the Son of God, when the noble city of Florence, which for its great beauty excels all others in Italy, was visited by the deadly pestilence. Some say that it descended upon the human race through the influence of the heavenly bodies, others that it was a punishment signifying God's righteous anger at our iniquitous way of life. But whatever its cause, it had originated

---

8 Vipers were thought the most villainous of creatures, and proverbially ungrateful – hence the expression (which derives from Aesop's *Fables*) to nourish a viper in one's bosom.

some years earlier in the East, where it had claimed countless lives before it unhappily spread westward, growing in strength as it swept relentlessly on from one place to the next.

In the face of its onrush, all the wisdom and ingenuity of man were unavailing. Large quantities of refuse were cleared out of the city by officials specially appointed for the purpose, all sick persons were forbidden entry, and numerous instructions were issued for safeguarding the people's health, but all to no avail. Nor were the countless petitions humbly directed to God by the pious, whether by means of formal processions or in any other guise, any less ineffectual. For in the early spring of the year we have mentioned, the plague began, in a terrifying and extraordinary manner, to make its disastrous effects apparent. It did not take the form it had assumed in the East, where if anyone bled from the nose it was an obvious portent of certain death. On the contrary, its earliest symptom, in men and women alike, was the appearance of certain swellings in the groin or the armpit, some of which were egg-shaped whilst others were roughly the size of the common apple. Sometimes the swellings were large, sometimes not so large, and they were referred to by the populace as *gavòccioli*. From the two areas already mentioned, this deadly *gavòcciolo* would begin to spread, and within a short time it would appear at random all over the body. Later on, the symptoms of the disease changed, and many people began to find dark blotches and bruises on their arms, thighs, and other parts of the body, sometimes large and few in number, at other times tiny and closely spaced. These, to anyone unfortunate enough to contract them, were just as infallible a sign that he would die as the *gavòcciolo* had been earlier, and as indeed it still was.

Against these maladies, it seemed that all the advice of physicians and all the power of medicine were profitless and unavailing. Perhaps the nature of the illness was such that it allowed no remedy; or perhaps those people who were treating the illness (whose numbers had increased enormously because the ranks of the qualified were invaded by people, both men and women, who had never received any training in medicine), being ignorant of its causes, were not prescribing the appropriate cure. At all events, few of those who caught it ever recovered, and in most cases death occurred within three days from the appearance of the symptoms we have described, some people dying more rapidly than others, the majority without any fever or other complications.

But what made this pestilence even more severe was that whenever those suffering from it mixed with people who were still unaffected, it would rush upon these with the speed of a fire racing through dry or oily substances that happened to be placed within its reach. Nor was this the full extent of its evil, for not only did it infect healthy persons who conversed or had any dealings with the sick, making them ill or visiting an equally horrible death upon them, but it also seemed to transfer the sickness to anyone touching the clothes or other objects which had been handled or used by its victims.

It is a remarkable story that I have to relate. And were it not for the fact that I am one of many people who saw it with their own eyes, I would scarcely dare to believe it, let alone commit it to paper, even though I had heard it from a person whose word I could trust. The plague I have been describing was of so contagious a nature that very often it visibly did more than simply pass from one person to another. In other words, whenever an animal other than a human being touched anything belonging to a person who had been striken or exterminated by the disease, it not only caught the sickness, but died from it almost at once. To all of this, as I have just said, my own eyes bore witness on more than one occasion. One day, for instance, the rags of a pauper who had died from the disease were thrown into the street, where they attracted the attention of two pigs. In their wonted fashion, the pigs first of all gave the rags a thorough mauling with their snouts after which they took them between their teeth and shook them against their cheeks. And within a short time they began to writhe as though they had been poisoned, then they both dropped dead to the ground, spreadeagled upon the rags that had brought about their undoing.

These things, and many others of a similar or even worse nature, caused various fears and fantasies to take root in the minds of those who were still alive and well. And almost without exception, they took a single and very inhuman precaution, namely to avoid or run away from the sick and their belongings, by which means they all thought that their own health would be preserved.

Some people were of the opinion that a sober and abstemious mode of living considerably reduced the risk of infection. They therefore formed themselves into groups and lived in isolation from everyone else. Having withdrawn to a comfortable abode where there were no sick persons, they locked themselves in and settled down to a peaceable existence, consuming modest quantities of delicate foods and precious wines and avoiding all excesses. They refrained from speaking to outsiders, refused to receive news of the dead or sick, and entertained themselves with music and whatever other amusements they were able to devise.

Others took the opposite view, and maintained that an infallible way of warding off this appalling evil was to drink heavily, enjoy life to the full, go round singing and merrymaking, gratify all of one's cravings whenever the opportunity offered, and shrug the whole thing off as one enormous joke. Moreover, they practised what they preached to the best of their ability, for they would visit one tavern after another, drinking all day and night to immoderate excess; or alternatively (and this was their more frequent custom), they would do their drinking in various private houses, but only in the ones where the conversation was restricted to subjects that were pleasant or entertaining. Such places were easy to find, for people behaved as though their days were numbered, and treated their belongings and their own persons with equal abandon. Hence most houses had become common property, and any passing stranger could make himself at home as naturally as though he were the rightful owner. But for all their riotous manner of living, these people always took good care to avoid any contact with the sick.

In the face of so much affliction and misery, all respect for the laws of God and man had virtually broken down and been extinguished in our city. For like everybody else, those ministers and executors of the laws who were not either dead or ill were left with so few subordinates that they were unable to discharge any of their duties. Hence everyone was free to behave as he pleased.

There were many other people who steered a middle course between the two already mentioned, neither restricting their diet to the same degree as the first group, nor indulging so freely as the second in drinking and other forms of wantonness, but simply doing no more than satisfy their appetite. Instead of incarcerating themselves, these people moved about freely, holding in their hands a posy of flowers, or fragrant herbs, or one of a wide range of spices, which they applied at frequent intervals to their nostrils, thinking it an excellent idea to fortify the brain with smells of that particular sort; for the stench of dead bodies, sickness, and medicines seemed to fill and pollute the whole of the atmosphere.

Some people, pursuing what was possibly the safer alternative, callously maintained that there was no better or more efficacious remedy against a plague than to run away from it. Swayed by this argument, and sparing no thought for anyone but themselves, large numbers of men and women abandoned their city, their homes, their relatives, their estates and their belongings, and headed for the countryside, either in Florentine territory or, better still, abroad. It was as though they imagined that the wrath of God would not unleash this plague against men for their iniquities irrespective of where they happened to be, but would only be aroused against those who found themselves within the city walls; or possibly they assumed that the whole of the population would be exterminated and that the city's last hour had come.

Of the people who held these various opinions, not all of them died. Nor, however, did they all survive. On the contrary, many of each different persuasion fell ill here, there, and everywhere, and having themselves, when they were fit and well, set an example to those who were as yet unaffected, they languished away with virtually no one to nurse them. It was not merely a question of one citizen avoiding another, and of people almost invariably neglecting their neighbours and rarely or never visiting their relatives, addressing them only from a distance; this scourge had implanted so great a terror in the hearts of men and women that brothers abandoned brothers, uncles their nephews, sisters their brothers, and in many cases wives deserted their husbands. But even worse, and almost incredible, was the fact that fathers and mothers refused to nurse and assist their own children, as though they did not belong to them.

Hence the countless numbers of people who fell ill, both male and female, were entirely dependent upon either the charity of friends (who were few and far between) or the greed of servants, who remained in short supply despite the attraction of high wages out of all proportion to the services they performed. Furthermore, these latter were men and women of coarse intellect and the majority were unused to such duties, and they did little more than hand things to the invalid when asked to do so and watch over him when he was dying. And in performing this kind of service, they frequently lost their lives as well as their earnings.

As a result of this wholesale desertion of the sick by neighbours, relatives and friends, and in view of the scarcity of servants, there grew up a practice almost never previously heard of, whereby when a woman fell ill, no matter how gracious or beautiful or gently bred she might be, she raised no objection to being attended by a male servant, whether he was young or not. Nor did she have any scruples about showing him every part of her body as freely as she would have displayed it to a woman, provided that the nature of her infirmity required her to do so; and this explains why those women who recovered were possibly less chaste in the period that followed. Moreover a great many people died who would perhaps have survived had they received some assistance. And hence, what with the lack of appropriate means for tending the sick, and the virulence of the plague, the number of deaths reported in the city whether by day or night was so enormous that it astonished all who heard tell of it, to say nothing of the people who actually witnessed the carnage. And it was perhaps inevitable that among the citizens who survived there arose certain customs that were quite contrary to established tradition.

It had once been customary, as it is again nowadays, for the women relatives and neighbours of a dead man to assemble in his house in order to mourn in the company of the women who had been closest to him; moreover his kinsfolk would forgather in front of his house along with his neighbours and various other citizens, and there would be a contingent of priests, whose numbers varied according to the quality of the deceased; his body would be taken thence to the church in which he had wanted to be buried, being borne on the shoulders of his peers amidst tl e funeral pomp of candles and dirges. But as the ferocity of the plague began to mount, this practice all but disappeared entirely and was replaced by different customs. For not only did people die without having many women about them, but a great number departed this life without anyone at all to witness their going. Few indeed were those to whom the lamentations and bitter tears of their relatives were accorded; on the contrary, more often than not bereavement was the signal for laughter and witticisms and general jollification – the art of which the women, having for the most part suppressed their feminine concern for the salvation of the souls of the dead, had learned to perfection. Moreover it was rare for the bodies of the dead to be accompanied by more than ten or twelve neighbours to church, nor were they borne on the shoulders of worthy and honest citizens, but by a kind of gravedigging fraternity, newly come into being and drawn from the lower orders of society. These people assumed the title of sexton, and demanded a fat fee for their services, which consisted in taking up the coffin and hauling it swiftly away, not to the church specified by the dead man in his will, but usually to the nearest at hand. They would be preceded by a group of four or six clerics, who between them carried one or two candles at most, and sometimes none at all. Nor did the priests go to the trouble of pronouncing solemn and lengthy funeral rites, but, with the aid of these so-called sextons, they hastily lowered the body into the nearest empty grave they could find.

As for the common people and a large proportion of the bourgeoisie, they presented a much more pathetic spectacle, for the majority of them were constrained, either by their poverty or the hope of survival, to remain in their houses. Being confined to their own parts of the city, they fell ill daily in their thousands, and since they had no one to assist them or attend to their needs, they inevitably perished almost without exception. Many dropped dead in the open streets, both by day and by night, whilst a great many others, though dying in their own houses, drew their neighbours' attention to the fact more by the smell of their rotting corpses than by any other means. And what with these, and the others who were dying all over the city, bodies were here, there and everywhere.

Whenever people died, their neighbours nearly always followed a single, set routine, prompted as much by their fear of being contaminated by the decaying corpse as by any charitable feelings they may have entertained towards the deceased. Either on their own, or with the assistance of bearers whenever these were to be had, they extracted the bodies of the dead from their houses and left them lying outside their front doors, where anybody going about the streets, especially in the early morning, could have observed countless numbers of them. Funeral biers would then be sent for, upon which the dead were taken away, though there were some who, for lack of biers, were carried off on plain boards. It was by no means rare for more than one of these biers to be seen with two or three bodies upon it at a time; on the contrary, many were seen to contain a husband and wife, two or three brothers and sisters, a father and son, or some other pair of close relatives. And times without number it happened that two priests would be on their way to bury someone, holding a cross before them, only to find that bearers carrying three or four additional biers would fall in behind them; so that whereas the priests had thought that they had only one burial to attend to, they in fact had six or seven, and sometimes more. Even in these circumstances, however, there were no tears or candles or mourners to honour the dead; in fact, no more respect was accorded to dead people than would nowadays be shown towards dead goats. For it was quite apparent that the one thing which, in normal times, no wise man had ever learned to accept with patient resignation (even though it struck so seldom and unobtrusively), had now been brought home to the feeble-minded as well, but the scale of the calamity caused them to regard it with indifference.

Such was the multitude of corpses (of which further consignments were arriving every day and almost by the hour at each of the churches), that there was not sufficient consecrated ground for them to be buried in, especially if each was to have its own plot in accordance with long-established custom. So when all the graves were full, huge trenches were excavated in the churchyards, into which new arrivals were placed in their hundreds, stowed tier upon tier like ships' cargo, each layer of corpses being covered over with a thin layer of soil till the trench was filled to the top.

But rather than describe in elaborate detail the calamities we experienced in the city at that time, I must mention that, whilst an ill wind was blowing through Florence itself, the surrounding region was no less badly affected. In the fortified towns, conditions were similar to those in the city itself on a minor scale; but in the scattered hamlets and the countryside proper, the poor unfortunate peasants and their families had no physicians or servants whatever to assist them, and collapsed by the wayside, in their fields, and in their cottages at all hours of the day and night, dying more like animals than human beings. Like the townspeople, they too grew apathetic in their ways, disregarded their affairs, and neglected their possessions. Moreover, they all behaved as though each day was to be their last, and far from making provision for the future by tilling their lands, tending their flocks, and adding to their previous labours, they tried in every way they could think of to squander the assets already in their possession. Thus it came about that oxen, asses, sheep, goats, pigs, chickens, and even dogs (for all their deep fidelity to man) were driven away and allowed to roam freely through the fields, where the crops lay abandoned and had not even been reaped, let alone gathered in. And after a whole day's feasting, many of these animals, as though possessing the power of reason, would return glutted in the evening to their own quarters, without any shepherd to guide them.

But let us leave the countryside and return to the city. What more remains to be said, except that the cruelty of heaven (and possibly, in some measure, also that of man) was so immense and so devastating that between March and July of the year in question, what with the fury of the pestilence and the fact that so many of the sick were inadequately cared for or abandoned in their hour of need because the healthy were too terrified to approach them, it is reliably thought that over a hundred thousand human lives were extinguished within the walls of the city of Florence? Yet before this lethal catastrophe fell upon the city, it is doubtful whether anyone would have guessed it contained so many inhabitants.

3. The plague in Padua

Cortusii Patavini Duo, sive Gulielmi et Abrigeti Cortusiorum, Historia de Novitatibus Paduae et Lombardiae ab anno MCCLVI usque ad MCCCLXIV, in L. A. Muratori (ed), *Rerum Italicarum Scriptores* XII, Milan, 1728, cols 926-7.

Almighty God, who does not desire the death of a sinner, but that he may be converted and live, first threatens and secondly strikes to reform the human race, not to destroy it.[9] Wishing to assail the human race with enormous and unprecedented blows, his terrifying judgement began firstly in the furthest part of the world, in the countries of the East. After he had struck at the Tartars, Turks and all the other unbelievers, there was on 25 January 1348, at the 23rd hour, a great earthquake to terrify the Christians, which lasted for half an hour. After which the unprecedented plague crossed the sea and so came to the Veneto, Lombardy, the March, Tuscany, Germany, France and spread through virtually the whole world. It was carried by some infected people who had travelled from the East and who, by sight alone, or by touch, or by breathing on them, killed everyone. The infection was incurable; it could not be avoided. The wife fled the embrace of a dear husband, the father that of a son, and the brother that of a brother. Even the houses or clothes of the victims could kill. Those burying, carrying, seeing or touching the infected often died suddenly themselves. Just as one infected sheep infects the whole flock, so one death within a household was always followed by the death of all the rest, right down to the dogs. The bodies even of noblemen lay unburied. Many, at a price, were buried by poor wretches, without priests or candles. Indeed in Venice, where 100,000 died, boats were hired at great expense to carry bodies to the islands and the city was virtually deserted.

A single stranger carried the infection to Padua, to such effect that perhaps a third of the people died within the region as a whole. In the

---

9 The reference, which will recur repeatedly in these texts, is to Ezechiel 33.11: 'Say to them: As I live, saith the Lord God, I desire not the death of the wicked, but that the wicked may turn from his way and live'.

hope of avoiding such a plague, cities banned the entry of all outsiders, with the result that merchants were unable to travel from city to city. Cities and settlements were left desolate by this calamity. No voices could be heard, except in mourning and lamentation. The voice of the bride and groom ceased, and so did music, the songs of young people and all rejoicing. The plagues in the days of Pharoah, David, Ezechiel and Pope Gregory now seemed nothing by comparison, for this plague encircled the whole globe.[10] In the days of Noah God did not destroy all living souls and it was possible for the human race to recover.

As described above, some were infected very badly by this plague and died suddenly from blood poisoning, others from a malignant tumour, or from worms. A certain sign of death, found on almost everyone, were incurable tumours near the genitals, or under the armpits, or in some other part of the body, accompanied by deadly fevers. People with these died on the first or second day; after the third day, although rarely, there was some hope of recovery. Some people fell asleep and never woke up, but passed away. Doctors frankly confessed that they had no cure for the plague, and the most accomplished of them died of it. During the plague Guerra Sambonifacio, *podestà* of Siena, died with virtually all his household. There was also terrible mortality at Florence, Pisa and throughout the whole of Tuscany. The plague generally lasted for six months after its outbreak in each area. The noble man Andrea Morosini, *podestà* of Padua, died in July in his third term of office. His son was put in office, but died immediately. Note, however, that amazingly during this plague no king, prince, or ruler of a city died.

4. The plague in Sicily

This account comes from the *Cronaca* of the Franciscan Michele da Piazza, edited by Rosarius Gregorio, *Bibliotheca Scriptorum qui res in Sicilia gestas sub Aragonum imperio retulere* I, Palermo, 1791, pp. 562-8. I have checked some of the readings against a more recent edition of the text, published by the Istituto di Storia Medievale of the University of Palermo, 1980.

10 These four exemplars recur regularly in fourteenth-century discussions of the plague. Three are biblical: the plague which killed the first born of Egypt (Exodus 12); the plague in the reign of David which was halted by the king's prayers (2 Kings 24); and the various manifestations of God's vengeance described by Ezechiel. The plague in Rome in the 590s was halted at the intercession of Pope Gregory – for whom see the introduction to Part Two.

In October 1347, at about the beginning of the month, twelve Genoese galleys, fleeing from the divine vengeance which Our Lord had sent upon them for their sins, put into the port of Messina. The Genoese carried such a disease in their bodies that if anyone so much as spoke with one of them he was infected with the deadly illness and could not avoid death. The signs of death among the Genoese, and among the Messinese when they came to share the illness with them, were as follows. Breath spread the infection among those speaking together, with one infecting the other, and it seemed as if the victim was struck all at once by the affliction and was, so to speak, shattered by it. This shattering impact, together with the inhaled infection, caused the eruption of a sort of boil, the size of a lentil, on the thigh or arm, which so infected and invaded the body that the victims violently coughed up blood, and after three days' incessant vomiting, for which there was no remedy, they died – and with them died not only anyone who had talked with them, but also anyone who had acquired or touched or laid hands on their belongings.

The people of Messina, realising that the death racing through them was linked with the arrival of the Genoese galleys, expelled the Genoese from the city and harbour with all speed. But the illness remained in the city and subsequently caused enormous mortality. It bred such loathing that if a son fell ill of the disease his father flatly refused to stay with him, or, if he did dare to come near him, was infected in turn and was sure to die himself after three days. Not just one person in a house died, but the whole household, down to the cats and the livestock, followed their master to death. Because of the scale of the mortality, many Messinese looked to make confession of their sins and to make their wills, but priests, judges and notaries refused to visit them, and if anyone did visit their houses, whether to hear confession or draw up a will, they were soon sure to die themselves. Indeed the Franciscans and Dominicans, and others who were willing to visit the sick to hear their confession and impose penance, died in such large numbers that their priories were all but deserted. What more is there to say? Corpses lay unattended in their own homes. No priests, sons, fathers or kinsmen dared to enter; instead they paid porters large sums to carry the bodies to burial. The houses of the dead stood open, with all the jewels, money and treasure in full view, and if someone wanted to enter there was nothing to stop them; for the plague struck so suddenly that at first there weren't enough officials and then there were none at all.

The Messinese, observing this terrible and unnatural event, chose to leave the city rather than stay and die. Not only did they refuse to enter the city; they did not want to be anywhere near it, but camped with their families in the open air among the vineyards outside the city. Some, indeed the majority, went to the city of Catania, believing that the blessed virgin Agatha of Catania would save them from the disease. From Catania Queen Elisabetta of Sicily ordered her son Federico, who was then in Messina, to join her quickly and he arrived promptly with Venetian galleys.[11]

Several of the Messinese in Catania addressed pious requests to the Patriarch, all begging that he would personally carry the relics of the virgin Agatha to Messina with all due honour. 'For we believe', they said, 'that if the relics come to Messina the city will be saved completely from this disease.' The Patriarch, deeply moved by their prayers, agreed that he would come in person to Messina with the relics. This was about the end of November, 1347. The holy virgin Agatha, aware of the deep seated deceit and cunning of the Messinese (who have always wanted to keep the virgin's relics at Messina and were capable of exploiting the calamity to that end), directed her prayers to God, who arranged it that the whole body of citizens took themselves off to the Patriarch, clamouring and shouting that they did not like this plan at all; and, wresting the keys from the keeper of the church, they roundly abused the Patriarch, declaring that they would see him dead before they let the relics go to Messina.

Confronted by this uproar the Patriarch could not carry out his plan, and accordingly he entered the place where the relics were kept, with all possible devotion and honour, and to the accompaniment of religious chants and prayers he laved some of the holy relics with pure water, and announced that he would take the holy water with him when he travelled to Messina.

What a stupid idea on the part of you Messinese – to attempt, under cover of devotion, to steal the relics of the blessed virgin Agatha in such a furtive and underhand manner. How could you forget that when the virgin's body was at Constantinople and she wanted to come home, she appeared in dreams to Ghisbert and Agoselm and ordered them to

11 Elisabetta di Tirolo, widow of Pietro II of Sicily (d.1342). At the time of the plague her son Ludovico was nominal ruler of Sicily, with his uncle Giovanni (Pietro's brother) as regent. Federico succeeded in 1355.

carry her body to Catania?[12] Don't you think that if she had wanted to make her home in Messina she would have said so?

What more is there to say? The Patriarch duly arrived in Messina with the holy water and cured all sorts of sick people in great numbers by sprinkling them with the water and making the sign of the cross. The citizens of Messina flocked to see him, hastening to him with great rejoicing and offering many thanks to him and to God. For demons were manifesting themselves in the city in the likeness of dogs, which inflicted great harm on the bodies of the Messinese. Numb with terror, no man dared leave home. However, at the bidding of the Archbishop of Messina, and with general approval, they all agreed to process around the city with devout litanies. Just as all the people were entering the city a black dog appeared in their midst, carrying a naked sword in its paw. It rushed raging into the church, and broke and smashed all the silver vessels, lamps and candlesticks on the altars. At this sight everyone, half dead with terror, prostrated themselves. When, after some hesitation, they got up again they saw the dog leaving the church, but no one dared to follow it or go near it.

The Messinese, appalled by this incredible sight, were now all panic-stricken. They accordingly decided to go in procession, barefoot and accompanied by priests, to Santa Maria della Scala, six miles from Messina. As they drew near the Virgin they all knelt as one, tearfully calling upon the help of God and the Virgin. They then entered the church with devout prayers, the priests chanting the psalm *miserere nostri Deus*, and laid hands upon a carving of the Mother of God, which had been placed there in ancient times and which they had chosen to take back to Messina, because they thought that upon its arrival the sight of it would drive out the demons from the city and deliver it from the mortality. Accordingly they chose a suitable priest to ride carrying the statue in his arms with due respect and so made their way back to the city with it.

As the holy Mother of God approached the city and saw it before her, all bloody with its sins, it was so hateful to her that she turned her back on it – she not only did not want to enter the city, but could not

---

12 According to the *Life* of St Agatha, she had been martyred and buried in Catania, but when Sicily fell under Moslem influence her body, with those of other saints, was removed to Constantinople. In 1126 she appeared in a vision to Gislebert, a western Christian living in Constantinople, and announced her desire to return to Catania. Gislebert, with the help of Goselin, stole the body and returned it to Sicily: *Acta Sanctorum, Februarii* I, pp. 637-42.

bear to look upon it. Therefore the earth gaped wide and the horse upon which the statue of the Mother of God was being carried became as fixed and immovable as a rock and could not be made to go either forwards or backwards. When the people of Messina saw these miracles they begged the Virgin, making their lamentations with sad sighs and frequent tears, that she would not take new revenge for their past sins. At their prayers the Virgin, the holy Bride of Christ, added her holy petitions to God to their humble prayers; whereupon the horse sets off again, the earth which had opened closes, and in a short time they had passed through the gate of the city into which the holy Mother of God had refused to enter. At last, accompanied by pious prayers to her, she made her entry into Santa Maria la Nuova, the main church of Messina, where the women of Messina smothered the statue with silk cloths and precious jewels.

But could not the holy Mother of God have remained in her church, she who totally refused to enter the city? Are we suggesting that she was carried unwillingly from her place? Indeed she could have remained there, since there is no power that could remove her – she to whom all mercy, all might, all goodness is granted by God's power – but it was so that the people, frantic with terror, might cleanse themselves completely of worldly allurements.

What more is there to say? The arrival of the statue profited nobody. On the contrary, the mortality raged even more, so that no one could help anyone else. Most of the citizens left Messina and scattered, some going to Calabria, others to various parts of Sicily, and especially to Catania. But what did this resort to flight avail them, given that the illness, already carried within them, was consuming their bodies? Of those who fled some collapsed in the roadway, in fields, on the sea shore, at sea, in the huts of Mascali, in woods, in ditches and in all manner of unlikely places. Those who made it to Catania breathed their last in lodgings – and they died in the city in such numbers that the Patriarch, in response to a demand by the citizens of Catania, ordered that no one from Messina should be buried within the city on pain of excommunication, but should instead be buried outside the city in good deep graves. What more is there to say? The Messinese were so loathed and feared that no man would speak with them, or be in their company, but hastily fled at the sight of them, holding his breath. And all the Catanians turned this into a sour joke, so that if anyone made to speak to someone that person would reply, in the vernacular, 'Don't talk to me if you're from Messina'. No one would give them shelter, so that they could not find houses in which to live, and unless other Messinese already established in the city gave them shelter secretly they were virtually without help.

And thus the Messinese were dispersed across the whole island. In going to Syracuse their illness infected the Syracusans so thoroughly that it was the death of a great many people. The regions around Sciacca and Trapani and the city of Agrigento also shared the pestilence with the Messinese in the same way – and especially Trapani, which has remained almost bereft of people. And what can we say about Catania, which has been delivered to oblivion? So strongly did the plague spring up there that not only the pustules commonly called *antrachi* but also a sort of tumour would erupt in various parts of the body – some on the chest, others on the legs, arms or throat. These tumours were at first the size of hazel nuts, and were accompanied by a marked stiffness and coldness. They so weakened and tormented the human body that at last the victim, unable to stay on his feet, had to take to his bed, by which stage he would be burning with a very high fever and suffering profound depression. These tumours grew to the size of a walnut and then to the size of a hen or goose egg, and their intense pain, and the accompanying putrefaction of humours, caused the victim to cough up blood, and this sputum, in passing from the infected lungs into the throat, corrupted the whole body. And it was from this corruption, and from the imperfection of the humours, that the victims died. The illness lasted three days; on the fourth day at the latest the victims went the way of all flesh.

The Catanians were well aware that the illness quickly proved fatal, and when they felt the depression and the cold stiffness coming over them their immediate priority was to make full confession of their sins to a priest and then make their wills. But the mortality was so great in the city that judges and notaries refused to go and draw up wills; and if they did visit a sick man they stood well away from him. Even priests were afraid to visit the sick for fear of death. And the mortality was so great that the judges and notaries were unable to meet the demand for wills, or the priests for hearing confession. Accordingly the Patriarch, concerned for the souls of the Catanians, bestowed upon every priest, however lowly, the same power to absolve sins which he enjoyed as bishop and patriarch. As a result, it is believed on the best authority that all those who died passed without fail safely to God.

Duke Giovanni, afraid of death and not wanting to come near cities or other settlements because of the infected air, ranged ceaselessly through wild and uninhabited places. And as he roamed here and there like a fugitive – now at *aqua mili* in the forest of Catania, now at a tower called *lu blancu* six miles from Catania, now at the church of San Salvatore *de blanchardu* in the forest of Catania – he came at last to a church or place called Sant'Andrea, newly built by him within the woods of Mascali, where, while he was living safe and sound, illness came upon him and he died. His body was buried in the main church of Catania, in the tomb where the former king Federico, his father, was buried. And this was in April 1348.

The mortality lasted from September more or less until the time of the duke's death. The mortality was so heavy that sex and age made no difference, but everyone died alike.... The Patriarch died in this mortality and was buried in the main church in Catania, may his soul rest in peace.

5. The plague in Avignon

The following letter, sent from the papal court at Avignon, was copied into the chronicle of an unknown Flemish cleric as part of his account of the plague. It is not entirely clear where paraphrase ends and direct quotation begins, perhaps as early as the sentence beginning 'On the first day' in the first paragraph. The letter's author was Louis Heyligen [*Sanctus*] of Beeringen, one of a group of northern musicians in the service of Cardinal Giovanni Colonna, who died of the plague on 3 July.[13] Louis was a close friend of Petrarch, some of whose comments on the plague are printed below [76].

Breve Chronicon Clerici Anonymi, ed J-J de Smet, *Recueil des Chroniques de Flandre*, III, Brussels, 1856, pp. 14–18

A huge mortality and pestilence started in September 1347, as I have seen in a copy of a letter written by a canon and cantor of St Donatian, who was at the time in the company of a cardinal, his master, at the Roman Curia and sent the letter to his colleagues in Bruges, to give them the news by way of warning. It recounts how terrible events and unheard of calamities had afflicted the whole of a province in eastern India for three days. On the first day it rained frogs, snakes, lizards, scorpions and many other similar poisonous animals. On the second day thunder was heard, and thunderbolts and lightning flashes mixed with hailstones of incredible size fell to earth, killing almost all the people, from the greatest to the least. On the third day fire, accompanied by stinking smoke, descended from heaven and consumed all

13 B. Guillemain, *La Cour Pontificale d'Avignon (1309-1376)*, Paris, 1962, pp. 214n, 261.

the remaining men and animals, and burnt all the cities and settlements in the region.

The entire province was infected by these calamities, and it is surmised that the whole coast and all the neighbouring countries caught the infection from it, by means of the stinking breath of the wind which blew southwards from the region affected by plague; and always, day by day, more people died. Now, by God's will, it has reached our coasts and, as some people believe, in this way. On 31 December 1347 three galleys loaded with spices and other goods put into the port of Genoa after being storm-driven from the East. They were horribly infected and, when the Genoese realised this, and that other men were dying suddenly without remedy, the ships were driven from the port with burning arrows and other engines of war. For there was no one who had dared to touch them or do business with them who did not immediately die. And thus, driven from port to port, one of the galleys at last put in at Marseilles, and at its arrival the same thing happened: men were infected without realising it, and died suddenly, and the inhabitants thereupon drove the galley away. It joined up with the other two ships, which were wandering about the sea, and it is said that they are heading towards the Atlantic along the Spanish coast, and that they will therefore, if they can, put in at the ports further south to conclude their trading. The infection that these galleys left behind along their whole route, particularly in coastal cities and regions – first in Greece, then in Sicily and Italy (especially in Tuscany) and subsequently in Marseilles and then as a result throughout Languedoc – was so great that its duration and horror can scarcely be believed, let alone described.

It is said that the disease takes three forms. In the first people suffer an infection of the lungs, which leads to breathing difficulties. Whoever has this corruption or contamination to any extent cannot escape, but will die within two days. Anatomical examinations, in which many corpses were opened, were carried out in many Italian cities, and also, on the pope's orders, in Avignon, to discover the origins of this disease, and it was found that all those who died suddenly had infected lungs, and had been coughing up blood. And this form is the most dangerous of all these terrible things, which is to say that it is the most contagious, for when one infected person dies everyone who saw him during his illness, visited him, had any dealings with him, or carried him to burial, immediately follows him, without any remedy.

There is another form of the disease which exists alongside the first one, in which boils erupt suddenly in the armpits, and men are killed by these without delay. And there is also a third form, which again co-exists with the other two, but takes its own course, and in this people of both sexes are attacked in the groin and killed suddenly. Because of the growing strength of this disease it has come to pass that, for fear of infection, no doctor will visit the sick (not if he were to be given everything the sick man owns), nor will the father visit the son, the mother the daughter, the brother the brother, the son the father, the friend the friend, the acquaintance the acquaintance, nor anyone a blood relation – unless, that is, they wished to die suddenly along with them, or to follow them at once. And thus an uncountable number of people died without any mark of affection, piety or charity – who, if they had refused to visit the sick themselves, might perhaps have escaped.

To be brief, at least half the people in Avignon died; for there are now within the walls of the city more than 7000 houses where no one lives because everyone in them has died, and in the suburbs one might imagine that there is not one survivor. Therefore the pope bought a field near Notre-Dame des Miracles[14] and had it consecrated as a cemetery. By 14 March 11,000 bodies had been buried there, and that is in addition to those buried in the churchyards of the Hôpital de Saint-Antoine[15] and the religious orders and in the many other churchyards in Avignon. And I should not pass over the neighbouring areas in silence. In Marseilles all the gates of the city save for two posterns were closed, for there four out of five people died. Nor did it help to flee, for it was believed that flight to healthier air only meant that people died more quickly. And I could tell you similar things about every city and settlement in Provence.

And now it has crossed the Rhône and devoured many cities and settlements as far as Toulouse, and always as it goes it spreads itself more widely. And the scale of the mortality means that for fear of death men do not dare to speak with anyone whose kinsman or kinswoman has died, because it has often been observed that when one member of a family dies, almost all the rest follow. And it is the

---

14 The chapel of Our Lady was situated in the extreme south west corner of the walled city, but the field is likely to have been outside the walls, near the gate named after the chapel.

15 The house of the Knights Hospitallers in Avignon.

common report among ordinary people that the sick are treated like dogs by their families – they put food and drink next to the sick bed and then flee the house. When they are dead, boorish yokels from the mountains of Provence – poor, half-naked men, with no finer feelings – will come, and (assuming they are paid enough) will carry the dead to burial. Neither kinsmen nor friends visit the sick. Priests do not hear the confessions of the sick, or administer the sacraments to them. Everyone who is still healthy looks after himself. So it happens every day that a rich man is carried to his grave by these ruffians, with just a few lights and no mourners apart from them, for while the corpse is going along the street everyone else hides away indoors. But these wretches do not escape, for they too die within a short time, infected by the contagion as well as oppressed by want. Virtually all the poor supported by *La Pignotte*[16] who performed these services for the better off died. I can sum it up by saying that whereas at *La Pignotte* they normally got through 64 measures of grain in a day, with one measure enough for 500 loaves, now no more than one measure (and sometimes only half) is needed.[17]

They say that in the three months from 25 January to the present day, a total of 62,000 bodies was buried in Avignon. Around the middle of March, after mature deliberation, the pope granted a plenary indulgence to all those dying confessed and contrite; the indulgence to be valid until Easter. He also commanded the performance of devout processions with the chanting of litanies on specified days of the week. It is said that these were attended by 2,000 people from all the region round about: men and women alike, many barefoot, others wearing hairshirts or smeared with ashes. As they processed with lamentations and tears, and with loose hair, they beat themselves with cruel whips until the blood ran. The pope himself took part in some of these processions, but later only those which took place in the precincts of his palace. God knows what the end will be – or what the beginning was, although some people fear that God is scourging the world with these evils in punishment for the death of King Andrew, who was butchered.[18]

16 The papal almonry, responsible for doles of food and clothing to the poor.

17 Guillemain pp. 556–7 suggests that this represents a drop from 4–5,000 poor to less than 70. The fall in the numbers being fed is not necessarily the same as the number of deaths, although the writer clearly intends the figures to be read in that light.

18 Andrew [András] of Hungary had married Jeanne I of Naples. He was murdered in September 1345 and Jeanne was suspected of complicity. She fled to Avignon, where Clement VI acquitted her of the charges and authorised her second marriage to Louis of Taranto.

Some wretched men were found in possession of certain powders and (whether justly or unjustly, God knows) were accused of poisoning the wells – with the result that anxious men now refuse to drink water from wells. Many were burnt for this and are being burnt daily, for it was ordered that they should be punished thus.

Also sea fish are now not generally eaten, men holding that they have been infected by the infected air. Moreover no kinds of spices are eaten or handled, unless they have been in stock for a year, because men are afraid that they might have come from the galleys of which I spoke. For on many occasions eating fresh spices or certain sea fish has been found to have extremely unpleasant results.

I am writing to you, most dearly beloved, so that you should know in what perils we are now living. And if you wish to preserve yourselves, the best advice is that a man should eat and drink moderately, and avoid getting cold, and refrain from any excess, and above all mix little with people – unless it be with a few who have healthy breath; but it is best to stay at home until the epidemic has passed. According to astrologers the epidemic takes ten years to complete its cycle, of which three have now elapsed, and so it is to be feared that in the end it will have encircled the whole world, although they say that it will affect cold regions more slowly.

You should know that the pope is reported to be leaving Avignon immediately and going to Étoile-sur-Rhône, two leagues from Valence. He is to remain there until things change, although the Curia wishes to remain in Avignon. Business has been suspended until Michaelmas; all the auditors, advocates and proctors have either left, or died, or plan to leave immediately. I am in the hands of God and I commend me to you. They say that my lord follows the pope and that I am to go with him. Since that place looks towards Mount Ventoux, where the plague has not yet come, it is the best place to be – or, anyway, so they say.

May Omnipotent and Merciful God grant that we all choose what is for the best.

Given at Avignon, Sunday 27 April, 1348.

6. The plague seen from Tournai

Gilles li Muisis, Abbot of St Giles at Tournai, wrote two accounts of the plague. The first, a brief summary written late in 1348, appears in his *Chronicle* and is printed as a below. Early in 1350 li Muisis supplemented his chronicle with a detailed description of the events of 1349 and his reflections upon them. The prologue and extracts are printed as b below.

(a) Gilles li Muisis from J-J. de Smet (ed), *Recueil des Chroniques de Flandre* II, Brussels, 1841, pp. 279-80.

In 1348 the most holy father, Pope Clement VI, ruled the holy and universal mother church, and the Curia was based in the city of Avignon in Provence, beyond the Rhône. In that year there were reportedly many storms and the air was unhealthy, and there was also a great mortality among both sexes. I have hunted out the most reliable account and the most accurate information I could find concerning the mortality, and here record it in writing so that future generations may have knowledge of it.

I heard that in the previous year, 1347, an innumerable horde of Tartars laid siege to a very strong city inhabited by Christians. The calamitous disease befell the Tartar army, and the mortality was so great and widespread that scarcely one in twenty of them remained alive. After discussing it among themselves, they came to the decision that such a great mortality was caused by the vengeance of God, and they resolved to enter the city which they were besieging and ask to be made Christians. Accordingly the most powerful of the survivors entered the city, but they found few men there for all the others had died. And when they saw that the mortality had broken out among the Christians as well as among themselves, because of the unhealthy air, they decided to keep to their own religion.

In the same year the Turks and all the other infidels and Saracens who currently occupy the Holy Land and possess the holy city of Jerusalem were so severely hit by the mortality that, according to the reliable report of merchants, not one in twenty survived. In that year also the mortality crossed the sea, carried by sailors and travellers, with almost everyone dying on board the ships. The Genoese sent eight ships to the aid of a force besieging a certain castle, and only two returned because everyone in the other six had died on the way back.

Also in 1347 the mortality grew strong in Rome, the Romagna, Sicily, Tuscany, Italy, Gascony, Spain and various other countries, at last entering France in 1348 according to the Roman reckoning, which dates the new year from Christmas. The death rate was unbelievable at Marseilles, where the illness arrived by land and sea, at Montpellier, throughout Provence and in Avignon, where the Roman Curia was then based, and throughout the whole country round about. Travellers, merchants, pilgrims and others who journeyed through the area reported that animals roamed freely through fields, towns and waste land, that barns and wine cellars stood open, houses empty, and that few people were to be seen. In many towns, cities and settlements, where there had originally been 20,000 people, scarcely 2000 remained; in many towns and villages 1500 people were reduced to barely 100; and in many regions the vineyards and farms were left uncultivated. I heard this from a knight learned in the law, who was one of the members of the Paris *Parlement* sent by King Philip of France on embassy to the King of Aragon with the Bishop of Maurienne. On their return they travelled through Avignon and he claimed that there and in Paris he was told these things by many people worthy of belief.

I heard the following story from a pilgrim who, in making his pilgrimage to the shrine of St James at Compostella, went via Our Lady of Rocamadour and Toulouse, because the wars prevented him going by the usual route. When he had completed his pilgrimage he returned through Galicia, and with his companion arrived at a sizeable town called Salvatierra, which had been so depopulated by the mortality that not one in ten remained alive. The pilgrim related that they dined with their host (who alone survived with two of his daughters and just one servant) and had no suspicion that any of them was ill. After they had negotiated the cost of their accommodation, and paid their host, they went to bed. In the morning the pilgrims got up and looked for their hosts to tell them of their departure, but could not make anybody hear. They finally found an old woman in bed and learnt from her that their host, his two daughters and their servant had all died in the night. Hearing this, the pilgrims beat a hasty retreat.

(b) Gilles li Muisis, ibid., pp. 305-7, 340-42, 378-82.

I Gilles, unworthy abbot of the Benedictine monastery of St Giles in Tournai, the 17th abbot since the restoration of the monastery after its destruction by the Vandals and Norsemen, was thinking after the Feast of All Saints [1 November] in 1349 that at the end of November I would have spent 60 years as a monk of the monastery, and that it would be the 78th year of my age and the 18th since I was promoted to abbot. I considered also that I had caused the writing of a book, which dealt in three sections with many events, but that since the beginning of 1349 the whole world has been encompassed by evil[19] and many new happenings have been reported from distant places throughout the world – now the seizure of Jews; now people performing public penance; now the mortality of men, women and children. There were great rumours of these things, but the people did not take much notice, and did not realise the connection with their sins, with the result that censures, words and sermons had little or no effect until the blow actually fell.

I have been thinking about the clerk Master Jean Haerlebech. He was a devout man, always studying some branch of knowledge, but especially astronomy, in which subject he was an expert – so much so that many regular and secular clergy from other countries, who were students of that science, would often come to visit him, for he was crippled and enfeebled by an illness he had had in his youth. And although he was so famous an astrologer, yet he commended the catholic faith and affirmed its truth, and until his death he led a religious life, always wearing a hair shirt and mortifying his flesh with fasting. He was very unwilling to speak of astrology, unless very briefly to close associates and friends, and then only in secret and without making specific predictions.[20] And when I was a young monk I was close to him, and he would often speak to me in secret of things which I afterwards saw come to pass.

In 1298, after the beginning of the Flemish wars, when Gui Count of Flanders renounced his homage to the King of France, Philip the Fat, it so happened that I and the said Master Jean were both involved in the negotiations during the whole of Lent. One day, seeing him in a better mood than usual, I begged him, if he would, to make some forecast for me about the war. He replied that, out of affection for me, he would look into it and tell me his findings, on condition that while he lived I would not reveal it to anyone, or disclose it or refer to it in any way.

He subsequently told me that the war would last a long time and that other wars would arise from it and many evils would befall, as afterwards I saw happen. He predicted that in 1345 major wars would begin in various places and countries, and that in 1346 and 1347 they

19 A reference to 1 Epistle John 5.19. The full verse, in the Reims/Douai translation, reads: 'We know that we are of God and the whole world is seated in wickedness'.

20 The church disapproved of specific predictions, which (with their implication that human action was determined by an external force) appeared to deny free will – a central tenet of medieval theology.

would spread everywhere, so that people would not know where to go or where to turn for safety; but that in 1348 the evils would begin to abate a little and the wars be partially halted, for the sake of trade. As far as 1349 was concerned, he told me that the people then alive would be more amazed by the transformation of evil into good than they had been by all the previous events from the beginning of the wars until that year. But he did not want to tell me anything about 1350, and I was not able to wring anything from him. However, I was young, and never dreamt that I would live so long, and so I took very little notice. But I was still alive in 1349, and so, just as I saw the events of the preceding years and recorded them in a book, I now propose to record the events of 1349 itself.

[Li Muisis introduces his discussion by citing the prediction of the astrologer Jean de Murs that the conjunction of three major planets in March 1345 would lead to the destruction of sects, changes of government, the appearance of prophets, unrest among the people, new rites, and finally winds of terrifying power.]

In 1345 and in the following years 1346, 1347 and 1348 it seemed that many of these things came to pass. Moreover in 1349 there was the destruction of the Jews, the death of people from an epidemic, the appearance of people who performed public penance and beat themselves, and many other events which I plan to mention later – not that I intend to put more trust in the sayings and prognostications of astrologers and mathematicians than faith allows, always saving the authority of the Papal See and the catholic faith....

In 1349 there came news of many happenings, and everywhere it was rumoured that the Jews were trying to destroy Christians by putting poison in springs, wells and rivers.

In addition there were persistent reports of a mortality which had begun in the East, and spread throughout India and all Christian and pagan countries from East, North and South, as was attested by the travellers and merchants who regularly visited those distant countries. The mortality was so great that in many places a third of the population died, elsewhere a quarter or a half, and in several areas only one or two people out of ten survived. And in many places the fields and vineyards remained untended. The astrologers said that this calamity was caused by the conjunction of certain stars and planets, because the conjunction corrupted the air and that generated a sickness which they called an epidemic.

It was also strongly rumoured that in Hungary, Germany and the duchy of Brabant, in cities, towns, settlements and villages, men were inciting one another and gathering in crowds of 200, 300, even 500 and more, depending on the size of the local population. They went through the countryside twice a day for thirty three days, barefooted and naked except for their drawers, wearing hoods and beating themselves with whips until the blood flowed. At last they arrived in Flanders....

In 1349 Jews were seized and put in chains and into prison everywhere, in all the places where they dwelt. The reason for this was a strong suspicion that they planned to destroy the Christians by means of poison, and that they had secretly put poison into wells, springs and rivers so that Christians would drink it. And the common report was that they had done this in various places. For there were some among the Jews who were cunning and learned astrologers and they had forecast the impending mortality from the course of the stars, and this encouraged them to put their evil intention into practice with more confidence and cunning. They also saw by the course of the stars that a religious sect was to be destroyed (and they hoped that this meant the Christians) and that men bearing red crosses would appear (and they were unsure whether this meant their sect would then be destroyed); and they said many other things which it would take too long to relate here.

Few or no Jews had lived in the kingdom of France since the days of St Louis; but in other kingdoms and countries where they were to be found they were all arrested and charged, and many denied the accusation, but some confessed that that had been their intention. I do not know the truth of what happened in distant countries, but the word was that throughout Germany and in other countries they were burnt, or beheaded, or killed by some other means. And certainly in Lotharingia and Bari all those who could be found were burnt.[21]

The see of Tournai was vacated by the death of the most reverent father and most pious lord Jean des Prés, the last bishop, a man who often travelled in search of healthy air. Accordingly, because the summer was hot and because there were rumours of deaths in the city, he arranged to go to the town of Guise, to the house of his retainer Sir Peter de Mocout, where he intended to stay for a while. He travelled

21 'Lotharingia' comprised the Low Countries, Luxembourg, Lorraine and Alsace. Bari was in southern Italy.

through Arras to Cambrai, where he was present on Corpus Christi day, which was also the feast of St Barnabas the apostle [11 June]. He performed divine service in the cathedral church there and in the general procession carried a very heavy vessel, in which the blessed Sacrament was reserved. This tired him out, and it was also very hot in the sun so that he sweated profusely in the extreme heat. Afterwards he celebrated mass. He stayed in the city all day, and at dinner in the evening seemed fit and in good spirits. In the morning he continued his journey towards Cateau-Cambrésis. However in the course of the journey he remarked to his companions and servants that he did not feel very well, and thought that he was sickening for something. After reaching the town, he stayed there for a whole day. The next morning, which was Saturday, he got up, heard mass and prepared the horses for departure, but he then returned to bed – it was God's will, which no man can go against – and shortly afterwards breathed his last. But it is written: 'The just man, if he be prevented with death, shall be in rest: and man knoweth not whether he be worthy of love, or hatred', therefore may his soul rest in peace.[22]

His whole household was terrified, but they had his body carried to the episcopal palace in Tournai, and on the Thursday of the following week he was honourably buried, as was fitting, lamented by all, churchmen and laymen alike.

After his burial, the dean and chapter, according to custom and as was their right, took responsibility for spiritual matters, the bishop's official and the rest performing their offices. However, the king's agents took possession of all the temporalities in the king's name; and, alas, they collected and carried away all the materials acquired for making repairs and undertaking new building within the diocese.

From this time until the begining of August, no other persons of authority died in Tournai; but after the feast of St John [29 August] the mortality began in the parish of St Piat in Merdenchon Street, and later it began in other parishes, so that every day the dead were carried into churches: now 5, now 10, now 15. And in the church of St Brice, sometimes 20 or 30. And in all the parishes the priests, the parish clerks and the grave diggers earned their fees by tolling the passing bells by day and night, in the morning and in the evening; and thus

22 Wisdom 4.7; Ecclesiastes 9.1. A reference to the belief that the souls of the righteous would spend the time between death and the last judgement (when they would go to heaven) 'in rest' [*in refrigerium*]: an intermediate, but still happy and blessed, state.

everyone in the city, men and women alike, began to be afraid; and no one knew what to do.

The civic authorities, seeing that the dean and chapter, and all the rest of the clergy, were doing nothing to find a solution (because inactivity was in their interests and was proving profitable), consulted together and made the following ordinances and had them publicly proclaimed.

The first public proclamation

Firstly, that everyone having a concubine ought either to marry her or put her away, and that the appointed constables in the neighbourhood should tell them to do so, and then make an inspection and if necessary remove the concubines; and they should be banished at the command of the *jurés* and council.

Item, that if anyone dies because of the mortality, at whatever hour of the day or the night, and regardless of his social standing, his grave should be dug immediately and he should be buried in a coffin or box, and should have the bell tolled in accordance with his status and the customary masses sung on Sundays.

Item, that graves should be six feet deep and the coffins not piled up;[23] and that in each parish there should always be three graves ready prepared.

Item, that during the vigils and funeral mass in church there should be a pall placed over the hearse, as is done in services, and lights commensurate with the means and wishes of the dead person's friends, and that on leaving the church the mourners should not gather in the houses of the dead, nor should banners or seats be placed in the streets, nor should other customary observances be performed.[24]

Item, that no one should wear black, except the father, brother, husband or child of the deceased; and no funeral feast should cost more than ten schilds.

---

23 *non elevati*, literally, not lifted up. This could refer back to the previous clause banning the reception of the coffined body into the church, but I have taken it to mean that coffins should not be stacked up vertically in a single grave but that each should be the full six feet under ground.

24 This emphasises the earlier requirement that the body should be buried immediately, and that it could therefore not, as was customary, rest in the church during the funeral mass. Instead its presence was to be symbolised (as it would be at a commemorative mass) by a pall spread over the hearse: a metal frame holding the candles which burnt in the dead person's name during mass.

Item, proclamation was made that no one should work at any trade after noon on Saturday, and should neither buy nor sell.

Item, that on Sundays nothing should be sold except foodstuffs.

Item that no one should make or sell dice, or play any sort of game which involves rolling or using dice. And that in such games, and in others, there should be none of the usual swearing by God or the saints. However, these ordinances were only in force for a short time. Later, when the calamitous mortality was growing much worse, a proclamation was made on St Matthew's Day [21 September] that nobody at all should wear black, or toll bells for the dead, that palls should not be placed over the bier, and that crowds should not be invited, as usual, to attend the funeral, but only two to pray for the dead and to attend the vigils and mass. The authorities had these things proclaimed, together with numerous other matters for the good of the city, under pain of certain penalties at the discretion of the *jurés* and council.

I dare to assert, and I have heard it from many people worthy of belief, that this proclamation caused a great many men to marry the women they had previously kept as concubines; and they also refrained from swearing and from the other forbidden things. Also I put it on record for future generations that I have learnt and heard that the craftsmen who make dice have turned evil into good, and to recoup their losses have begun to make prayer beads from the material from which they made dice.

I have recorded these things to the best of my knowledge and ability, and have enquired into the truth of all these things as far as possible. And when the mortality was so appalling in Tournai, who could conceive what was happening in all the other kingdoms and countries? For the rumour was that the mortality had begun in the East and had spread throughout the whole world. And future generations should know that in Tournai there was a staggering mortality at Christmas time, for I have heard from many people who said that they knew for a fact that in Tournai more than 25,000 people had died, and the strange thing is that most of the deaths were among the more influential and wealthy inhabitants. Few or none died among those who drank wine and who avoided bad air and visiting the sick. But others, who visited or lived among the sick, either became seriously ill or died; and they died especially in the streets in the market area, and more people died in narrow lanes than in broad streets and open squares. When one or two people had died in a house, the rest followed in a very short time, so that very often ten or more died in a single house; and in many houses the dogs and cats died as well. Thus no one, rich, middling or poor, was safe, but each one of them spent every day awaiting God's will. And certainly there were many deaths among the parish priests and chaplains who heard confessions and administered the sacraments, and also among the parish clerks and those who visited the sick with them.

While the mortality was at its height an enormous number of people (including those of noble birth, knights, matrons, ecclesiastics, canons and members of religious orders, as well as ordinary men and women) flocked to the monastery of St Peter at Hennegau, when it was discovered that there were relics of St Sebastian in a shrine there. Their devotion was wonderful to behold, but as the mortality began to abate after the feast of All Saints [1 November] the pilgrimages and devotion ceased.

While the pestilence raged in France pilgrims of both sexes and every social class also poured from all parts of France into the monastery of St Médard at Soissons, where the body of that martyr St Sebastian was said to lie. But when the disaster came to an end, the pilgrimage and devotion ended too.

The things written above relate to the period up to the beginning of March [1350], for there I have made an end of 1349. The winter was certainly very odd, for in the four months from the beginning of October until the beginning of February, although a hard frost was often expected, there was not so much ice as would support the weight of a goose. But there was instead such a lot of rain that the Scheldt and all the rivers round about burst their banks, so that meadows became seas, and this was so in our country and in France. Of distant countries I cannot speak with authority. Many wise men suspect that because of the lack of frost and the excess of water there will be much sickness in March and in summer.

7. The plague in France according to Jean de Venette

Jean de Venette was a Carmelite friar, who probably died in 1369. This section of his chronicle seems, from internal evidence, to have been written around 1359-60. For fuller details of his career, and an annotated translation of the whole chronicle, see Richard Newhall and Jean Birdsall, *The Chronicle of Jean de Venette*, Columbia University Press, New York, 1953. The translation which follows is my own.

H. Geraud (ed), *Chronique Latin de Guillaume de Nangis avec les continuations de cette chronique*, 2 vols, Paris, 1843, II pp. 210-16.

In 1348 the people of France, and of virtually the whole world, were assailed by something more than war. For just as famine had befallen them, as described in the beginning of this account, and then war, as described in the course of the account, so now pestilences broke out in various parts of the world. In the August of that year a very large and bright star was seen in the west over Paris, after vespers, when the sun was still shining but beginning to set. It was not as high in the heavens as the rest of the stars; on the contrary, it seemed rather near. And as the sun set and night approached the star seemed to stay in one place, as I and many of my brethren observed. Once night had fallen, as we watched and greatly marvelled, the great star sent out many separate beams of light, and after shooting out rays eastwards over Paris it vanished totally: there one minute, gone the next. Whether it was a comet or something else – perhaps something condensed from some sort of exhalations which then returned to vapour – I leave to the judgement of astronomers. But it seems possible that it presaged the incredible pestilence which soon followed in Paris and throughout the whole of France, as I shall describe.

As a result of that pestilence a great many men and women died that year and the next in Paris and throughout the kingdom of France, as they also did in other parts of the world. The young were more likely to die than the elderly, and did so in such numbers that burials could hardly keep pace. Those who fell ill lasted little more than two or three days, but died suddenly, as if in the midst of health – for someone who was healthy one day could be dead and buried the next. Lumps suddenly erupted in their armpits or groin, and their appearance was an infallible sign of death. Doctors called this sickness or pestilence an epidemic. Such an enormous number of people died in 1348 and 1349 that nothing like it has been heard or seen or read about. And death and sickness came by imagination, or by contact with others and consequent contagion; for a healthy person who visited the sick hardly ever escaped death. In many towns and villages the result was that the cowardly priests took themselves off, leaving the performance of spiritual offices to the regular clergy, who tended to be more courageous. To be brief, in many places not two men remained alive out of twenty. The mortality was so great that, for a considerable period, more than 500 bodies a day were being taken in carts from the Hôtel-Dieu in Paris for burial in the cemetery of the Holy Innocents.[25] The saintly sisters of the Hôtel-Dieu, not fearing death, worked sweetly and with great humility, setting aside considerations of earthly dignity. A great number of the sisters were called to a new life by death and now rest, it is piously believed, with Christ.

It is said that this mortality began among the infidel and then travelled to Italy. Afterwards it crossed the mountains and arrived in Avignon, where it attacked various cardinals and carried off their entire households. Then it gradually advanced through Gascony and Spain and into France, advancing town by town, street by street, and finally from house to house – or, rather, person to person. It then crossed into Germany, although it was less virulent there than with us. During the epidemic the Lord, of his goodness, deigned to confer such grace on those dying that, however suddenly they died, almost all of them faced death as joyfully as if they had been well prepared for it. Nor did anyone die without making confession and receiving the last sacrament. So that more of those dying would make a good end, Pope Clement mercifully gave the confessors in numerous cities and villages the power to absolve the sins of the dying, so that as a result they died the more happily, leaving much of their land and goods to churches or religious orders since their right heirs had predeceased them.

Men ascribed the pestilence to infected air or water, because there was no famine or lack of food at that time but, on the contrary, a great abundance. One result of this interpretation was that the infection, and the sudden death which it brought, were blamed on the Jews, who were said to have poisoned wells and rivers and corrupted the air. Accordingly the whole world brutally rose against them, and in Germany and in other countries which had Jewish communities many thousands were indiscriminately butchered, slaughtered and burnt alive by the Christians.[26] The insane constancy shown by them and their wives was amazing. When Jews were being burnt mothers would throw their own children into the flames rather than risk them being baptised, and would then hurl themselves into the fire after them, to burn with their husbands and children.

25 This figure is sometimes taken as an error for 50, but it is more likely that 500, although clearly exaggerated, was what the author intended to write. In the fifteenth century the Hôtel could house between 400 and 500 patients: Margaret Wade Labarge, *A Small Sound of the Trumpet*, London, 1986, p. 189.

26 The Jews had been expelled from France by Philip the Fair in 1322. For their persecution elsewhere in Europe see **6b** and **68-73**.

It was claimed that many wicked Christians were discovered poisoning wells in a similar fashion. But in truth, such poisonings, even if they really happened, could not have been solely responsible for so great a plague or killed so many people. There must have been some other cause such as, for instance, the will of God, or corrupt humours and the badness of air and earth; although perhaps such poisonings, where they did occur, were a contributory factor. The mortality continued in France for most of 1348 and 1349 and then stopped, leaving many villages and many town houses virtually empty, stripped of their inhabitants. Then many houses fell quickly into ruin, including numerous houses in Paris, although the damage there was less than in many places.

When the epidemic was over the men and women still alive married each other. Everywhere women conceived more readily than usual. None proved barren, on the contrary, there were pregnant women wherever you looked. Several gave birth to twins, and some to living triplets. But what is particularly surprising is that when the children born after the plague started cutting their teeth they commonly turned out to have only 20 or 22, instead of the 32 usual before the plague. I am unsure what this means, unless it is, as some men say, a sign that the death of infinite numbers of people, and their replacement by those who survived, has somehow renewed the world and initiated a new age. But if so, the world, alas, has not been made any better by its renewal. For after the plague men became more miserly and grasping, although many owned more than they had before. They were also more greedy and quarrelsome, involving themselves in brawls, disputes and lawsuits. Nor did the dreadful plague inflicted by God bring about peace between kings and lords. On the contrary, the enemies of the king of France and of the Church were stronger and more evil than before and stirred up wars by land and sea. Evil spread like wildfire.

What was also amazing was that, in spite of there being plenty of everything, it was all twice as expensive: household equipment and foodstuffs, as well as merchandise, hired labour, farm workers and servants. The only exception was property and houses, of which there is a glut to this day. Also from that time charity began to grow cold, and wrongdoing flourished, along with sinfulness and ignorance – for few men could be found in houses, towns or castles who were able or willing to instruct boys in the rudiments of Latin.

8. The plague in France according to the Great Chronicle

The great chronicle of France was kept by the monks of Saint-Denis, a project initiated by St Louis in the thirteenth century. For the early part of the reign of Philip VI their account is based on another chronicle (the continuation of the chronicle of Guillaume de Nangis), but from 1340 the Saint-Denis account is independent and, in the opinion of its editor, the description of the plague is that of an eye witness. The previous year's entry recounts the advance of the plague from Lombardy to Provence and Languedoc.

Jules Viard (ed), *Les Grandes Chroniques de France*, IX, Paris, 1937, pp. 314–16.

In the year of grace 1348 the aforementioned plague reached the kingdom of France, and lasted more or less one and a half years, with such vigour that in Paris 800 people were dying every day. The plague broke out in a country town named Roissy, near Gonnesse, some three leagues from Saint-Denis. It was most pitiful to see the bodies of the dead in such great quantities; for in the space of a year and a half, so it was said, the number of deaths in Paris rose to more than 50,000, and in the town of Saint-Denis to around 16,000. Yet despite the fact that people were dying in such numbers, nonetheless they all received confession and the other sacraments.

It happened that during this pestilence, two monks of Saint-Denis, being sent on a visitation at the command of their abbot, were riding through a town where they saw men and women dancing to the sound of drum and bagpipe and making merry. The monks asked the people why they were dancing, and they replied, 'We have seen our neighbours die, and are seeing them die daily, but since the plague has not entered our town, we hope that our merrymaking will keep it away, and this is why we are dancing'. So the monks left to carry out their mission. When they had accomplished their task, they set out on their return journey and passed through the same town, but found there very few people, all with sad faces. So the monks asked them, 'Where are the men and women who not long ago were making so merry in this town?' And they replied, 'Alas, good lords, the wrath of God came upon us in a hailstorm, for a great hailstorm came from the sky and fell on our town and all around, so suddenly that some people were killed by it, and others died of fright, not knowing where to go or which way to turn'.

9. The plague in Central Europe

This account is taken from the chronicle of the monastery of Neuberg in southern Austria.

Continuatio Novimontensis, ed. G. H. Pertz *Monumenta Germaniae Historica – scriptorum* IX, Hanover, 1851, pp. 674-6.

In 1348, on the feast of the Conversion of St Paul [25 January] at the hour of vespers, a terrible earthquake struck the whole region, although it can be shown to have been particularly severe in the city of Villach. For there, while people were assembled to worship in the churches, all of a sudden the buildings collapsed, killing the people in them on the spot. The shock virtually demolished the city wall and other buildings as well, and countless people who could not make their escape from the devastation quickly enough were killed. The fortifications of castles and towns were also thrown down all of a sudden.

In the same year there were immense upheavals in many parts of the world, as the result of a cruel pestilence which first broke out in countries across the sea and killed everyone in various horrifying ways. First, through the malignant influence of the planets and the corruption of the air, men and animals in those countries were struck motionless while going about their business, as if turned to stone. Then, in the countries where ginger comes from, a deadly rain fell, mixed with serpents and all sorts of pestilential worms, and instantly killed everyone it touched. Not far from that country dreadful fire descended from heaven and consumed everything in its path; in that fire even stones blazed like dry wood. The smoke which arose was so contagious that merchants watching from a long way off were immediately infected and several died on the spot. Those who escaped carried the pestilence with them, and infected all the places to which they brought their merchandise – including Greece, Italy and Rome – and the neighbouring regions through which they travelled.

As a result the inhabitants, frantic with terror, ordered that no foreigners should stay in the inns, and that the merchants by whom the pestilence was being spread should be compelled to leave the area immediately. The deadly plague reigned everywhere, and once populous cities, because of the death of their inhabitants, now kept their gates firmly shut so that no one could break in and steal the possessions of the dead. In Venice the death toll was so heavy that scarcely a quarter of the people remained alive. The pestilence thrust forward through Carinthia and then brutally took possession of Styria, driving men almost mad with despair.[27]

Scholars could not decide whether such a deadly year was due to the vagaries of the planets or the corrupted air, but could only commit everything to God's will. Accordingly people began to make public demonstrations of their penitence, in the hope that God would look mercifully upon the human race. Men gathered together from cities and towns and went devoutly in procession from church to church, walking two by two, totally naked except for a white cloth covering them from their loins to their ankles, singing beautiful hymns in honour of the Passion in their mother tongue and beating themselves so hard with knotted whips that drops of blood spattered the roadway. When the chapels closed after vespers, women humbly followed them. This habit of flagellation lasted from Michaelmas to Easter. In addition regular and secular clergy frequently carried relics around their churches with prayers to avert the impending disaster, and the pope appointed special prayers, which it would be tiresome to itemise. But when prayers failed to prevent it, when indeed the misery increased daily to a pitch never before recorded in the history of the world, and when the efforts of physicians proved unable to cure or avert it, then all they could do was to commit everything to God.

The signs which generally preceded the pestilence were red apostumes dotted around the genitals or under the armpits, and those victims with no hope of recovery voided blood. From the latter there issued a pestilential stink, which infected those who visited them or attended their funeral. It was very common for the death of one person to be followed by the death of everyone else in the house, so that it was hardly possible to find anyone living there; and it seemed to be the natural course of things that those related by blood should die at the same time.

Because of this great and widespread devastation flocks wandered shepherdless in the fields, for no one was prepared to risk his life to gather them in, and the ravening wolves which sought to attack them turned tail and bolted after one look.[28] The goods and chattels bequeathed by the dead were given a wide berth by all, as if they too were infected. The mortality always peaked around the time of the new moon.

27 Carinthia is now Karnten, a province of southern Austria. Styria is represented by Steiermark in southern Austria and by Stajersko, across the border in Slovenia.

28 The implication appears to be that the wolves sensed the infection.

The pestilence descended on the Neuberg estates around the feast of St Martin[29] and killed many monks and tenants. People were deeply distressed by these terrible events, and thoughtful men resolved that they should try to cheer each other up with comfort and merrymaking, so that they were not overwhelmed by depression. Accordingly wherever they could they held parties and weddings with a cheerful heart, so that by rekindling a sort of half-happiness they could avoid despair.

In 1349 the kings and princes of our country, although previously at each others' throats, all allied in friendship. A great flood did extensive damage everywhere. The contagious plague came in due course to Vienna and all its territories, and as a result countless people died and scarcely a third of the population remained alive. Because of the stench and horror of the corpses they were not allowed to be buried in churchyards, but as soon as life was extinct they had to be taken to a communal burial ground in God's Field outside the city, where in a short time five big deep pits were filled to the brim with bodies. The pestilence lasted from Pentecost [31 May] to Michaelmas [29 September]. It cruelly attacked not only Vienna but other places round about, and it did not spare monks and nuns, for 53 monks died in Heiligenkreuz at that time. The hateful signs described above were no respecters of persons, but marked all those carrying the plague.

The best wine was easily come by, and all those who indulged in it to excess behaved as if they were mad, beating and abusing people for no reason. Survivors of the plague, apparently putting the terrible experience right out of their minds, embroiled themselves in many disputes and quarrels over the wealth of the dead, or shamelessly went beyond the bounds of decency and, in many cases, lived with no reference to the law.

Nobles and citizens, seeking to escape death, took themselves to safer places, but they had already been infected and so in spite of their efforts many were unable to escape and died.

29 There are two feasts of St Martin and the chronicler does not specify which is intended, but the chronology of his narrative suggests St Martin in winter is meant: 11 November. The word translated here as descended [*declinavit*] carries the sense of turning aside and could therefore be translated in the opposite sense: that the plague died down in November – a reading preferred by Cardinal Gasquet, *The Great Pestilence*, London, 1893, p. 62. There seems little doubt, however, that the chronicler is describing the plague's arrival rather than its departure.

II: The plague in the British Isles

10. The arrival of the plague at Bristol

This brief account comes from the Anonimalle Chronicle, which covers the period up to 1381.[1] It was written by an unknown author, probably in the north of England – although its author seems not to have been very interested in the spread of the plague northwards.

The Anonimalle Chronicle, ed. V. H. Galbraith, Manchester, 1970, p. 30.

In 1348, about the feast of St Peter in chains [1 August] the first pestilence arrived in England at Bristol, carried by merchants and sailors, and it lasted in the south country around Bristol throughout August and all winter. And in the following year, that is to say, in 1349, the pestilence began in the other regions of England and lasted for a whole year, with the result that the living were hardly able to bury the dead.

11. The arrival of the plague near Bristol

This is taken from the continuation of Ralph Higden's *Polychronicon*. Higden was a monk of the Benedictine monastery of St Werburgh's, Chester, who died in the early 1360s. His work is a history of the world from its creation until 1340. It was enormously popular, and many religious houses had their own copies, to which they added continuations. Indeed Higden himself added brief entries covering the period 1341-52, which were in turn incorporated into some of the other continuations.

C. Babington and J. R. Lumby (eds), *Polychronicon Radulphi Higden Monachi Cestrensis*, 9 vols, Rolls Series, 1865-86, VIII pp. 344-6, 355.

In 1348 there was inordinately heavy rain between Midsummer and Christmas, and scarcely a day went by without rain at some time in the day or night. During that time a great mortality of men spread across the world and was especially violent in and around the Roman Curia at Avignon, and around the coastal towns of England and Ireland.

This year around the feast of St John [24 June] the aforesaid pestilence attacked the Bristol area and then travelled to all the other

---

1 I have taken the details about each source from Antonia Gransden, *Historical Writing in England II: c.1307 to the early sixteenth century*, London, 1982.

parts of England in turn, and it lasted in England for more than a year. Indeed it raged so strongly that scarcely a tenth of mankind was left alive. A mortality of animals followed in its footsteps, then rents dwindled, land fell waste for want of the tenants who used to cultivate it, and so much misery ensued that the world will hardly be able to regain its previous condition. Few, virtually none, of the lords and great men died in this pestilence.

12. The arrival of the plague in Dorset

The following brief account comes from the chronicle compiled by the Franciscans of Lynn (now King's Lynn) in Norfolk.

Antonia Gransden (ed), 'A Fourteenth-Century Chronicle from the Grey Friars at Lynn', *English Historical Review* LXXII, 1957, p. 274.

In 1348 two ships, one of them from Bristol, landed at Melcombe in Dorset a little before Midsummer. In them were sailors from Gascony who were infected with an unheard of epidemic illness called pestilence. They infected the men of Melcombe, who were the first to be infected in England. The first inhabitants to die from this illness of pestilence did so on the Eve of St John the Baptist [23 June], after being ill for three days at most.

In 1349, at about Easter or a little earlier, pestilence broke out in East Anglia and lasted for the whole summer.

13. The plague spreads

The *Eulogium*, from which this extract is taken, was modelled on the *Polychronicon* [11] and surveys the history of the world from the creation. It was compiled at Malmesbury Abbey (Wiltshire) in the 1350s.

F. S. Haydon (ed), *Eulogium Historiarum sive Temporis*, 3 vols, Rolls Series, 1858-63, III pp. 213-14.

In 1348, at about the feast of the Translation of St Thomas the martyr [7 July], the cruel pestilence, hateful to all future ages, arrived from countries across the sea on the south coast of England at the port called Melcombe in Dorset. Travelling all over the south country it wretchedly killed innumerable people in Dorset, Devon and Somerset. It was, moreover, believed to have been just as cruel among pagans as Christians. Next it came to Bristol, where very few were left alive, and then travelled northwards, leaving not a city, a town, a village, or even, except rarely, a house, without killing most or all of the people there, so that over England as a whole a fifth of the men, women and children were carried to burial. As a result, there was such a shortage of people that there were hardly enough living to look after the sick and bury the dead. Most of the women who survived remained barren for many years. If any did conceive they generally died, along with the baby, in giving birth. In some places, because of the lack of burial grounds, bishops consecrated new sites. At that time a quarter of wheat sold for 12d; a quarter of barley for 9d; a quarter of beans for 8d; a quarter of oats for 6d; a strong ox for 40d; a good horse, once valued at 40s, for 6s; a good cow for 2s or 18d; and even at this price buyers were rarely found. And this pestilence reigned in England for two years and more before it was purged.

By the time the plague ceased at the divine command it had caused such a shortage of servants that men could not be found to work the land, and women and children had to be used to drive ploughs and carts, which was unheard of.

14. The plague spreads to London

This account comes from the chronicle of Robert of Avesbury, a secular clerk based in London and employed in the court of the archbishop of Canterbury at Lambeth. His chronicle is primarily concerned with the military campaigns of Edward III and he has relatively little to say about the plague, but his account of the arrival of the flagellants in London [53a] has the immediacy of an eye-witness account. Avesbury died at the beginning of 1359.

E. M. Thompson (ed), *Robertus de Avesbury de Gestis Mirabilibus Regis Edwardi Tertii*, Rolls Series, 1889, pp. 406-7.

The pestilence, which first began in the land inhabited by the Saracens, grew so strong that, sparing no lordship, it visited every place in all the kingdoms stretching from that land northwards, up to and including Scotland, striking down the greater part of the people with the blows of sudden death. It began in England in the county of Dorset, about the feast of St Peter in chains [1 August], and immediately progressed without warning from place to place. It killed a great many healthy people, removing them from human concerns in the course of a morning. Those marked for death were scarcely permitted to live longer than three or four days. It showed favour to no one, except for a very few of the wealthy. On the same day 20, 40, or 60 bodies, and on many occasions many more, might be committed for burial together in the same pit.

The pestilence arrived in London at about the feast of All Saints [1 November] and daily deprived many of life. It grew so powerful that, between Candlemas [2 February, 1349] and Easter [12 April], more than 200 corpses were buried almost every day in the new burial ground made next to Smithfield, and this was in addition to the bodies buried in other churchyards in the city.[2] It ceased in London with the coming of the grace of the Holy Spirit, that is to say at Pentecost [31 May], proceeding uninterupted towards the north, where it also stopped about Michaelmas [29 September] 1349.

15. The plague in York

This account is taken from the continuation of the chronicle of the archbishops of York written by Thomas Stubbs in c.1373 (the year the continuation ends). From his northern perspective Stubbs, who was probably a Dominican friar, set the arrival of the plague in England considerably later than was in fact the case.

J. Raine (ed), *Historians of the Church of York*, 3 vols, Rolls Series, 1879-94, II p. 418.

In 1348, about Michaelmas, there began a mortality of men in England. After Christmas, on 31 December, the river Ouse flooded and burst its banks at the bridge towards Micklegate, a state of affairs which persisted until Lent. And after this, at around Ascensiontide [21 May], the mortality began in the city of York and raged until the feast of St James the Apostle [25 July].

16. The plague according to Thomas Walsingham

Walsingham, a monk of St Albans Abbey, completed the first versions of his two chronicles in the 1390s, although he produced continuations of them both before his death in c.1422. His treatment of the first three outbreaks of pestilence is fairly cursory, but his account of the period 1376-92 was written more or less contemporaneously with the events it describes and includes much fuller descriptions of the fourth and fifth pestilences [27b and 28].

H. T. Riley (ed), *Historia Anglicana, 1272-1422*, 2 vols, Rolls Series, 1863-4, I pp. 272-4.

---

2 For a fuller account of one of the new London burial grounds see **83**.

[1348] This year there was a great downpour which lasted from Midsummer to the following Christmas, and it was speedily followed by a mortality in the east among the Saracens and other unbelievers. It was so great that scarcely a tenth of the Saracens were left alive, and they, thinking that the plague had been sent to them because of their unbelief, converted to the Christian faith. But when they discovered that the same plague raged among Christians they returned to their unbelief like dogs to their vomit.

In 1349, that is in the 23rd year of the reign of King Edward III, a great mortality of men advanced across the globe, beginning in the southern and northern zones. Its destruction was so great that scarcely half mankind was left alive. Towns once packed with people were emptied of their inhabitants, and the plague spread so thickly that the living were hardly able to bury the dead. In some religious houses no more than two survived out of twenty. It was calculated by several people that barely a tenth of mankind remained alive. A murrain of animals followed on the heels of this pestilence. Rents dwindled and land was left untilled for want of tenants (who were nowhere to be found). And so much wretchedness followed these ills that afterwards the world could never return to its former state.

Meanwhile, as the plague raged in England, Pope Clement granted – because of the epidemic – full remission of penance to all those thoughout the kingdom who died truly contrite and after making confession.

17. The plague seen from Lincolnshire

This brief account comes from the chronicle of the Cistercian abbey of Louth Park, which ends in 1413.

E. Venables (ed), *Chronicon Abbatiae de Parco Ludae: The Chronicle of Louth Park Abbey*, Horncastle, 1891, pp. 38-9.

In the year of the Lord 1349 the hand of Almighty God struck the human race a deadly blow, which, beginning in the southern regions, passed on to the northern countries and attacked all the kingdoms of the world. This stroke felled Christians, Jews and infidels alike. It killed confessor and penitent together. In many places it did not leave a fifth of the people alive. This blow struck the whole world with immense terror. So great a pestilence had not been seen, or heard, or written about, before this time. For it is thought that so great a multitude of people were not killed in Noah's Flood. A greater number of the dead were carried to the grave after dinner than were buried before it.

In this year many of the monks of Louth Park died, among them, on 13 July, Dom Walter de Louth, the abbot, who had endured great harassment on account of the manor of Cockerington and was buried before the high altar beside Sir Henry le Vavasour, knight. Dom Richard de Lincoln succeeded him, and was elected properly, rightly and canonically on the same day, as ordained by the Lord and by the Order.

18. The plague at Meaux Abbey

Meaux was a Cistercian abbey in the East Riding of Yorkshire. Its chronicle was written by one of its monks, Thomas Burton, between c.1388 and 1396, the year in which he became abbot. The chronicle has three separate entries on the plague and some repetition has been omitted in the third section.

E. A. Bond (ed), *Chronica Monasterii de Melsa*, 3 vols, Rolls Series, 1866-68, III pp. 35-7, 40, 72.

Hugh the fifteenth abbot caused a new crucifix to be made in the lay brothers' choir. The craftsman only sculpted anything of beauty and note on Fridays, on which day he fasted on bread and water. He worked from a nude model standing before him and from him copied the beautiful image to adorn the crucifix. The Almightly constantly performed manifest miracles through this crucifix. It was accordingly thought that if women had access to the crucifix it would increase popular devotion and also bring great benefit to our monastery. The abbot of Citeaux, in response to our request, thereupon gave us permission to admit men and honest women to see the said crucifix; although women were not allowed to enter the cloisters, dormitory or any other buildings. An exception was made for the foundress, and for the wife, daughter or daughter-in-law of the founder, but they, and the others, were not allowed to spend the night within the abbey precinct or to be there before prime or after compline. If we were to do otherwise, then the abbot's licence would be revoked. With the authority of this licence women often came to the crucifix, especially when devotion had grown cold in them. But it was to our damage, for they came in such numbers to see the church that entertaining them increased our expenses.

Dom Adam, the predecessor of Abbot Hugh, had begun the construction of a chapel above the main gateway, because it was usual to have a chantry of six monks at a chapel outside the gate, but the work was left unfinished at his death. Abbot Hugh, whether unimpressed by the work, or not thinking it worth completion, demolished that part of the foundations of the chapel, which could still be seen just as they had been left, and carried away almost all the materials. From the stone prepared for the construction of the chapel he had made, among other things, a beautiful stone vessel next to the malt kiln in which we used to malt our barley. After this, with the help of Brother John de Wandesforth, he had the monks' dormitory roofed with lead.

When Abbot Hugh had ruled the monastery for 9 years, 11 months and 11 days (at which time there were 42 monks and 7 lay brothers, not counting himself), he died in the great pestilence, along with 32 monks and lay brothers. This pestilence grew so strong in our monastery, as it did in other places, that within the month of August the abbot, 22 monks and 6 lay brothers died; of whom the abbot and 5 monks were buried together on a single day. Other deaths followed, so that when the pestilence ceased only 10 monks and no lay brothers were left alive out of the 50 monks and lay brothers. From this time the rents and goods of the monastery began to dwindle, largely because the majority of our tenants had died, and because after the abbot, prior, cellarer, bursar and other experienced men and officials had died, the survivors made misguided grants of the goods and possessions of the monastery.

The abbot died on 12 August 1349 and was buried in the lay brothers' choir before the crucifix which he had had put up. In addition he left the house a debt of more than £500 and the monastery unprovided with any supplies of grain.

At the beginning of 1349, during Lent on the Friday before Passion Sunday [27 March],[3] an earthquake was felt throughout England. Our monks of Meaux were at vespers and had come to the verse 'He hath put down the mighty' in the Magnificat, when they were thrown from their stalls by the earthquake and sent sprawling on the ground. The earthquake was quickly followed in this part of the country by the pestilence.

In 1349 there befell that great and universal pestilence. The pope accordingly sent to England a general absolution, to last for 3 months

---

3 In medieval English reckoning the year began on Lady Day, March 25. March 27 is thus indeed 'at the beginning' of the year.

from its publication, for all who died of the pestilence within those three months. He instituted a new mass for assuaging the plague, and within the papal curia he took part in person in solemn processions of the clergy and people.[4] In addition he had a beautiful silver statue made in honour of the Blessed Virgin Mary and had it carried in these processions, until the pestilence was laid to rest in the Curia by the merits of the Blessed Virgin.

It was said that the pestilence had first broken out strongly among the infidel. As a result the Saracens who survived, believing that the judgement of God had blasted them because they had not adopted the Christian faith, were inclined to believe in Christ. They sent men into Christendom to investigate whether the pestilence was as strong there as it was among them, but when the messengers returned and announced that there was the same general pestilence among the Christians as among the Saracens, they again refused to believe in Christ.

This pestilence held such sway in England at that time that there were hardly enough people left alive to bury the dead, or enough burial grounds to hold them. During that time two closes or crofts were consecrated for the burial of the dead in London, and two monasteries were afterwards founded in them, one of the Cistercian order, the other of the Carthusians. The pestilence grew so strong that men and women dropped dead while walking in the streets, and in innumerable households and many villages not one person was left alive. However, God's providence ensured that, in most places, chaplains survived unharmed until the end of the pestilence in order to perform the exequies of those who died. But, after the funerals of the laymen, chaplains were swallowed by death in great numbers, as others had been before....

In the year before the pestilence came to dominate England, the nobility of England held tournaments and hastiludes in various cities and towns throughout the realm, to which ladies, matrons and other gentlewomen were invited.[5] But scarcely any married woman attended with her own husband, but had instead been chosen by some other man, who used her to satisfy his sexual urges. And, shortly before this time, there was a certain human monster in England, divided from the navel upwards and both masculine and feminine, and joined in the

4 The mass *Recordare Domini*, for which see **38b**.

5 For these tournaments see **43**.

lower part. When one part ate, drank, slept or spoke, the other could do something else if it wished. One died before the other, and the survivor held it in its arms for three days. They used to sing together very sweetly. They died, aged about 18, at Kingston upon Hull a short time before the pestilence began.[6]

19. The plague seen from Rochester

This contemporary account is taken from the *Historia Roffensis*, the chronicle of the cathedral priory of Rochester, which covers the period 1314-50. An abridged version (omitting most of the detail about the plague) was printed by Henry Wharton, *Anglia Sacra*, 2 vols, London, 1691, where its composition is credited to William Dene.

British Library, Cottonian MS, Faustina B V fos 96v-101.

[1348]
A great mortality of men began in India and, raging through the whole of infidel Syria and Egypt, and also through Greece, Italy, Provence and France, arrived in England, where the same mortality destroyed more than a third of the men, women and children. As a result there was such a shortage of servants, craftsmen, and workmen, and of agricultural workers and labourers, that a great many lords and people, although well-endowed with goods and possessions, were yet without all service and attendance. Alas, this mortality devoured such a multitude of both sexes that no one could be found to carry the bodies of the dead to burial, but men and women carried the bodies of their own little ones to church on their shoulders and threw them into mass graves, from which arose such a stink that it was barely possible for anyone to go past a churchyard.

As remarked above, such a shortage of workers ensued that the humble turned up their noses at employment, and could scarcely be persuaded to serve the eminent unless for triple wages. Instead, because of the doles handed out at funerals, those who once had to work now began to have time for idleness, thieving and other outrages, and thus the poor and servile have been enriched and the rich impoverished. As a result, churchmen, knights and other worthies have been forced to thresh their corn, plough the land and perform every other unskilled task if they are to make their own bread.

6 Matteo Villani, the chronicler of the plague in Florence, juxtaposes a similar description of a human 'monster' with his account of the plague: F. G. Dragomanni (ed), *Cronica di Matteo Villani*, 2 vols, Florence, 1846, I p. 14.

From his modest household the Bishop of Rochester [Hamo Hethe] lost 4 priests, 5 squires, 10 household servants, 7 young clerks and 6 pages, leaving no one in any office who should have served him. At Malling he appointed two abbesses who promptly died. No one remained alive there except 4 professed nuns and 4 novices, and the bishop committed custody of the temporalities to one of them and the spiritualities to another, since no adequate person could be found to fill the post of abbess.[7]

This want was strongly felt both in Kent and throughout the whole of England, among the clergy and the people, religious and others alike. Because of it, the prelates and leading men of the kingdom appeared before the king and asked for some remedy to be ordained for these problems. Therefore, by the counsel of the prelates and leading men of the whole of England, they ordained remedy for these things in the following manner: [The ordinance of labourers follows, for which see 98].

After the death of the Archbishop of Canterbury [John Stratford], the pope, acting on the request of the king, gave the archbishopric to the Chancellor of England, Master John Offord – an infirm and paralysed man. Offord borrowed a great sum of money from all sides to give to the pope – but he might as well not have bothered for he died soon afterwards and thereby lost the lot. He died on Ascension Day [21 May] and was buried without ceremony in the church of Canterbury; elected to the see but not yet consecrated. Thus he was the ruin of a great many creditors, who were reduced to poverty. For in these days juicy benefices come expensive, and as a result their buyers can scarcely recover the cost, but languish in poverty during their whole time in office. Thus in our day we see many holders of benefices existing in permanently straitened circumstances. The Dominican, Brother Thomas of London, the Bishop of Ely, was one example, and there are numberless others. But in spite of such great poverty, buyers can always be found, to the confusion and destruction of the church.

This time the Canterbury chapter chose, for a second time, Master Thomas Bradwardine of Cowden, a native of the diocese of Rochester, who had also been their choice immediately after the death of Archbishop Stratford. And on that occasion the pope gave Master Thomas the archbishopric in the usual way before Offord could reach him, choosing rather to have thanks than insisting on his right to make

7 The documents describing the situation at Malling are printed below, 80.

the appointment. But after his collation, the king wrote on Offord's behalf and hindered the proceedings in other ways.[8] Sad to relate, the archbishopric has been so damaged by the number of vacancies, as a result of bad custody and the payments made at the Roman Curia, that there seems no hope of its recovering in our days. Since the time of St Thomas [Becket] the church of Canterbury has never been as impoverished and so damaged by unaccustomed burdens as it is now.

Master Thomas, after returning to the Roman Curia for consecration, hurried to London, but died in the hostel of the Bishop of Rochester at *La Place*, where he had lain sick for four days. Then the Canterbury chapter quickly chose Master Simon Islip, a royal clerk, and the pope, at the king's request, sent his bulls of consecration and confirmation to England, making the usual charges. He was consecrated at St Paul's, London, by the bishops of London, Winchester and Worcester. This offended the monks of Canterbury, who grumbled indignantly about his action. The archbishop, finding his diocese spoiled and wasted and stripped of all its possessions, did not know where to turn.

The shortage of labourers and of workers in every kind of craft and occupation was then so acute that more than a third of the land throughout the whole kingdom remained uncultivated. Labourers and skilled workers became so rebellious that neither the king nor the law and the judges who enforced it were able to correct them, and more or less the whole population turned to evil courses, became addicted to all forms of vice and stooped to more than usually base behaviour, thinking not at all of death or of the recently-experienced plague, nor of how they were hazarding their own salvation by uniting in rebellion; and priests, making light of the sacrifice of a contrite spirit, took themselves to where they might receive a stipend greater than the value of their benefices. As a result, many benefices remained unserved by parish priests, whom neither prelates nor ordinaries were powerful enough to bridle.[9] Thus spiritual dangers sprouted daily

8 When Stratford died, the Canterbury chapter elected Bradwardine without first securing the king's licence. To maintain his rights in the matter the king thereupon asked the pope to set aside Bradwardine in favour of Offord. When Offord's death necessitated a second election the chapter asked for a royal licence, which came with a recommendation to elect Bradwardine.

9 Dene's use of the verb to bridle [*refrenare*] is a reference to Simon Islip's 1350 attempt to limit the wages of the clergy, known, from its opening word, as *Effrenata* [unbridled]. It is printed below, **108**.

among the clergy and laity. At that time the king spent Christmas at Orsett, a manor of the Bishop of London.

[1349]

For the whole of that winter and summer, the aged and infirm Bishop of Rochester stayed at Trottiscliffe, made ill and miserable by the sudden change in the world. For in all the manors of the diocese, buildings and walls were crumbling, and the manors barely yielded £100 that year. Moreover in the monastery of Rochester there was such a shortage of food that the monks were obliged to grind their own bread. The prior, however, had plenty of good things....

At that time there was such a shortage of fish, that men were obliged to eat flesh on Wednesdays and it was ordered in England that 4 herring should sell for a penny.[10] In Lent, indeed, there was such a lack of fish that many people who had been accustomed to live daintily had to make do with just pastry, bread and potage. But the threshers, labourers and workmen were so well supplied with cash that they did not need to worry about paying the full price for such foods. And thus, by an inversion of the natural order, those who were accustomed to have plenty and those accustomed to suffer want, fell into need on the one hand and into abundance on the other.

[1350]

In this year the harvest was late, the crops scanty, barns empty and haystacks small – all the grain gathered did not suffice to meet the expenses of the manors. And this want and the harshness of the days began to stiffen men's malice. No workman or labourer was prepared to take orders from anyone, whether equal, inferior or superior, but all those who served did so with ill will and a malicious spirit. It is therefore much to be feared that Gog and Magog have returned from hell to encourage such things and to cherish those who have been corrupted.[11]

---

10 Fridays, Wednesdays and Saturdays were days of abstinence, on which no meat or other animal product should be eaten. The requirement seems to have been generally observed on Fridays but rather more loosely on other days.

11 In Ezechiel 38-39 Gog and the land of Magog are described as the enemies of Israel. The names were accordingly used to refer to anyone perceived as an enemy of God's people and were regularly applied to Jews and Moslems in the middle ages. More specifically, as here, the reference is to the belief that the reign of Antichrist would be heralded by the return of Gog and Magog (Apocalypse 20.7-9). For the chronology of the Last Days, see the introduction to Part Two, below.

20. The plague according to John of Reading

Reading was a monk of Westminster, who died in 1368/9. His chronicle covers the period 1346-67, and was apparently all written towards the end of that period. As this and the other extracts from his chronicle show, he was a savage critic of contemporary behaviour.

James Tait (ed), *Chronica Johannis de Reading et Anonymi Cantuariensis 1346-1367*, Manchester, 1914, pp. 106-10.

In 1348 rain poured down in the south and west country from Midsummer to Christmas, scarcely stopping by day or night but still drizzling. It was followed by the mortality of men, which grew throughout the world but especially around the Roman Curia and other coastal and watery places. It left hardly enough people alive to give the dead a decent burial; instead they dug broad, deep pits and buried the bodies together and, reducing everyone to the same level, threw them into the ground – treating everyone alike except the more eminent.

In this year, and in the next immediately following, a fierce mortality devoured men from east to west by pestilence. Ulcers broke out in the groin and the armpit, which tortured the dying for three days. To those dying of the disease in England Pope Clement of his clemency granted a plenary indulgence for confessed sins. Among those who died was Master John Offord, Chancellor of England and Archbishop-elect of Canterbury. The diocese had been left empty by the death of Archbishop John Stratford and Offord had been confirmed but not consecrated. Master Thomas Bradwardine succeeded him and was canonically elected, confirmed and consecrated at Avignon. Offord was succeeded as chancellor by Master John Thoresby.

Brother Simon Bircheston, Abbot of Westminster, died in the same pestilence. He left Westminster greatly burdened with debt, the result of his own extravagence and the fraudulent depredations of his household and kinsmen. Brother Simon Langham, the prior there, succeeded him, after a harmonious and canonical election.... Thomas de la Mare, Prior of Tynemouth, succeeded Michael Abbot of St Albans.

And there was in those days death without sorrow, marriage without affection, self-imposed penance, want without poverty, and flight without escape. How many who fled from the face of the pestilence were already infected and did not escape the slaughter. As Isaiah says: 'He that shall flee from the noise of the fear shall fall into the pit: and he that shall rid himself out of the pit shall be taken in the snare' [24.18]. In the end the plague devoured a multitude of people, who left behind them all their worldly riches. Scarcely a tenth of the population survived. However, for a long time afterwards all these worldly goods were not enough for those few who remained alive, although before, when everyone was still alive, they had been enough for sustenance and dignity. It was believed that this Mammon of iniquity wounded the regular clergy very much, but wounded the mendicants fatally. The superfluous wealth poured their way, through confessions and bequests, in such quantities that they scarcely condescended to accept oblations. Forgetful of their profession and rule, which imposed total poverty and mendicancy, they lusted after things of the world and of the flesh, not of heaven. Superfluous finery was everywhere: in their chambers, at table, in riding – all contrary to the requirements of their order and prompted by the devil. They maintained in their sermons that Jesus Christ and his disciples were poor and begged in this world; and upheld various errors which we shall pass over as beneath notice.

In the same year a remarkable thing was noticed for the first time: that everyone born after the pestilence had two fewer teeth than people had had before.

The year of grace 1350, the 8th year of Pope Clement and the 24th year of the reign of King Edward in England and his 12th in France, was a year of jubilee, and one of divine, not human, remission of penance. But alas, how quickly people forget the vengeance of God. It was because of the sins of men, or so it was believed, that God allowed the human race to be poisoned and destroyed by the said pestilence to such an extent that there were scarcely enough survivors to bury the bodies, but people did not turn away from their despicable crimes. Many sinners absolved in Rome returned to their countries abstaining from none of these things; on the contrary .... Among such people the traditional respect due to superiors was weakened so that this prophecy came true: 'As with the people, so with the priest: and as with the servant, so with his master: as with the handmaid, so with her mistress' [Isaiah 24.2]. Their greed, scorn and malice were asking to be punished.

21. The plague according to Henry Knighton

Knighton was an Augustinian canon of Leicester, who produced his chronicle in the early 1390s. He died in c.1396.

J. R. Lumby (ed), *Chronicon Henrici Knighton vel Cnitthon monachi Leycestrensis*, 2 vols, Rolls Series, 1889-95, II pp. 58-65.

In that year and the following year there was a universal mortality of men throughout the world. It began first in India, then in Tarsus, then it reached the Saracens and finally the Christians and Jews. According to the opinion current in the Roman Curia, 8000 legions of men,[12] not counting Christians, died a sudden death in those distant countries in the space of one year, from Easter to Easter. When the King of Tarsus saw this sudden and unprecedented ruin of his people, he set out to travel to the pope at Avignon, accompanied by a great multitude of noblemen. He intended to become a Christian and to be baptised by the pope, for he believed that the vengeance of God had weakened his people because of their wicked unbelief. However, when he had completed 20 days of his journey, he heard that the fatal plague was as strong among Christians as among other nations, and turning from the path he went no further on that journey but hastened back to his own country. The Christians, however, who had been following in the rear, killed about 2000 of them.

On a single day 1312 people died in Avignon, according to a calculation made in the pope's presence. On another day more than 400 died. 358 of the Dominicans in Provence died during Lent. At Montpellier only seven friars survived out of 140. At Magdalen seven survived out of 160, which is quite enough. From 140 Minorites at Marseilles not one remained to carry the news to the rest – and a good job too. Of the Carmelites of Avignon, 66 had died before the citizens realised what was causing the deaths; they thought that the brothers had been killing each other. Not one of the English Augustinians survived in Avignon – not that anyone will be upset by that.[13] At the same time the plague raged in England. It began in the autumn in various places and after racing across the country it ended at the same time in the following year. In Corinth and Achaia at that time many citizens were buried when the earth swallowed them. Castles and towns cracked apart and were thrown down and engulfed. In Cyprus mountains were levelled, blocking rivers and causing many citizens to drown and towns to be destroyed. At Naples it was the same, as a friar had predicted. The whole city was destroyed by an earthquake and storms, and the earth was suddenly overwhelmed, like a stone thrown into water. Everyone died, including the friar who had foretold it,

12 A legion was 4200-6000 men.

13 This uncharitable treatment of the mortality among the friars reflects the dislike felt towards them by other religious orders. See also Walsingham's account of the events in Cambridge which preceded the outbreak of 1390 [28] where a reliquary holding the Host began to behave strangely as it passed an Augustinian friary.

except one friar who fled and hid in a garden outside the town. And all those things were brought about by the earthquake.

Then the pope sent letters urging that peace be restored between kingdoms in order to avert the just punishment of God. He asserted that all these things were happening because of the sins of mankind. The king accordingly sent the earls of Lancaster and Norfolk with other magnates to Calais to treat for peace. The leading men of France waited at St Omer. But while this was going on the commons of Flanders, with the French and some Flemings, entered Bruges by guile and beheaded and hanged those Flemings who had sided with the King of England. King Edward, intending to go to Flanders to destroy the deserters, gathered his people and set out, but the Earl of Lancaster hastened to meet him with the news that the Flemings would return to the king under certain conditions, as will be shown below. It was agreed that certain people from England and France would negotiate peace between the kingdoms until September, and if agreement could not be reached by then the crown of France should be taken to a place within France agreed by both sides and the matter be settled by a pitched battle, without any further rebellion.

Then the most lamentable plague penetrated the coast through Southampton and came to Bristol, and virtually the whole town was wiped out. It was as if sudden death had marked them down beforehand, for few lay sick for more than 2 or 3 days, or even for half a day. Cruel death took just two days to burst out all over a town. At Leicester, in the little parish of St Leonard, more than 380 died; in the parish of Holy Cross more than 400; in the parish of St Margaret 700; and a great multitude in every parish. The Bishop of Lincoln sent word through the whole diocese, giving general power to every priest (among the regular as well as the secular clergy) to hear confession and grant absolution with full and complete authority except only in cases of debt. In such cases the penitent, if it lay within his power, ought to make satisfaction while he lived, but certainly others should do it from his goods after his death. Similarly the pope granted plenary remission of all sins to those at the point of death, the absolution to be for one time only, and the right to each person to choose his confessor as he wished. This concession was to last until the following Easter.

In the same year there was a great murrain of sheep throughout the realm, so much so that in one place more than 5000 sheep died in a single pasture, and their bodies were so corrupt that no animal or bird would touch them. And because of the fear of death everything fetched a low price. For there were very few people who cared for riches, or indeed for anything else. A man could have a horse previously valued at 40*s* for half a mark, a good fat ox for 4*s*, a cow for 12*d*, a bullock for 6*d*, a fat sheep for 4*d*, a ewe for 3*d*, a lamb for 2*d*, a large pig for 5*d*, a stone of wool for 9*d*. And sheep and cattle roamed unchecked through the fields and through the standing corn, and there was no one to chase them and round them up. For want of watching animals died in uncountable numbers in the fields and in bye-ways and hedges throughout the whole country; for there was so great a shortage of servants and labourers that there was no one who knew what needed to be done. There was no memory of so inexorable and fierce a mortality since the time of Vortigern, king of the Britons, in whose time, as Bede testifies in his *De gestis Anglorum*, there were not enough living to bury the dead. In the following autumn it was not possible to hire a reaper for less than 8*d* and his food, or a mower for 12*d* with his food. For which reason many crops rotted unharvested in the fields; but in the year of the pestilence, as mentioned above, there was so great an abundance of all types of grain that no one cared.

The Scots, hearing of the cruel plague of the English, declared that it had befallen them through the revenging hand of God, and they took to swearing 'by the foul death of England' – or so the common report resounded in the ears of the English. And thus the Scots, believing that the English were overwhelmed by the terrible vengeance of God, gathered in the forest of Selkirk with the intention of invading the whole realm of England. The fierce mortality came upon them, and the sudden cruelty of a monstrous death winnowed the Scots. Within a short space of time around 5000 died, and the rest, weak and strong alike, decided to retreat to their own country. But the English, following, surprised them and killed many of them.

Master Thomas Bradwardine was consecrated as Archbishop of Canterbury by the pope, and on his return to England he went to London, where he died within two days. He was renowned above all other clerks in Christendom, especially in theology but also in the other liberal arts. At that time there was such a great shortage of priests everywhere that many churches were widowed and lacked the divine offices, masses, matins, vespers, and the sacraments and sacramentals.[14] A man could scarcely get a chaplain for less than £10

14 Sacramentals are objects blessed by a priest (such as water or candles) which, as well as having ecclesiastical functions, can be taken away and used by the laity. There is a good brief discussion of them, and their popularity among the laity, in R.W. Scribner, *Popular Culture and Popular Movements in Reformation Germany*, London, 1987, pp. 32-4, 39-41.

or 10*m* to minister to any church, and whereas before the pestilence there had been a glut of priests, and a man could get a chaplain for 4 or 5 marks, or for 2*m* with board and lodging, in this time there was scarcely anyone who would accept a vicarage at £20 or 20*m*. But within a short time a great crowd of men whose wives had died in the pestilence rushed into priestly orders. Many of them were illiterate, no better than laymen – for even if they could read, they did not understand what they read.[15]

The hide of an ox was priced at a mere 12*d*, a pair of shoes at 10*d*, 12*d* or 14*d*, a pair of boots at 3*s* or 4*s*. Meanwhile the king sent commands into every county that reapers and other workers should not take more than they were accustomed to take, under penalties laid down by the statute which he had introduced to this end. But the workers were so above themselves and so bloody-minded that they took no notice of the king's command. If anyone wished to hire them he had to submit to their demands, for either his fruit and standing corn would be lost or he had to pander to the arrogance and greed of the workers. When it was brought to the king's attention that people were not obeying his orders, but were giving higher wages to the workers, he levied heavy fines on abbots, priors, greater and lesser knights, and on others, of both greater and lesser standing, in the country; taking 100*s* from some, 40*s* or 20*s* from others, depending on their ability to pay. And he took 20*s* from each ploughland nationwide, and in this way raised as much as a fifteenth.[16] Then the king had numerous workers arrested and sent to prison, and many of these escaped and took to the woods and if they were captured they were heavily fined. And most took oaths that they would not take more than their old daily wages, and thereby secured their release from prison. The same was done to artisans in boroughs and towns.

In the same year, on 25 October, the body of St Thomas of Hereford was translated.[17] After the aforesaid pestilence many buildings of all

---

15 Knighton is using the word *illiteratus* in its usual medieval sense, to denote an inability to read or write Latin.

16 Direct taxation in this period was in theory assessed on an individual's movable goods: a tenth of their value in towns, a fifteenth elsewhere. By this period 'a fifteenth' was a lump sum, to which local communities had to contribute a fixed amount. In the 1340s a fifteenth yielded £38,000 (information I owe to Dr Mark Ormrod).

17 Thomas Cantilupe. His translation (the removal of his body to a new shrine) was later credited with halting the plague in Hereford: W. H. Frere and L. E. G. Brown, *The Hereford Breviary* II, Henry Bradshaw Society XL, 1911 p. 382.

sizes in every city fell into total ruin for want of inhabitants. Likewise, many villages and hamlets were deserted, with no house remaining in them, because everyone who had lived there was dead, and indeed many of these villages were never inhabited again. In the following winter there was such a lack of workers in all areas of activity that it was thought that there had hardly ever been such a shortage before; for a man's farm animals and other livestock wandered about without a shepherd and all his possessions were left unguarded. And as a result all essentials were so expensive that something which had previously cost 1*d* was now worth 4*d* or 5*d*. Confronted by this shortage of workers and the scarcity of goods the great men of the realm, and the lesser landowners who had tenants, remitted part of the rent so that their tenants did not leave. Some remitted half the rent, some more and some less; some remitted it for two years, some for three and some for one – whatever they could agree with their tenants. Likewise those whose tenants held by the year, by the performance of labour services (as is customary in the case of serfs), found that they had to release and remit such works, and either pardon rents completely or levy them on easier terms, otherwise houses would be irretrievably ruined and land left uncultivated. And all victuals and other necessities were extremely dear.

22. The plague according to Geoffrey le Baker

Baker was a clerk of Swinbrook in Oxfordshire, whose chronicle covers the period 1303-56 and was probably begun in the 1340s.

E. M. Thompson (ed), *Chronicon Galfridi le Baker de Swynebroke*, Oxford, 1889, pp. 92, 98-100.

In 1347, after the capture of Calais, there began in those parts that universal pestilence, which had poured in waves out of the east, of which a great multitude of people died in every part of the world.

In 1349, in the 23rd year of the king's reign, an unexpected and universal pestilence from the eastern lands of the Indians and Turks infected the centre of the world and slaughtered the Saracens, Turks, Syrians, Palestinians and finally the Greeks with such butchery that they, driven by terror, resolved to receive the Christian faith and sacraments, having heard that the Christians beyond the Greek Sea were not dying more suddenly or in greater numbers than usual. At last fierce destruction came to the countries beyond the Alps, and from there, in stages, to western France and Germany, and, in the seventh year since its beginning, to England. First it virtually stripped a Dorset seaport and then its hinterland of their inhabitants, and then it ravaged Devon and Somerset up to Bristol. As a result, the people of Gloucester denied admission to people from Bristol, believing that the breath of those who had lived among the dying would be infectious. But in the end Gloucester, and then Oxford and London too, and finally the whole of England were so violently attacked that scarcely a tenth of either sex survived. When the churchyards proved inadequate, fields were designated for the burial of the dead. The Bishop of London bought the croft called *Nomanneslond* by the Londoners, and Sir Walter Marney that called *the new chierche hawe*, where he founded a house of religion to bury the dying. Cases in the courts of King's Bench and Common Pleas inevitably came to a stop.

A few noblemen died, among whom were Sir John Montgomery (the Captain of Calais) and the lord of Clisteles – who died in Calais and were buried in the church of the Carmelite friars in London. Numberless commoners and a multitude of religious and other clerics, who are known only to God, departed this life. This disaster chiefly overwhelmed the young and strong; the elderly and weak it generally spared. Hardly anyone dared to have anything to do with the sick. They fled from the things left by the dead, which had once been precious but were now poisonous to health. People who one day had been full of happiness, on the next were found dead. Some were tormented by boils which broke out suddenly in various parts of the body, and were so hard and dry that when they were lanced hardly any liquid flowed out. Many of these people escaped, by lancing the boils or by long suffering. Other victims had little black pustules scattered over the skin of the whole body. Of these people very few, indeed hardly any, recovered life and health. The pestilence, which began in Bristol on the feast of the Assumption of the Virgin [15 August] and in London around Michaelmas [29 September], raged for more than a year in England and completely emptied many rural settlements of human beings.

With such a disaster laying England waste, the Scots gleefully swore that they would beat the English. They used to swear this jokingly (and blasphemously) 'by the foul death of the English'. But their joy was replaced by grief. The sword of the wrath of God, withdrawn from the English, punished the Scots with madness and leprosy no less than it had punished the English with boils and pustules. In the following year it laid waste the Welsh as well as the English; and then it took ship to Ireland, where the English residents were cut down in great numbers but the native Irish, living in the mountains and uplands, were scarcely touched until 1357 when it took them unawares and annihilated them everywhere.

23. The plague in Ireland

The plague arrived in the Pale, the area of English settlement in the east of Ireland, in 1348, and advanced across the rest of the country in the following year. The only detailed description is the one which follows, by John Clynn, a Franciscan friar, who was himself apparently a victim of the plague. After the material printed here there is a brief eulogy of Sir Fulk de la Frene, who died in 1349, and then a note in the copyist's hand: 'Here it seems the author died'.

R. Butler (ed), *Annalium Hibernae Chronicon*, Irish Archaeological Society, 1849, pp. 35-7.

In 1348, particularly during the months of September and October, bishops and prelates, ecclesiastics and members of religious orders, nobles and others, everybody in fact, women as well as men, gathered in droves from all over Ireland to make the pilgrimage to Tech-Moling and wade in the water,[18] with the result that on many days you might have seen thousands of people assembled. Some came out of devotion; others, the majority in fact, came because of their fear of the plague which was then raging. It first began near Dublin, at Howth, and at Drogheda, and virtually wiped out those cities, emptying them of inhabitants. In Dublin alone 14,000 people died between the beginning of August and Christmas. This pestilence was said to have arisen in the east and to have killed some forty million people as it swept through the Saracens and unbelievers. In Avignon in Provence, where the Roman Curia was then based, it began in the previous January, in the pontificate of Clement VI. There were not enough churches and burial grounds in the city to hold all the dead bodies, and the pope himself ordered a new burial ground to be consecrated for the burial of those killed by the pestilence. From May to the Translation of St Thomas [3 July] more than 50,000 bodies were buried there.

It was said that in the previous year, that is in 1347, an amazing vision

18 Tech-Moling (the house of Moling) was on the river Barrow. St Moling, the founder of an important monastic house there, had built a watermill nearby, utilising a spring to feed the millstream. Pilgrims waded up the stream to the wellhouse at its head: D. D. C. Pochin Mould, *Irish Pilgrimage*, Dublin, 1955, pp. 36-8, 127.

concerning this pestilence was vouchsafed in the Cistercian monastery at Tripoli.[19] A monk was celebrating mass before his abbot, with another official present, when between the ablution and the communion of the mass a hand appeared, writing on the corporal cloth on which the monk had consecrated the elements. 'The lofty cedar of Lebanon shall be set ablaze, and Tripoli destroyed and Acre taken, and a borderer[20] will conquer the world, and Saturn will ambush Jove, and the bat will put the duke of the bees to flight. Within fifteen years there will be one faith and one God, and the others will vanish away, the sons of Jerusalem will be delivered from captivity, a race will arise without a head. The bark of Peter will be tossed in mighty waves, but will escape and will have dominion at the end of the day. Woe to the clergy and to sterility.[21] There will be many battles and great slaughter, fierce hunger and mortality, and political upheaval; the land of the Barbarians will be converted; the mendicant orders will surely oppose many people; the eastern beast and the western lion will subjugate the whole world by their power; and for fifteeen years there will be peace throughout the whole earth and an abundance of crops. Then all the faithful will pass to the Holy Land over the parted waters and the city of Jerusalem will be glorified and the Holy Sepulchre honoured by all. In this tranquillity there will be heard news of Antichrist. Be watchful.'

Since the beginning of the world it has been unheard of for so many people to die of pestilence, famine or other infirmity in such a short time. Earthquakes, which extended for many miles, threw down cities, towns and castles and swallowed them up. Plague stripped villages, cities, castles and towns of their inhabitants so thoroughly that there was scarcely anyone left alive in them. This pestilence was so contagious that those who touched the dead or the sick were immediately infected themselves and died, so that penitent and confessor were carried together to the grave. Because of their fear and horror men

19 This prophecy, with various changes of date and content, had been circulating throughout Europe since the mid 13th century. It has been studied in detail by Robert E. Lerner, *The Powers of Prophecy*, University of California, 1983. I have used the variants of the prophecy collected in his appendices to clarify some doubtful readings in the Clynn version.

20 *Marchionatus*; other versions have the planet Mars or Mercury here. In the context of the Black Death, Mars would make most sense. Taken with the references to Saturn and Jupiter which follow it could be interpreted as a reference to the conjunction of the three planets in 1345, which was thought to have caused the plague.

21 *Sic*; other versions, rather more plausibly, have 'woe to Christianity'.

could hardly bring themselves to perform the pious and charitable acts of visiting the sick and burying the dead. Many died of boils, abscesses and pustules which erupted on the legs and in the armpits. Others died in frenzy, brought on by an affliction of the head, or vomiting blood. This amazing year was outside the usual order of things, exceptional in quite contradictory ways – abundantly fertile and yet at the same time sickly and deadly. Among the Franciscans at Drogheda 25 brothers died before Christmas, and 23 died at Dublin.... At Kilkenny the pestilence was strong during Lent, and eight Dominicans died between Christmas and 6 March. It was very rare for just one person to die in a house, usually husband, wife, children and servants went the same way, the way of death.

And I, Brother John Clynn, of the Friars Minor of Kilkenny, have written in this book the notable events which befell in my time, which I saw for myself or have learnt from men worthy of belief. So that notable deeds should not perish with time, and be lost from the memory of future generations, I, seeing these many ills, and that the whole world is encompassed by evil, waiting among the dead for death to come, have committed to writing what I have truly heard and examined; and so that the writing does not perish with the writer, or the work fail with the workman, I leave parchment for continuing the work, in case anyone should still be alive in the future and any son of Adam can escape this pestilence and continue the work thus begun.

24. The plague in Scotland

This account is taken from the *Scotichronicon* by John of Fordun, a clerk of Aberdeen who died in 1384. His chronicle ends in the previous year.

W. F. Skene (ed), *Chronica Gentis Scotorum*, Edinburgh, 1871, I pp. 368-9.

In 1350 there was a great pestilence and mortality of men in the kingdom of Scotland, and this pestilence also raged for many years before and after this in various parts of the world, indeed, throughout the whole globe. So great a plague has never been heard of from the beginning of the world to the present day, or been recorded in books. For this plague vented its spite so thoroughly that fully a third of the human race was killed. At God's command, moreover, the damage was done by an extraordinary and novel form of death. Those who fell sick of a kind of gross swelling of the flesh lasted for barely two days. This sickness befell people everywhere, but especially the middling and lower classes, rarely the great. It generated such horror that children did not dare to visit their dying parents, or parents their children, but fled for fear of contagion as if from leprosy or a serpent.

25. The second pestilence, 1361

(a) Henry Knighton, p. 116.

In 1361 a general mortality oppressed the people. It was called the second pestilence and both rich and poor died, but especially young people and children. Eleven canons of our house died.

(b) Anonimalle Chronicle, p. 50.

In 1361 there was a second pestilence within England, which was called the mortality of children. Several people of high birth and a great number of children died.

(c) Thomas Walsingham, *Historia Anglicana 1272–1422*, I p. 296.

Also in 1361 there was a great pestilence, which devoured men rather than women. There died at this time Reginald, Bishop of Worcester, Michael, Bishop of London and Thomas, Bishop of Ely .... Among the nobility Henry, Duke of Lancaster, Reginald Cobham, William Fitzwaryn and John Mowbray died.

(d) Continuation of the Polychronicon of Ralph Higden, pp. 360, 411-12.

About Easter 1361 a great pestilence of men began in London and then it steadily advanced from the south of England to the rest of the country, killing many men but few women.

In 1361 there was a great human mortality, particularly of men. Their widows, as if degenerate and not restrained by any shame, took as their husbands foreigners and other imbeciles or madmen. For it is a failing of some women, forgetful of their own honour, to couple with their inferiors – turning away from the more eminent and lowering themselves to baser men. In this year there died numerous men of standing, of whom Henry, Duke of Lancaster, Reginald Cobham and William Fitzwaryn deserve special mention as men of particular worth.

(e) Chronicle of Louth Park Abbey, pp. 40-1.

In AD 1361 there was a mortality of men, especially of adolescents and boys, and as a result it was commonly called the pestilence of boys. In the same year, about the feast of St Maurus the abbot [15 January 1362][22] a strong gale blew from the north so violently for a day and a night that it flattened trees, mills, houses and a great many church towers.

(f) Grey Friars of Lynn, p. 275.

At about Michaelmas 1360 the pestilence began in London, where at first it killed infants in huge numbers, and then after the following Easter men and women died in huge numbers.

In 1361 there was a great pestilence in the south of England, with the death of children and adolescents, and of the wealthy. However, this pestilence was considerably less than that of thirteen years earlier. In the same year by English reckoning, on 15 January [1362] there was a violent wind which destroyed bell towers, took the roofs off churches and houses, and uprooted trees.

(g) An anonymous Canterbury chronicle.

This chronicle, not hitherto cited, covers the period 1346-67.

J. Tait (ed), *Chronica Johannis de Reading et Anonymi Cantuariensis,* Manchester, 1914, p. 212.

In 1361 a grave pestilence and mortality of men began throughout the whole world. At the Roman Curia in Avignon about seven cardinals and other prelates and clerics of various nationalities died suddenly. In other parts of the world scarcely a third of the population survived. In England the pestilence began in June that year. Children and adolescents were generally the first to die, and then the elderly. Members of religious orders and parish clergy and others died suddenly without respect of persons when the first spots and the other signs of death appeared on their bodies, as on the bodies of the victims everywhere. Many churches were then left unserved and empty through lack of priests. The plague lasted for more than four months in England.

(h) John of Reading, pp. 148-50.

On 6 May 1361, that is on the vigil of Ascension Day,[23] there was an eclipse of the sun at noon. A damaging drought followed, and because

22 In medieval England the new year was dated from Lady Day, March 25. 1 January
     to 24 March *1362*, by our reckoning, was thus considered part of 1361.
23 6 May 1361 was Ascension Day, not its vigil.

of the lack of rain there was a great shortage of fruit and hay. And in the same month, on 27th, a bloody rain fell in Burgundy and a bloody cross appeared over the sky in Bologna from early in the morning until the sixth hour, when it moved away and fell into the sea. Afterwards foxes and wolves came out of the woods in those countries in search of villages, where they seized and ate living men.

And at the same time in France, England and other countries (as many who saw it can testify) two castles appeared from nowhere on level, empty ground, and two troops of warriors issued from them, one apparelled in the trappings of knighthood and the other all in black. When they met the knights defeated the blacks, and then in their second encounter the blacks defeated the knights. And then they returned to their castles and everything vanished. Immediately after Michaelmas [29 September] a rose tree produced blossoms of perfect colour and fragrance. Also ravens, geese and other birds produced young.

In this year the diocese of London fell empty through the death of Master Michael Northburgh, and Master Simon Sudbury, who was then auditor at the Roman Curia, was provided to the see by the pope. After the death of Master Thomas Lisle, the pope provided Brother Simon Langham to the diocese of Ely, his choice coinciding with the king's wishes. Langham was Abbot of Westminster at the time, and in that capacity had previously been a shepherd to the Londoners. Master John Barnet was elected in succession to Reginald Bryan as Bishop of Worcester, and Master Lewis Charlton in place of Master John Trilleck at Hereford.

The abbots of Bury, Reading and Abingdon also died, as did numerous prominent men from all the religious orders, together with the lord Henry, Duke of Lancaster, Reginald Cobham, William Fitzwaryn, John Mowbray, and Margaret and Mary, daughters of the King of England, who were buried at Abingdon. For this year the mortality was particularly of males, who were devoured in great numbers by the pestilence. However, the greatest cause of grief was provided by the behaviour of women. Widows, forgetting the love they had borne towards their first husbands, rushed into the arms of foreigners or, in many cases, of kinsmen, and shamelessly gave birth to bastards conceived in adultery. It was even claimed that in many places brothers took their sisters to wife. And there was at this time death without sorrow — just as there was in 1349. Afterwards many, regardless of status, class or degree, no longer worried about sexual lapses, for they now regarded fornication, incest or adultery as a game rather than a sin.

(i) John of Fordun, *Chronica Gentis Scotorum*, pp. 380-1.

In 1362 the mortality of men raged amazingly throughout the whole realm of Scotland, and the form of the disease and the number of deaths were just the same as in the first outbreak in the jubilee year [1350].

26. The third pestilence, 1369

(a) Anonimalle Chronicle, p. 77.

In 1369 there was a third pestilence in England and in several other countries. It was great beyond measure, lasted a long time and was particularly fatal to children.

(b) Thomas Walsingham, *Historia Anglicana 1272-1422*, I p. 309.

This year [1369] there was a great pestilence, which also affected larger animals. It was followed by floods and a great blight of corn, so that in the following year a measure of grain sold for 3s.

27. The fourth pestilence, 1374-9

(a) Anonimalle Chronicle, pp. 77, 79, 124.

In 1374 the fourth pestilence began in England in several towns in the south of the country and lasted for a long time. In the following year a large number of Londoners, from among the wealthier and more eminent citizens, died in the pestilence. Several well-placed clerks of the Chancery, Common Pleas and Exchequer also died.

In 1375 the fourth pestilence arrived in the north country.

In 1378 the fourth pestilence arrived in York and was particularly fatal to children. It began there before Michaelmas [29 September] and lasted for over a year.

(b) Thomas Walsingham, *Historia Anglicana 1272-1422*, I pp. 319, 409-11.

In 1375 the weather was scorching, and there was a great pestilence which raged so strongly in England and elsewhere that infinite numbers of men and women were devoured by sudden death. The lord

pope, at the instigation of the cardinal of England,[24] accordingly
granted (in two bulls which were to be valid for six months) full
remission of penance to everyone dying in England who was contrite
for their sins and had made confession.

In the summer of 1379, due to a hostile configuration of the planets,
plague broke out in the north country on a scale never seen before.
The mortality waxed so powerful that almost the whole region was
rapidly stripped of its best men; and among the middle classes it was
said that nearly every house was deprived of its residents and left
standing empty. Even large families were wiped out by the plague,
with not one person left alive. But this was nothing compared with
what followed.

For the hand of God was so heavy on us that villages and towns, which
had once been packed with warlike, provident and wealthy men, and
with settlers, were emptied of their inhabitants and left desolate and
abandoned. And on top of everything, the Scots (showing themselves
to be enemies of the human race), feeling no pity for the deaths of so
many of their neighbours, forgot that such disasters demand sympathy
for the wretched victims; and above all they failed to respect the hand
of God manifest so near them, but instead, like inhuman brutes or
ravening beasts, brutalised by their cruel nature, thought that it was
a suitable time to move against a people weakened by sickness and
plague. Those whom the Lord had beaten, they hunted down, and
added wounds to existing misery, putting to the sword all the able-
bodied men who had not yet died of plague or disease. They beheaded
many people and then – carried away by their savage nature – were
not ashamed to kick the heads backwards and forwards as though
playing football with them.

When they realised that nothing stood in the way of such evil actions,
and that they were meeting with no resistance, they grew bolder,
believing that they could get away with anything. They overran the
countryside, looted settlements, carried off the plunder, drove away
farm animals and oxen. They even drove before them whole herds of
pigs, which was a type of animal the Scots had not previously
attempted to take away.

But when the Scots first thought of plundering the countryside –
before they marched into the area – they had anxiously tried to learn

24 Simon Langham, who had resigned as Archbishop of Canterbury when he became
   cardinal priest of St Sixtus in 1368.

from some of the inhabitants why so great a plague had afflicted them more than the Scots, or other neighbouring races. The people summoned by the Scots replied simply that they did not know, for the divine judgements in such matters were hidden. But as one man they doggedly asserted that every disaster, every death, indeed every misfortune which had befallen them, had come to pass through the special grace of God; that it was because of their sins, so that they would atone during this life for the sins which they had already committed, and be deterred from further wrongdoing by the fear of death. Further, it was in order to test the just, so that they would have more faith in God, as it is written: the just will fear and hope in the Lord.[25] And it was because of many other reasons which it was not proper for the Scots to know.

When the Scots heard from the inhabitants that the plague seemed to them an expression of God's grace, they, who had never been afraid before, trembled with a sort of fear which, like brutes, they had not previously experienced. As a result, when they entered the country, and every morning after they had entered it, they signed themselves with the cross, as though blessing themselves – a ritual which they had devised with much care and which they thought essential. It went like this. The eldest or most highly born of them would say, 'Bless – ' and would be answered, ' – the Lord'. Then the first speaker would continue, 'God and St Kentigern, St Romanus and St Andrew, save us this day, and every day, from God's grace and from the foul death which is killing the English'. And after this blessing they used to think themselves adequately protected and defended from all the evil things which might befall them. The blessing sounds even more ridiculous in their own language and I therefore think it appropriate to record it here: *Gode and Seynt Mango, Seynt Romayne and Seynt Andreu, scheld us this day fro Goddis grace, and the foule deth that Yngleesh men dyene upon.* It is to be hoped that, at least in the future if not now, they feel the effect of their prayer, and receive the due reward for the inhuman cruelty which they showed towards a people humbled under the flails of God – by which I mean struggling under the plague. For although divine severity advances by slow steps, yet it makes up for that delay by its harshness.

---

25 A paraphrase of Ps 39.4: 'many shall see and shall fear: and they shall hope in the Lord'.

28. The fifth pestilence, 1390-3

Thomas Walsingham, *Historia Anglicana 1272-1422*, II pp. 185-6, 197, 203, 213.

In Cambridge in 1389, on the feast of the Commemoration of St Paul [30 June], which was also kept as the feast of the dedication of the church of St Mary there, the feast was marked by carrying the Body of Christ in procession through the parish on the shoulders of two priests. The shrine was not heavy; on the contrary, it was so light that a boy of seven could have carried it without difficulty. The procession went on its way through the town, led by the two priests carrying the Body of Christ, until they passed the Augustinian friary, which stands near the market place. Suddenly the shrine, which until then had been balanced comfortably on their shoulders, reared up, as if an unseen force was pushing it from their shoulders, and at the same time became so heavy that the priests could barely support it. They could neither put it down nor keep it steady. They struggled, sweating and panting with the effort, and calling for help from the laity. They came running and put their hands under the shrine but, amazingly, could feel no weight. The priests' difficulties lasted while they passed in front of the friary, but when they had got past the shrine immediately settled itself on their shoulders again.

But then a silly wretch began to dance and caper grotesquely in front of the Host. He was instantly struck by a terrible vengeance, for in the midst of his foolery he suddenly fell to the ground and in a few minutes gave up the ghost. All sorts of explanations were adduced for these amazing events, but we have preferred to come to our own decision, and would rather ignore the opinions of others than trust blindly in people we don't know. Accordingly we are prepared to hazard the explanation that this was an *exemplum*[26] of the great and terrible pestilence which ensued at Cambridge, and which – so it was said – suddenly attacked healthy men, who then died raving, out of their minds and without receiving the viaticum.

In 1390 a great plague ravaged the country. It especially attacked adolescents and boys, who died in incredible numbers in towns and villages everywhere. The epidemic was soon followed by a dearth of foodstuffs, so that in some places a measure of grain sold for 23*d*.

In 1391 such a great mortality arose in Norfolk and in many other

---

26 An *exemplum* is a story with a moral. Medieval preachers used them extensively to enliven their sermons; for the technique in action see **48-9**.

counties that it was thought as bad as the great pestilence. To take only one example, in a short space of time 11,000 bodies were buried at York.

In September 1393 many died in Essex from an outbreak of plague.

PART TWO:
EXPLANATIONS AND RESPONSES

All contemporary commentators were agreed that the plague was an act of God, sent to punish mankind for its sinfulness and to frighten it into repentance and future good behaviour. It followed, therefore, that the only effective hope of averting the plague was to turn to God for help, backing up the appeal with contrition and penance. In England Edward III instructed the Archbishop of Canterbury to order prayers throughout his province [34], although by the time the orders were transmitted some bishops had already taken action on their own initiative and arranged penitential processions and masses [29-33]. They would all have been familiar with the precedent for the efficacy of such processions from the pontificate of Gregory the Great. In 590, when Rome was ravaged by plague, Gregory had led a procession through the city chanting the great litany, which he had devised. As the procession went on its way, the Archangel Michael appeared on the top of the mausoleum of Hadrian sheathing his sword, as a sign that God's anger had been appeased – an event commemorated by the renaming of the mausoleum as the Castel Sant'Angelo, and by the great statue of the archangel placed on its top.[1]

Orders for public penance continued to be issued throughout the first pestilence, although by December 1349 their tone was beginning to shift, and Simon Islip's letter of that month [35] urges people to give thanks to God for their own survival, as well as praying for the divine anger to be averted. Similar commands were repeated in subsequent outbreaks, and the letters tended to become standardised. In 1361 John Thoresby's letter to his official, his executive agent at York [36], is a virtual recapitulation of Archbishop Zouche's 1348 letter [29]. In 1375, however, Simon Sudbury struck a new note with his explicit rejection of political and intellectual solutions to current problems; an approach which perhaps implies that the drive towards expiation was beginning to lose some of its urgency [37].

Ordinary men and women, as well as participating in the organised processions and masses, expressed their fear and penitence in other

1 The story was familiar to medieval readers from Jacobus de Voragine's *Golden Legend*. It was the great litany which the Bishop of Winchester specifically ordered to be used in processions in his diocese [33].

ways. John Clynn noted how anxieties about the approaching plague triggered an urge to go on pilgrimage [23], and the treasurers' accounts of Canterbury cathedral reveal a surge in the offerings made there in 1350.[2] The papacy recognised the phenomenon and declared 1350 a Jubilee Year, in which a pilgrimage to the churches of Rome would earn pilgrims a plenary indulgence – the full remission of the penance due for their sins.[3] In 1361, as the second plague threatened the West Midlands, the number of pilgrims to Merevale (Warks) was causing anxiety [50]. This response seems to have been less marked in the fifteenth century, and although in the plague year of 1471 it was reported that 'the king and the queen and much other people are ridden and go to Canterbury, never so much people seen in pilgrimage heretofore at once, as men say', this probably had more to do with the king's wish to give thanks for his restoration to the throne than anxieties about the resurgent plague.[4]

Elsewhere in Europe penitence might take other forms. A number of Italian cities saw the formation of fraternities dedicated to tending and burying the plague victims. This was a public-spirited work of charity, given the extreme unwillingness of most people to have anything to do with the dead and dying, but it was also a penitential act of self-abasement. More showy self-abasement was practised by the flagellants [52-3], an extreme penitential movement which gained a large popular following in the aftermath of the Black Death. Unusually, the group which arrived in England late in 1349 seems to have generated no more than mild curiosity, perhaps in part because the tide of official approval had by then turned decisively against the movement. Although clerical observers had initially been rather impressed by the flagellants' penitential fervour, and the pope himself had participated in some of their processions at Avignon [5], the movement's growing contempt for the church's authority, coupled with the virulent anti-semitism which its exponents stirred up, led Pope Clement VI to outlaw it in October 1349.[5]

2 C. E. Woodruff, 'The financial aspect of the cult of St Thomas of Canterbury', *Archaeologia Cantiana* XLIV, 1932, p. 20.

3 J. Sumption, *Pilgrimage: an image of mediaeval religion*, London, 1975, pp. 231-42.

4 N. Davis (ed), *Paston Letters and Papers of the fifteenth century*, 2 vols, Oxford, 1971-6, I p. 443 (spelling modernised). For the fifteenth-century fall in offerings: R. C. Finucane, *Miracles & Pilgrims: popular beliefs in medieval England*, London, 1977, pp. 193-4.

5 S. Simonsohn (ed), *The Apostolic See and the Jews:* I *Documents 492-1404*, Toronto, 1988, pp. 399-401. For a survey of the movement: P. Ziegler, *The Black Death*, Harmondsworth, 1970, pp. 87-98.

One of the hymns which the flagellants used as a marching song was the *Stabat Mater*, the thirteenth-century poem evoking the sufferings of Mary as she beheld the crucifixion of her son, in which the poet begs to share the pain of Christ and be intoxicated by his suffering.[6] Mary was regularly invoked against the plague and its terrors [39], and the image of her as the Mother of Mercy, shielding mankind with her cloak, became popular in the century and a half after the plague's arrival, with the figures clustering around her sometimes represented with the characteristic plague buboes.[7] The plague also had its special patron saints. The best known was St Sebastian, who was invoked throughout Europe. His relics in Flanders [6] and Italy drew pilgrims throughout the epidemic, and a Scottish chronicler considered that the best hope of safety from the plague lay in devotion to the saint.[8] Sebastian was reputedly a member of the imperial guard martyred by the emperor Diocletian in the third century. He was shot with arrows and left for dead, but was healed by Irene, the widow of another Christian martyr. When his survival was discovered the emperor had him bludgeoned to death. Throughout the epidemic, the onslaught of plague was described as arrows fired at the victims; and the saint's naked body, pierced by the arrows of his first, abortive, martyrdom, accordingly came to symbolise Sebastian's power to resist plague.[9] By the early fifteenth century, plague victims had acquired another patron, St Roche, who had contracted the plague while nursing the sick in northern Italy, but recovered; only to die later while falsely imprisoned as a spy.

When bishops urged their flocks to penitence they generally left unspecified the nature of the sins for which God was punishing the world. Chroniclers and moralists were less reticent. In England a number of commentators linked the plague's arrival in 1348 with divine disapproval of the tournaments staged in the previous year and the behaviour of those attending them [18, 43]. One aspect of that

---

6 M. Warner, *Alone of All Her Sex: the myth and cult of the Virgin Mary*, London,1985, p. 215; F. Brittain (ed), *The Penguin Book of Latin Verse*, Harmondsworth, 1962, pp. 246-9, especially stanza 7: 'cause me to be wounded by his blows, intoxicated by this Cross'.

7 P. Perdrizet, *La Vierge de la Miséricorde*, Paris, 1908.

8 J. B. Friedman, '"He hath a thousand slayn this pestilence": the iconography of the plague in the late middle ages' in F. X. Newman (ed), *Social Unrest in the late Middle Ages*, Binghamton, 1986, p. 76.

9 *Ibid*, pp. 85-6; J. Polzer, 'Aspects of the fourteenth-century iconography of death and the plague' in D. Williman (ed), *The Black Death: the impact of the fourteenth-century plague*, Binghamton, 1982, pp. 113-15.

behaviour which came in for particular disapproval was the clothing of
the participants. The new fashions of the 1340s and 1350s were
criticised across Europe for their indecency. Several English writers
held them responsible for the first two outbreaks of plague [44-5],
while at least one French writer blamed them for his country's defeats
at the hands of the English.[10] Other moralists had different candidates.
The disproportionate death rate among children in later outbreaks was
taken by one writer as evidence of, and punishment for, children's
disobedience to their parents [46] – for which parental indulgence
was held partly responsible; a theme also taken up by Langland in the
sermon which he put into the mouth of Reason in *Piers Plowman* [47].
Reason, however, is more concerned to emphasise the general depravity of the times than to insist on the primacy of a single cause, and the
same sense of the times being out of joint is to be found in other
literary treatments [41].

This emphasis on the universal sinfulness of mankind, which merited
a universal punishment, implicitly denied that plague strikes only the
individually guilty. But clearly the indiscriminate nature of the plague
did cause some uneasiness, and Thomas Brinton felt it necessary to
address the issue explicitly in one of his sermons [49]. Admitting that
the innocent do die, he argued that death is to their advantage, since
it saves them from future sin which might earn eternal damnation, and
that their death is also a way of increasing the pressure on the guilty,
who suffer grief for the death of friends and family. Plague is thus a
spiritual blessing and a sign of God's mercy, since it prompts men to
repent in this life and be spared the pains of hell in the next. This was
the point Thomas Walsingham was making when he mocked the
incomprehension of the Scots who prayed daily to be saved from God's
grace [27b]. It is made more explicitly, and more poignantly, by
Matteo Villani, whose brother Giovanni died of the plague in 1348. As
Matteo began his continuation of his brother's History of Florence he
noted: 'my mind is stupefied as it applies itself to write the sentence
that divine justice *in its great pity* sent on mankind, worthy by
corruption of sin of the final judgement'.[11]

For many observers, that final judgement seemed to have come one
step nearer in 1348. Medieval Christians believed that the second
coming of Christ to judge the world would be the climax of a whole

10 S. M. Newton, *Fashion in the Age of the Black Prince*, Woodbridge, 1980, pp. 9-10.
11 T. S. R. Boase, *Death in the Middle Ages: mortality, judgement and remembrance*,
   London, 1972, p. 98 (my italics).

series of apocalyptic events.[12] The detailed chronology of the Last Days was disputed, but it was believed that they would see the emergence of a great leader, the Emperor of the Last Days, who would destroy the heathen and institute a period of harmonious rule on earth. During his reign, however, the hosts of Gog and Magog, the enemies of Christ, would be unleashed from hell, bringing drought, famine, war, plague and universal destruction. At this sign the Emperor would journey to Jerusalem, where he would surrender his crown and die, ushering in the reign of Antichrist – the last triumph of evil before the coming of Christ in judgement.

Antichrist was a potent figure in the medieval (and later) popular imagination. He was envisaged not only as the arch-enemy of Christ, but as his total opposite; his life a blasphemous inversion or parody of the life of Christ. Thus, for example, as Christ was begotten on a virgin by the holy spirit, so Antichrist would be the son of a whore by the devil. The reign of Antichrist would see a vicious persecution of Christians and the apostasy of many of them, leaving only a faithful remnant. The prophets Enoch and Elias would then appear and reconvert the apostates, and the Jews, before being killed. They would then be resurrected and ascend into heaven. Antichrist – still parodying the life of Christ – would then attempt his own ascension from the Mount of Olives, tricking his disciples by being borne aloft by invisible devils. In a moment of high comedy, much enjoyed by the medieval artists who portrayed it, the devils would drop him, and he would fall to his death. There would then follow the fifteen signs of the end of the world, culminating in the coming of Christ in majesty.

For many contemporaries the plague fitted easily into the chronology of the Last Days. Its horrors – along with the earthquakes and wars which had preceded it – were identified with the devastation which would follow the unleashing of Gog and Magog. William Dene of Rochester made the connection explicitly [19], and it is implicit in the biblical phrases used by other writers in their descriptions of the plague. Against this background of disaster, Antichrist's coming seemed imminent, and rumours circulating in Rome claimed that he had already been born and was a beautiful child of ten in 1349 [54]. The same rumours also spoke of his predecessor: the last great ruler who would defeat the heathen. The Cedar of Lebanon prophecy quoted by John Clynn [23] also focuses on the last ruler, whose triumphs

---

12 For a detailed discussion see R. K. Emmerson, *Antichrist in the Middle Ages: a study of medieval apocalypticism, art and literature*, Manchester, 1981.

would precede the coming of Antichrist; while in Germany the plague gave a new impetus to the long-standing belief that Frederick II would be resurrected as the Emperor of the Last Days, and initiate a golden age of social justice [55].

The view of the plague as an act of divine intervention did not preclude attempts to explain it scientifically. God was the ultimate cause of all natural phenomena, since he had established the laws by which the universe functioned; and it was therefore possible to discuss the immediate causes of the plague without denying God his role as primary cause. Moralists like Brinton might disparage any explanation which seemed to lift responsibility for the plague off man's own shoulders [49], but most writers did not feel that the explanations were mutually exclusive. The author of a brief fifteenth-century plague treatise [63] was insistent that sin was the cause of plague, but distinguished that from what he calls its physical cause, which he considered to be the corruption of the air by poisonous matter from the sea.

Scientists were agreed that the physical cause of plague was the corruption of the air – or, rather, since air was an element and could not change its substance – the mixing of air with corrupt or poisonous vapours, which when inhaled would have a detrimental effect on the human body. Where they differed was in the explantions they gave for the corruption. Some causes were obvious. Everyone agreed that the air could be poisoned by rotting matter, including dead bodies, or by excrement or stagnant water. Naturally enough, suspicion was extended to anything which smelt unpleasant – such as slaughter houses or the processes of the tanning industry. Most sanitary regulations of the period therefore concentrated on removing such things safely beyond populated areas, or on cleaning up those which could not be moved. Those of Florence noted that pestilence could proceed from corrupt and infected air, which was itself mainly caused by decomposing substances, including human corpses.[13]

This belief in the dangers of corrupted air explains why suggested precautions against plague always include a recommendation to surround oneself with pleasant smells. No one could avoid breathing, and therefore it was sensible to try and create a barrier of aromatic vapours through which the bad air could not penetrate. This could be achieved indoors by burning spices or wood, such as juniper, which

13 F. Carabellese, *La Peste del 1348 e le condizione della sanità pubblica in Toscana*, Rocca S. Casciano, 1897, pp. 45-6 (n.2).

produce aromatic smoke. Those who had to leave the safety of their own rooms were advised to carry something fragrant with them, a nosegay of herbs or, for the wealthy, a ball of ambergris, and to hold it close to their nostrils at all times.[14] It was also prudent to try and minimise the amount of air entering the body by other routes, and people were therefore urged to avoid any activity which would make them hot and open the pores of their skin, such as bathing, strenuous physical exertion, sexual intercourse, or excessive eating and drinking. One dissident voice argued that, on the contrary, the best defence against corrupt air was to have one's body already full of the strong vapours generated by eating rich food and drinking alcohol [60]; a view firmly rejected by the medical profession, although Boccaccio's account of the plague in Florence suggests that it may have commanded some popular belief, even if only as a rationalisation of the desire to enjoy oneself while there was still time [2].

Domestic sources of bad air, such as rubbish heaps and dirty streets, were clearly dangerous, and were the first target of those attempting to control the spread of plague. But no one believed that they could have caused the mortality sweeping across Europe. To explain the scale of the epidemic, a universal corruption of the atmosphere was called for. One German writer of the fourteenth century blamed the epidemic on the corrupt vapours released from the bowels of the earth by the earthquakes which had preceded the first pestilence in central Europe [60]. Most writers preferred to blame changes to the atmosphere brought about by planetary configurations, particularly the 1345 conjunction of Mars, Saturn and Jupiter.

Belief in the influence of the planets was central to medieval science. The universe was seen as an integrated system in which, as in the human body, the condition of one part had a bearing on the health of the others. The earth stood at its centre, with seven planets circling it: the moon, Mercury, Venus, the sun, Mars, Jupiter and Saturn. The moon was the nearest planet to earth, Saturn the furthest away, and beyond Saturn were the fixed stars: the constellations against whose backdrop the planets moved across the heavens. The circle of the heavens was divided into twelve – the twelve signs of the zodiac – and as the planets travelled round their orbits they moved through the signs in turn.

14 Ambergris is a fragrant waxy secretion of the intestinal tract of the sperm whale, often found floating in the sea. For its medicinal use: J. M. Riddle. 'Pomum ambrae: amber and ambergris in plague remedies', *Sudhoff's Archiv für Geschichte der Medizin und der Naturwissenschaften* XLVIII, 1964, pp. 111-22.

Astrologers saw the planets as exerting a direct influence on men.
Each planet had its own characteristics, which it transmitted to
anything which came within its power. Broadly speaking, those
characteristics were analogous to those of the classical deities which
had given their names to the planets. Thus Mars was the planet
associated with war and stirred people to anger and violence. People
born under Mars – that is, when the planet was in a dominant position
in the heavens – were inclined to be short tempered and aggressive,
and might well die by violence. They were likely to become soldiers,
swordsmiths, butchers or barbers – the latter because barbers used
sharp blades.[15] As this suggests, Mars was seen as a malevolent planet,
second only to Saturn in its evil influence. The most beneficent planet,
by contrast, was Jupiter, followed by Venus. The influence of each
planet could not, however, be assessed in isolation. Its impact varied
depending on its place in the heavens – it might be strengthened by
the sign of the zodiac in which it found itself, for instance – and its
position relative to the other planets. Thus astrologers had to decide
which of the three planets in the 1345 conjunction was likely to be
dominant – a question of some importance when the conjunction
involved the best of the planets (Jupiter) and the two evil planets
(Mars and Saturn). Most astrologers at the time suggested that Jupiter
would probably dominate the situation, but their colleagues writing
after the arrival of the plague naturally gave more weight to the
malignant powers of Saturn and Mars.

Critics of astrology liked to point out that it clearly did not work,
because otherwise everyone would be influenced by the heavens in the
same way and at the same time, which was clearly not the case. Not
everyone went down with the plague, for instance. But the astrologers
themselves were insistent that the impact could not be expected to be
uniform. They pointed out that every inch of the earth's surface was in
a slightly different position relative to the position of the planets in the
sky, and would therefore experience the planets' influence differently.
More important, each individual would react to that influence in
different ways. Someone born under Saturn would naturally be more
susceptible to its influence in later life than someone born under
Jupiter, in many ways Saturn's opposite. In any case, planetary
influence could only predispose, it could not compel. As Geoffrey de
Meaux put it in his treatise on the 1325 conjunction: 'The celestial

---

15 The list of occupations is from Chaucer's description of the Temple of Mars in the
Knight's Tale, *The Canterbury Tales*, lines 2025-6.

bodies may create a disposition in us, but they cannot make us do much, if anything, against our will.'[16] The church insisted on this, since to argue otherwise would be to deny free will (a central tenet of medieval christianity) and make man no more than the puppet of forces outside his control. The church was accordingly opposed to the practice of judicial astrology – the making of specific predictions about what would befall an individual – although it was never able to stamp it out altogether, since that was precisely what the clients of astrologers most wanted to hear. But, with that proviso, the church had no difficulty in accepting the reality of planetary influence in general terms. After all, as the astrologers themselves were quick to point out, the universe was God's creation, and its configuration was therefore his design. Geoffrey de Meaux put it forcefully in the same treatise:

Holy scripture testifies, in the fourth book of
Deuteronomy: 'God created the sun and the moon and
the stars of heaven, that they should be in the
service of all the peoples who are under heaven'.[17]
And in the first book of Genesis it says that God
made them so that they should be a sign [Gen. 1.14].

Medieval astrologers sometimes give the impression that they saw planetary influence as occult. One of their favourite images is that the planets stamped their impression on human beings like a seal on soft wax – and, some added, the more self-indulgent or irrational the individual the more readily he would take the impression.[18] But this is slightly misleading. There was a scientific explanation for the effects of the planets and other heavenly bodies on earth and its inhabitants.[19] For medieval scientists everything on the earth and within its atmosphere was made up of a combination of the four elements: earth, water, air and fire. The elements in turn each consisted of two of the

16 H. Pruckner (ed), *Studien zu den Astrologischen schriften des Heinrich von Langenstein*, Berlin, 1933, p. 216. Pruckner mistakenly identifies this treatise as referring to the 1345 conjunction.

17 A misleading paraphrase of Deuteronomy 4.19, which in fact forbids men to worship or serve the sun, moon and stars, and says nothing about their service to man.

18 Pruckner, *Studien* p. 216.

19 The basics of medieval astrology are clearly set out in C. S. Lewis, *The Discarded Image*, Cambridge, 1964. More detailed accounts, in ascending order of complexity, are J. C. Eade, *The Forgotten Sky*, Oxford, 1984; J. Tester, *A History of Western Astrology*, Woodbridge, 1987; J. C. North, *Chaucer's Universe*, Oxford, 1988.

four contraries: hot and cold, wet and dry. Thus earth was cold and
dry; water cold and wet; air hot and wet; fire hot and dry. The planets,
too, were thought to have their own combinations of contraries; thus,
for example, Saturn was cold and dry, Mars hot and dry. The potency
of their contraries varied. Mars was excessively hot and dry, but
Jupiter was only moderately warm and moist. Each sign of the zodiac
also had an affinity with a particular element, giving three signs [a
trigon] to each of the four elements, as Geoffrey de Meaux details in
58.

Each human being, like everything else on earth, was made up of an
uneven mix of the four elements, with one predominating. This
mixture was known as the individual's *complexion*, and was believed to
derive from the configuration of the heavens at the time of the
individual's birth. Thus if Mars were dominant – a hot/dry planet –
the individual's complexion would be hot and dry. This imbalance
determined the individual's psychology, and in this context the
elements were known as *humours*. Someone with an excess of the cold/
dry humour would be melancholic – in modern terms a depressive. An
excess of the cold/wet humour produced someone who was phlegmatic; the hot/wet humour someone who was sanguine; and the hot/
dry humour someone who was choleric. As this terminology implies,
doctors came to equate the humours with body fluids: black bile,
phlegm, blood and yellow bile (choler) respectively. A serious imbalance of the humours in part of the body could also produce physical
illness, in which case the balance needed to be restored to achieve
health. In the case of an excess of the hot/wet humour this could be
achieved by bleeding the patient, but usually the balance was read-
justed by what the patient ate or drank. All substances displayed a
preponderance of one humour, and therefore a man suffering an excess
of the cold/wet humour, manifesting itself perhaps in what would now
be considered a heavy cold, ought to take medicinal substances which
were hot and dry.

When it came to explaining an outbreak of plague, scientists looked
first to the balance of contraries associated with the configuration of
the heavens, since this would determine the condition of the earth and
its atmosphere. In later outbreaks of plague the blame was often placed
on comets, which were believed to be excessively hot and dry and
therefore vitiated the atmosphere.[20] But there had been no comets
before the epidemic of 1347-50 and astrologers turned their attention

20 Friedman, 'Iconography', pp. 83-84.

instead to the triple conjunction of 1345. They argued that Jupiter drew up vapours – which were themselves hot and wet and therefore had an affinity with the planet – from the earth. The vapours were then ignited by Mars, an excessively hot, dry planet, and in burning produced poisonous fumes. These fumes were blown about the world by the strong southerly winds generated by Jupiter, killing men, animals and plants – whose putrefaction in turn generated more poisonous vapours to be carried on the wind. The intense cold of Saturn made matters worse by condensing the warm vapours into fogs which stayed close to the surface of the earth, where they would do most damage. Even so, as numerous writers pointed out, this could not be the whole story, since such conjunctions occurred every twenty years without triggering universal epidemics. It was necessary to look for an intensifying factor.

One explanation was that the 1345 conjunction took place in Aquarius. This is an air sign (hot and wet) and therefore intensified the force of Jupiter. This could not, however, be the full answer because the conjunction of Saturn, Mars and Jupiter in 1325 had also been in an air sign – Gemini – without leading to an epidemic. But Aquarius is also the 'mansion' of Saturn – that is, the zodiac sign in which Saturn's power is greatest – and Gemini is not the mansion of any of the planets involved in 1325. Most important, however, was the lunar eclipse which occurred during the period of the 1345 conjunction and which, according to astrologers like Geoffrey de Meaux [58], enormously enhanced the force of the planets concerned.

The impact of the planets, and of the atmospheric changes they brought about, varied depending on the complexion of the individual, as all astrologers emphasised. But the physical condition of the individual's body was at least as important. Doctors were agreed that poisonous vapours would be most likely to take hold on a body which already contained evil humours. The humours (phlegm, blood, black and yellow bile) were good things, essential to the body's nutrition, but they could be corrupted into a bad form, which was injurious to health. One way in which this could occur was by the humours becoming poisoned by 'superfluities'. These were the by-products of the digestive process. Food was broken down in the stomach into chyle, which then passed to the liver where it was 'concocted' [cooked] to produce the four humours.[21] Each stage of this process produced waste products, the superfluities, which, if not excreted or

21 N. G. Siraisi, *Medieval and Early Renaissance Medicine*, Chicago, 1990, p. 106.

egested, would build up in the body and produce corrupt or evil humours. Anyone who wanted to stay healthy, therefore, was told to avoid food which was difficult to digest or which produced excessive superfluities, especially when, as during a plague epidemic, corrupt air was looking for a foothold in the human body. For the same reason it was prudent to take purgatives or vomits regularly, certainly at the first sign of any illness, to make sure that any superfluities were thoroughly and promptly expelled from the body.

Once corrupt air had entered the body it generated toxic humours, which the body tried desperately to expel before they reached any of the vital organs: heart, brain, lungs or liver. Although most lay observers regarded the appearance of the plague buboes as an infallible token of death, doctors thought that they offered some hope of survival, showing that the body was putting up a fight and ejecting the poison to the surface; a process described in detail by John of Burgundy [62]. Doctors instructed that the buboes should be encouraged to ripen and then lanced, and the corrupt matter squeezed out. If the corrupt humours worked inwards, without venting themselves, the disease was sure to be fatal.

Most doctors felt that the action of corrupt air on the humours provided an adequate explanation of all aspects of the plague. It accounted for its near universality, and for the speed and virulence of its attack, since air was drawn deep into the body in breathing. It also provided an explanation of the way in which plague could apparently pass from person to person. This was the result of the intensified corruption of the air around the sick person. Doctors attending the sick were advised to stand near an open window, keep their nose in something aromatic, or hold a sponge soaked in vinegar in their mouth. This corruption of the air was not generally associated with the patient's breathing, but with the notoriously foetid body fluids characteristic of plague victims.[22] Plague sores were particularly dangerous, giving off a reek or smoke which corrupted the air around [59].

Not all observers were satisfied with this explanation. A doctor of Montpellier [61] argued that once plague had taken hold in a human body it could be transmitted by sight. His argument has come in for considerable ridicule, partly, one suspects, because he drew an analogy with the fatal powers of the mythical basilisk. But his argument made

22 Ziegler, *The Black Death*, p. 20.

perfectly good sense in the context of contemporary theories of sight. A prevalent theory was that sight entailed spirit passing from the eye of the observer to the thing observed.[23] The writer's only real problem, therefore, was to explain how the poisonous vapour could take on the characteristics of spirit, which was considerably lighter and thinner than air; a problem he slides over with the comment that the transformation is achieved 'amazingly'.

The Montpellier physician accepted that corrupt air was the starting point of an epidemic. Where he differed from his professional colleagues was in his evident sense that direct person to person transmission was taking place. Non-experts agreed. Most contemporaries were in no doubt that the disease killed by contact. Chronicles are full of accounts of whole households dying together, or lawyers drawing up a dying man's will and following him immediately to the grave. There was also a widespread belief that the possessions of the sick could kill, as in de' Mussis' story of the soldiers infected by sleeping under a stolen fleece [1], or Boccaccio's account of pigs which died while rooting among a pile of rags which had belonged to a plague victim [2].

Contact with the dying or their effects was not the only way to catch the disease. It was widely believed, by Jean de Venette among others [7], that the plague could be transmitted by imagination: that a person could be infected just by thinking about it. This was not unique to the plague. In the early sixteenth century it was reported that a thousand people had died of the sweating sickness in one night in London after they heard that the disease was prevalent in Sussex.[24] Physicians agreed that people brooding on the plague were more likely to be susceptible to its attack. Bengt Knutsson, in part of his treatise not printed here, assured his readers that 'to be merry in the heart is a great remedy for health of the body. Therefore in time of this great infirmity dread not death but live merrily and hope to live long.'[25] Others arrived at the same idea for themselves. The tenants of Neuberg 'resolved that they should try to cheer each other up with comfort and merrymaking, so that they were not overwhelmed by

23 Siraisi, *Medicine*, p. 108. For modern disparagement: A. Coville, 'Écrits contemporains sur la peste de 1348 à 1350', *Histoire Littéraire de la France* XXXVII, 1938, pp. 359-62.

24 S. Brigden, *London and the Reformation*, Oxford, 1991, p. 139.

25 *A Little Book for the Pestilence*, Manchester, 1911, fo. 7. For the early sections of this treatise see 59.

depression. Accordingly, wherever they could they held parties and weddings with a cheerful heart, so that by rekindling a sort of half-happiness they could avoid despair' [9].

It was the belief in contagion which did most to shape public efforts to control the plague. The doctors' elaborate regimens, predicated on the dangers of corrupt air, influenced contemporary practice to the extent that sanitary regulations aimed to remove sources of corruption and bad smells; although it should be noted that these attempts were not invariably prompted by the plague but, like the London butchery regulations [66], might see the risk of plague as a justification for a clean-up sought on public nuisance grounds. Regulations framed specifically to cope with the plague generally thought first in terms of segregating the sick and the healthy. The first clause of the Pistoia regulations [64] was an attempt to exclude persons from infected areas; and Gloucester reacted in the same way in 1348 [22]. The strategy of ejecting the afflicted took slightly longer to develop, probably because the speed with which the first epidemic took hold made any such attempt futile, if not impossible. In the third pestilence Bernabò Visconti, lord of Milan, ordered that the sick should be expelled from towns under his jurisdiction [65]. This was also normal practice in fifteenth-century Scottish towns. In 1456 (following a major plague outbreak in the previous year) the Scottish parliament fine-tuned the practice, ruling that it should not be obligatory for the well-to-do, who could choose to stay confined in their houses; although they would be ejected from the town if they wandered abroad. At the same time it was ordered that anyone removed to a place outside the town who tried to leave it should be brought back and punished.[26]

In the end, however, the best safeguard was flight; or, as a late fifteenth-century German manuscript put it: 'Clever doctors have three golden rules to keep us safe from pestilence: get out quickly, go a long way away and don't be in a hurry to come back'.[27] Not everyone was comfortable with the propriety of flight. Boccaccio [2] clearly felt that it was a selfish option, and jeered at the foolishness of those who thought they could avoid God's anger simply by shifting house. At the end of the fifteenth century Gabriel Biel of Speyer devoted a whole sermon to the morality of flight from the plague, and came to a similar conclusion. Although he conceded that flight could be seen as a form

26 J. Ritchie. 'The rule of pestilence', *Medical History* II, 1958, pp. 151-3.

27 *The Pest Anatomized: five centuries of the plague in Western Europe*, Wellcome Institute for the History of Medicine, 1985, p. 3.

of medicine, and therefore licit, he felt that it was never the less to be deprecated. Flight was contrary to charity, since it entailed abandoning the sick. It was also pointless, since God has set a limit on every human life; better, therefore, to recognise that plague is a divine punishment and seek spiritual regeneration.[28]

In arguing that it was proper for Christians to try and circumvent the plague by resorting to medicine, Biel was articulating received wisdom. But the propriety of seeking medical help was not entirely taken for granted. There had been a school of thought throughout the middle ages which saw the resort to medicine as impious (and doctors as no better than atheists for setting themselves against God's will); and plague, widely seen as God's direct intervention in human affairs, was particularly likely to prompt this response. It was an argument which the Paris medical faculty felt it necessary to rebut explicitly – and rather defensively – in 1348 [56], pointing out that God 'created earthly medicine, and although God alone cures the sick, he does so through the medicine which in his generosity he provided'.

For all the doubts about the propriety of medicine – and the competence of doctors – plague tractates survive in enormous numbers from the fourteenth and fifteenth centuries; testimony to the urgency with which people sought a cure, or, even better, a way of avoiding the disease altogether. Medical treatises, like public health regulations, at least gave the illusion that the plague could be controlled; but the overwhelming reaction of most people to the plague must have been one of helplessness. Perhaps that helps to explain contemporary claims that the plague had been caused by human agency. As well as meeting the familiar human need to find somebody to blame, the accusations may have made the plague seem more manageable, since what man caused could be halted by human efforts. In the panic caused by the epidemic feelings ran so high that accusations might be levelled against almost anyone perceived as an outsider, including foreigners, the poor, and, as the German mystic Heinrich Seuse found to his cost [75], travellers. But the most frequent scapegoats were the Jews. Local officials exchanged details of alleged Jewish enormities in their districts, and of confessions extorted under torture, creating an atmosphere of ready belief in which each piece of 'evidence' fired men to hunt out more offenders.

As the confessions from Savoy [71] demonstrate, the authorities were

28 G. Biel, *Sermones,* 2 vols in 1, Strassburg, 1619, I pp. 361- 7.

not interested only in extracting admissions of individual guilt, but in proving the existence of an international Jewish conspiracy. Even so, some contemporaries, including Jean de Venette [7], found it hard to reconcile the scale of the disaster with any purely human cause. This was the central argument in Pope Clement's letter of September 1348 forbidding the killing of Jews without legal process [73]. But in spite of intellectual reservations and papal disapproval, popular pressure to hunt out and slaughter the Jews usually proved irresistible. In January 1349 the civic officals of Cologne announced their continuing belief in Jewish innocence, and tried to persuade neighbouring cities not to sanction attacks on their Jewish communities [72]; but the city's own Jews were burnt on 23 August [69]. Similarly the efforts of the Duke of Austria to protect his Jewish subjects were overturned by popular protest [69].

The slaughter of thousands of Europe's Jews was not simply rooted in the belief that they were poisoning wells – an accusation which had been regularly levelled at outsiders, not only the Jews, throughout the middle ages. The plague seemed to many contemporaries to be the first act of an apocalyptic drama which would see the rule of Antichrist on earth, and finally the coming of Christ to judge the world. The Jews had a central role in that drama – as the enemies of Christ who must be converted, or murdered, before Christ would come in glory. As the flagellants showed, the passionate penitential desire to cleanse the individual soul of sin could easily become a desire to cleanse the world of the enemies of Christ.

III: The religious response

29. Intercessionary processions (1)

William Zouche, Archbishop of York, to his official at York, 28 July 1348. This is apparently the earliest episcopal reaction to the imminent threat of plague in England.

James Raine (ed), *Historical Letters and Papers from the Northern Registers*, Rolls Series, 1873, pp. 395-7.

Since the life of man on earth is a war, no wonder if those fighting amidst the miseries of this world are unsettled by the mutability of events: now favourable, now contrary. For Almighty God sometimes allows those he loves to be troubled while their strength is perfected in weakness by an outpouring of spiritual grace. There can be no one who does not know, since it is now public knowledge, how great a mortality, pestilence and infection of the air are now threatening various parts of the world, and especially England; and this is surely caused by the sins of men who, while enjoying good times, forget that such things are the gifts of the most high giver. Thus, since the inevitable human fate, pitiless death, which spares no one, now threatens us, unless the holy clemency of the Saviour is shown to his people from on high, the only hope is to hurry back to him alone, whose mercy outweighs justice and who, most generous in forgiving, rejoices heartily in the conversion of sinners; humbly urging him with orisons and prayers that he, the kind and merciful Almighty God, should turn away his anger and remove the pestilence and drive away the infection from the people whom he redeemed with his precious blood.

Therefore we command, and order you to let it be known with all possible haste, that devout processions are to be held every Wednesday and Friday in our cathedral church, in other collegiate and conventual churches, and in every parish church in our city and diocese, with a solemn chanting of the litany, and that a special prayer be said in mass every day for allaying the plague and pestilence, and likewise prayers for the lord king and for the good estate of the church, the realm and the whole people of England, so that the Saviour, harkening to the constant entreaties, will pardon and come to the rescue of the creation which God fashioned in his own image.

And we, trusting in the mercy of Almighty God, and the merits and prayers of his mother, the glorious Virgin Mary, and of the blessed apostles Peter and Paul, and of the most holy confessor William and of all the saints, have released 40 days of the penance enjoined by the gracious God on all our parishioners and on others whose diocesans have approved and accepted this our indulgence, for sins for which they are penitent, contrite and have made confession, if they pray devoutly for these things, celebrate masses, undertake processions or are present at them, or perform other offices of pious devotion. And you are to ensure that these things are speedily put into effect in every archdeaconry within our diocese by the archdeacons or their officials. Farewell.

30. Intercessionary processions (2)

Ralph of Shrewsbury, Bishop of Bath and Wells, to the archdeacons of his diocese, 17 August 1348. Although chronicle accounts suggest that the plague had arrived on the Dorset coast by 1 August, if not earlier, the bishop's letter (written at Evercreech, Somerset, about 45 miles away) refers to it only as having reached a 'neighbouring kingdom' – presumably France.

Register of Bishop Ralph of Shrewsbury, Somerset Record Society X, 1896, pp. 555-556.

Almighty God uses thunder, lightning and the other blows which issue from his throne to scourge the sons whom he wishes to redeem. Accordingly, since a catastrophic pestilence from the East has arrived in a neighbouring kingdom, it is very much to be feared that, unless we pray devoutly and incessantly, a similar pestilence will stretch its poisonous branches into this realm, and strike down and consume the inhabitants. Therefore we firmly order each and every one of you to expound the present order in English in your churches at a suitable time, and then urge the regular and secular clergy and laity subject to you (or see that they are so urged by others) in the bowels of Jesus Christ to come before the presence of the Lord in confession, reciting psalms and performing other works of charity.[1]

Remember the ruin which was justifiably prophesied to the people of Ninevah – who were then mercifully rescued from the extermination threatened by God's judgement after they had performed penance. For

---

1 Based on a version of Psalm 94.2: 'Let us come before his presence in confession'. The more usual version ends 'with thanksgiving'.

they said: 'Who can tell if God will turn and forgive and will turn away
from his fierce anger: and we shall not perish'. And it continues: 'And
God saw their works, that they were turned from their evil way, and
God had mercy on them' [Jonas 3.9-10] and therefore the most kindly
Lord mercifully and wholesomely translated his anger into mildness,
and destruction into construction, for the sake of a penitent people; but
he has done the opposite for obstinate men and for hard hearted people
unwilling to repent, as is proved by the stories of Pharoah, of the five
cities of Sodom, and of others who, impenitent to the end, perished
eternally.

You should arrange for processions and stations[2] (in which you should
lead the people) to be performed at least every Friday in every
collegiate, conventual and parish church, so that, abasing themselves
humbly before the eyes of divine mercy, they should be contrite and
penitent for their sins, and should not omit to expiate them with
devout prayers, so that the mercies of God may speedily prevent us
and that he will, for his kindness sake, turn away from his people this
pestilence and the other harsh blows, and grant peace between
Christian countries and send healthy air saying, with the Psalmist:
'Remember not our former iniquities. Let thy mercies speedily prevent
us for we are become exceeding poor' [Ps 78.8].

31. The importance of prayer

Edward III had asked John Stratford, the Archbishop of Canterbury, to
arrange prayers against the plague throughout the province of Canterbury.
Stratford died on 23 August 1348, and responsibility for arranging the
prayers accordingly devolved on the Prior of Christchurch, Canterbury. In
this letter of 28 September 1348 the prior asks the Bishop of London to
transmit the order to the other bishops of the southern province. The letter
is generally known, from its opening word, as *Terribilis.*

D. Wilkins, *Concilia Magnae Britanniae et Hiberniae,* 4 vols, 1739, II p. 738.

Terrible is God towards the sons of men, and by his command all
things are subdued to the rule of his will. Those whom he loves he
censures and chastises; that is, he punishes their shameful deeds in
various ways during this mortal life so that they might not be
condemned eternally. He often allows plagues, miserable famines,
conflicts, wars and other forms of suffering to arise, and uses them to
terrify and torment men and so drive out their sins. And thus, indeed,

2 Stations: points at which the procession halted for prayers and readings.

the realm of England, because of the growing pride and corruption of its subjects, and their numberless sins, has on many occasions stood desolate and afflicted by the burdens of the wars which are exhausting and devouring the wealth of the kingdom, and by many other miseries. And it is now to be feared that the same kingdom is to be oppressed by the pestilences and wretched mortalities of men which have flared up in other regions.

Our most excellent prince and lord, Edward by the grace of God the illustrious King of England and France, after giving serious consideration to these things, accordingly sent letters requesting John Stratford, formerly Archbishop of Canterbury, to have prayers said throughout the province of Canterbury for the peace of the church and of the realm of England, and so that Almighty God, of his ineffable mercy, might save and protect the king's realm of England from these plagues and mortality. But death stopped the archbishop putting the royal requests into practice. We, therefore, wishing, insofar as it pertains to us, to make good what he left unfinished, command and order you, on our authority as metropolitan of the church of Canterbury, to give strict instructions in all haste to every suffragan of our church of Canterbury that they, on our authority, urge and encourage those subject to them (or see that they are urged and encouraged) to intercede with the most high by devout prayers for these things. Bishops and others in priests' orders should celebrate masses and should organise, or have organised, sermons at suitable times and places, along with processions every Wednesday and Friday; and should perform other offices of pious propitiation humbly and devoutly, so that God, pacified by their prayers, might snatch the people of England from these tribulations, of his grace show help to them and, of his ineffable pity, preserve human frailty from these plagues and mortality.

And, so that those subject to you, and others within the province of Canterbury, should be made the more eager to do these things, you should arrange to grant indulgences to every one of your flock undertaking the things specified above. You should also, on our authority and that of our said church of Canterbury, tell all the other bishops to add indulgences on their own account, as seems best to them. You, meanwhile, are to see that all these things are effectively observed within your own city and diocese of London. Inform us in writing before Epiphany next when you received these letters and what action you took, and also tell your fellow-bishops to notify us in writing by the same date of the action they have taken.

32. The response in Exeter

The Bishop of London duly transmitted the king's orders to his fellow bishops. John Grandisson, Bishop of Exeter, forwarded them to the Dean of Exeter with the following note of the local action to be taken.

F. C. Hingeston-Randolph (ed), *The Register of John de Grandisson, bishop of Exeter*, 2 vols, 1894-9, II pp. 1069-70.

Therefore we direct and order you or another to make a solemn announcement of these letters and their contents during the procession and sermon in the cathedral on the Sunday after All Saints [2 November], and then speedily have them expounded in English to our subjects within the city and suburbs of Exeter; exhorting them with salutary admonitions that those in priests' orders should celebrate mass devoutly and that the rest should hastily prepare themselves by devout confession to come into the presence of the Lord, and to hymn him with psalms and other devout prayers, so that our Lord God, softened by these prayers, should (once the sins of mankind have been expelled) transmute his just judgement into mercy, and might deign, of his ineffable pity, to change his wrath into clemency. We also beseech and order you, for the same purpose, to arrange solemn public processions through the said city every Wednesday and Friday until Christmas, summoning all the clergy within the city and suburbs: possessioners and mendicants, also rectors, vicars and parish chaplains. To each of our parishioners, being in a state of grace, who is present at these processions, celebrates mass or says other devout prayers and performs other placatory offices for these reasons, we mercifully release 30 days of penance, by the authority of the Lord, trusting in the grace and immense mercy of God Almighty, and in the merits and prayers of the most blessed and glorious Mary, always virgin, his mother, of the blessed apostles Peter and Paul, our patrons, and of all the saints. And tell us by letters patent before the feast of the Circumcision [1 January] what you have done about this.

33. A Voice in Rama

William Edendon, Bishop of Winchester, sent copies of this letter (known, from its opening, as *Vox in Rama*) to the prior and chapter of Winchester and to all abbots, priors, chaplains, rectors and vicars in the diocese. Edendon wrote it on 24 October 1348 at his palace in Southwark, and his belief that the plague had not yet reached his diocese may therefore be out of date.

Hampshire Record Office, Reg. Edyngdon, 21M65 A1/9 fo. 17.

A voice has been heard in Rama and much lamentation and mourning has echoed through various parts of the world.[3] Nations, bereft of their children, alas, in the abyss of unprecedented pestilence, refused to be comforted. For, what is terrible to hear, cities, towns, castles and villages, which until now rejoiced in their illustrious residents (their wisdom in counsel, their splendid riches, their great strength, the beauty of their womenfolk), which rang with the abundance of joy, to which crowds of people poured from far and wide for succour, pleasure and comfort, have now been suddenly and woefully stripped of their inhabitants by this most savage pestilence, more cruel than a two-edged sword. As a result no one dares to enter these places, but instead flees far from them, as if from the caves of wild animals, so that all joy within them ceases, all sweetness is dammed up and the sound of mirth silenced, and they become instead places of horror and desolate wastelands. Broad, fruitful acres lie entirely abandoned now that their farmers have been carried off, and might as well be barren.

We report with anguish the serious news which has come to our ears: that this cruel plague has now begun a similarly savage attack on the coastal areas of England. We are struck by terror lest (may God avert it!) this brutal disease should rage in any part of our city or diocese.

Although God often strikes us, to test our patience and justly punish our sins, it is not within the power of man to understand the divine plan. But it is to be feared that the most likely explanation is that human sensuality – that fire which blazed up as a result of Adam's sin and which from adolescence onwards is an incitement to wrong doing – has now plumbed greater depths of evil, producing a multitude of sins which have provoked the divine anger, by a just judgement, to this revenge. But because God is benign and merciful, long-suffering, and above malice, it may be that this affliction, which we richly deserve, can be averted if we turn to him humbly and with our whole hearts, and we therefore earnestly urge you to devotion. We beg you in God's name, and firmly command you by the obedience which you owe us, that you present yourselves before God through contrition and the proper confession of your sins, followed by the making of due satisfaction through the performance of penance, and that every Wednesday and Sunday, assembled in the choir of your monastery, you humbly and devoutly recite the 7 penitential psalms and the 15

3 A reference to Matthew 2.18: 'A voice in Rama was heard, lamentation and great mourning; Rachel bewailing her children and would not be comforted, because they are not.' The passage echoes Jeremiah 31.15 and is a reference to the Massacre of the Innocents.

psalms of degrees on your knees.[4] We also order that every Friday you should go solemnly in procession through the marketplace at Winchester, singing these psalms and the great litany instituted by the fathers of the church for use against the pestilence and performing other exercises of devotion, together with the clergy and people of the city, whom we wish to be summoned to attend. They are to accompany the procession with bowed heads and bare feet, fasting, with a pious heart and lamenting their sins (all idle chatter entirely set aside), and as they go they are to say devoutly, as many times as possible, the Lord's Prayer and the Hail Mary. They are to remain in earnest prayer until the end of the mass which we wish you to celebrate in your church at the end of each procession, trusting that if they persevere in their devotions with faith, rectitude and firm trust in the omnipotence and mercy of the Saviour they will soon receive a remedy and timely help from heaven.

[The letter ends with the grant of an indulgence of 40 days to those taking part in the procession and mass and praying there for a successful expedition for the king, the safety of his family and subjects and of all Christians, the peace of the Church, England and Christendom, and for the end of the plague; and 30 days indulgence to those making similar prayers elsewhere.]

34. Edward III to the bishops, 5 September 1349

C. Johnson (ed), *Registrum Hamonis Hethe, diocesis Roffensis*, Canterbury and York Society XLVIII, 1948, pp. 894–5.

During the pestilences and many evil tribulations with which, by way of warning, a just God now visits the sons of men and lashes the world – showing harshness to his people so that they, in fear and penitence, might call upon his name more humbly – we have been turning the matter over in our mind with intense concentration, and we are amazed and appalled that the few people who still survive have been so ill-fated, so ungrateful towards God and so stiff-necked that they are not humbled by the terrible judgments and lessons of God. For, if their works[5] are any guide, sinfulness and pride are constantly increasing in the people, and charity has grown more than usually cold

---

4 The penitential psalms are numbers 6, 31, 37, 50, 101, 129, 142; the psalms of
   degrees numbers 119-133.

5 *operibus*, a reference to the ordinance of labourers of 18 June [98] which attempted
   to peg wage levels.

in them. This seems to presage a much greater calamity (not, I hope, total ruin), and it is to be feared that this will really happen unless God, who has been offended by their guilt, is pacified by the performance of penance for sin and by the prayers of the faithful.

Therefore, since there is nothing that prayer cannot achieve when accompanied by entreaty, humility, fasting and the other defences of virtue, we have come hastening back devoutly to the weapons of prayer, humbly commending us and our people to the divine mercy. But since we have little trust in our own merits, from the depth of our heart we beseech you, who have been chosen to make offerings and sacrifices for sins on behalf of mankind, to offer God devout prayers and sacrifices for our salvation and that of the people; and to cause others to do likewise, urging your parishioners and others with wholesome admonitions, so that, mindful of God's kindness, they repent their sins and give themselves up to prayer, fasting and the exercise of virtue, and turn away from evil, so that merciful God might repel the plague and illness, and confer peace and tranquillity, and health of body and soul. For we hope that if, by God's grace, the people drive out this spiritual wickedness from their hearts, the malignancy of the air and of the other elements will also depart.

35. Causes for gratitude

From a letter of Simon Islip, Archbishop of Canterbury, to the Bishop of London, written on 28 December 1349.

Wilkins, *Concilia* II p. 752.

When we recall the amazing pestilence which lately attacked these parts and which took from us by far the best and worthiest men, those of us who have survived and have been mercifully spared by Providence (although we do not deserve it), must break forth in praises and devout expressions of gratitude. And we are now under an even greater obligation to praise the Lord with all our might, having received encouraging proofs of his goodwill. For certain enemies of our magnificent king hatched grievous plots which, by the protection of divine grace, they were unable to bring off. They endeavoured, through treachery, to seize the town of Calais, notwithstanding that it was protected by a truce to which they were party. But they have now fallen into the snare which, unwittingly, they set for themselves; for the king, in accordance with God's wishes, has subdued them wonderfully to his authority, conquering the great host by his military skill and putting it to flight.

Therefore we require and order you, our most loving brother in the Lord, and firmly urge you, to bring the king's victory and the remembrance of the pestilence to your people's notice so that everyone can ask for the safety of the realm with proper reverence, and at the same time advance the general rejoicing. For these reasons, order the seven penitential psalms and the litany to be specially recited twice every week in parish churches for the peace of the realm, for the lord king and for the obedience of the people, and the usual processions around the churches and churchyards to be carried out on the same days, by which means the people, sincerely contemplating the past and present gifts of God, should be better able to serve and please him. And thus those of us who remain alive should pray for the good state of the world, for the lord king, for us and for you, so that God, having mercy on the prayers of the just, should turn away his anger and in response to our prayers show us how to serve him more devotedly.

36. Processions against the plague in 1361

John Thoresby, Archbishop of York, modelled this letter of 12 July 1361 closely on that of Archbishop Zouche [29] and only the preamble has been printed here.

York, Borthwick Institute of Historical Research, Reg. 11 fo. 48.

Since the life of man on earth is a war, no wonder if those fighting amidst the miseries of this world are unsettled by the mutability of events: now favourable, now contrary. For Almighty God scourges every son he accepts and commonly shows harshness to his people, sending many evil infirmities and sufferings to those who are straying and heaping humiliations on their heads, so that they may repent and seek his name with more humility. Indeed, the kingdom of England has been assailed with the whirlwinds of war and with pestilences and other misfortunes, directed at driving away the sins of men, on such a scale and for such a long time that it has now come to public notice, and the kingdom is bound to be assailed in the same way in the future unless divine mercy, looking down from heaven, sees the prayers and penance of the faithful and is inclined to mercy. Therefore we believe it important to urge, more devoutly and insistently, suffrages of devout prayer and other offices of pious propitiation, so that our Lord and God, pitying his people, may drive away all sickness, bestow health, and grant quiet, concord and peace in earth as in heaven.

37. A call for prayers in 1375

The preamble to a letter requesting penitential processions and prayers written by Simon Sudbury, Archbishop of Canterbury, on 15 July 1375.

Wilkins, *Concilia* III pp. 100-1.

Would that those who profess themselves zealous for peace, who give their attention to the mortality, pestilence or epidemic now reigning in England and to the unwonted frequency of current wars with subtle scheming, politic judgement and deep study, could be persuaded to pour out unceasing prayers to the most high for the cessation of this pestilence or epidemic and for the tranquillity of peace, and to entreat mercy of him with a humble heart. For prayer is an immediate defence, an immolation of the enemy, a solace to angels and a pleasing sacrifice to God, and assiduous appeals for mercy made by a just man very often carry great power; for we read of Moses, praying with hands raised to heaven that his people would conquer, of the city of Ninevah saved from destruction by prayers, and of the prophet who achieved the lengthening of his allotted lifespan.[6]

But in our modern times, alas, we are mired in monstrous sin and the lack of devotion among the people provokes the anger of the great king to whom we should direct our prayers. As a result we are assailed by plagues or epidemics, by the horrors of war, the unhealthiness of the air, the scarcity of crops and the diminishing of livestock, all of which leaves us more than usually bewildered and depressed. We cannot even take pleasure in our independence, for foreigners find ingenious excuses to plunder our possessions and make frequent attacks on our men, and other troubles increase daily – as is perfectly obvious to informed observers.

38. Masses to be said in time of plague

The medieval church had two masses against the pestilence, both printed here. The first, *Salus populi*, was ordered to be said throughout the province of Canterbury in 1382.[7] The second, as the rubric relates, was reputedly composed by Pope Clement VI and was credited with prophylactic powers.

6 In their battle with Amalek the Israelites were successful as long as Moses kept his hands raised: Exodus 17.8-13. The people of Ninevah dressed in sack cloth and ashes after listening to the preaching of Jonah, and their penitence averted God's anger: Jonas 3 (an example also cited by Ralph of Shrewsbury: 30). The prayers of the prophet Ezekiah were met by the grant of a further 15 years of life: 4 Kings 20.

7 F. C. Hingeston-Randolph (ed), *The Register of Thomas de Brantyngham, bishop of Exeter* pt 1, 1901, pp. 464-5.

Missale ad usum insignis et praeclarae ecclesiae Sarum, ed F. H. Dickinson, cols
810*-812*, 886*-890*.

(a) A Mass against Plague: *Salus populi*

Office: I am the safety of the people, says the Lord; when they shall
have cried to me from tribulation I will hear them, and I shall be their
Lord for ever.

Psalm 77: Attend, O my people, to my law: incline your ears to the
words of my mouth.

Prayer: O God, who of your sole mercy removed the danger which
hung over the people of Ninevah; to whom, so that you could show
your mercy, you gave penitence and conversion; look, we beseech you,
on your people prostrate before your mercy; for your mercy's sake, do
not allow the people whom you redeemed with the blood of your only
begotten son to die of pestilence [*mortalitatis*].

The Lesson (Jeremiah 14.7-8): If our iniquities have testified against
us, O Lord, do thou it for thy name's sake, for our rebellions are many:
we have sinned against thee. O expectation of Israel, the Saviour
thereof in time of trouble .... But thou, O Lord, art among us, and thy
name is called upon by us: forsake us not.

Gradual: Be kind, O Lord, to our sins; lest the people should say,
'Where is our God?'

Verse: Help us, O Lord our salvation; and for the honour of your name,
O Lord, free us.

Alleluia: Lord, you are our refuge, from generation to generation.

The Gospel (Luke 11.9-13): At that time Jesus said to his disciples:
Ask, and it shall be given you; seek, and you shall find; knock and it
shall be opened to you. For everyone that asketh receiveth; and he that
seeketh findeth; and to him that knocketh it shall be opened. And
which of you, if he ask his father bread, will he give him a stone? Or
a fish, will he for a fish give him a serpent? Or if he shall ask an egg,
will he reach him a scorpion? If you then, being evil, know how to give
good gifts to your children, how much more will your Father from
heaven give the good Spirit to them that ask him?

Offertory: All who know your name, O Lord, trust in you; because you
do not abandon those seeking you; sing unto the Lord who lives in
Sion, for the cry of the poor is not forgotten.

Secret: Almighty God, look, we beseech you, favourably upon the gift of your church, and come before us in your mercy rather than your anger, for if you choose to take notice of our iniquities, no creature could survive it; but for the sake of the wonderful kindness with which you made us, do not let the works of your hand perish.

Communion: Amen I say to you: whatever you seek with prayers, believe that you will receive it; and be it done to you.

Post communion: Almighty and merciful God, look upon the people subject to your majesty; and may the receiving of your sacrament prevent the fury of cruel death from coming upon us.

(b) Mass: *Recordare Domini*

A mass for turning away plague, which was made by Pope Clement and ordained with the approval of all the cardinals. And he granted 260 days of indulgence to all penitents, being truly contrite and confessed, who heard the following mass. And all those hearing the following mass should hold a burning candle while they hear mass on the five following days and keep it in their hand throughout the entire mass, while kneeling; and sudden death shall not be able to harm them. And this is certain and proved in Avignon and neighbouring regions.

Office: Remember, O Lord, your covenant, and say to the scourging angel, 'Now hold your hand', so that the earth is not laid waste and you do not lose every living soul.

Psalm 79: Give ear, O thou that rulest Israel: thou that leadest Joseph like a sheep.

Prayer: O God, who does not desire the death but the penitence of sinners, we beseech you graciously to turn your people to you, and that in as much as they are devoted to you you should mercifully withdraw the flail of your anger from them.

The Lesson (2 Kings 24.15-19): In those days the Lord sent a pestilence upon Israel, from the morning unto the time appointed. And there died of the people from Dan to Bersabea seventy thousand men. And when the angel of the Lord had stretched out his hand over Jerusalem to destroy it, the Lord had pity on the affliction and said to the angel that slew the people: It is enough. Now hold thy hand. And the angel of the Lord was near the threshing floor of Areuna the Jebusite. And David said to the Lord, when he saw the angel striking the people: It is I. I am he that have sinned: I have done wickedly.

These that are the sheep, what have they done? Let thy hand, I beseech thee, be turned against me and against my father's house. And Gad, the prophet of the Lord, came to David that day, and said: Go up, and build an altar to the Lord in the threshing floor of Areuna the Jebusite. And David went up according to the word of Gad, which the Lord had commanded him.

Gradual: The Lord sent his word and healed them, and snatched them from their ruin.

Verse: They should acknowledge before the Lord his mercy and his marvellous deeds for the sons of men.

Alleluia: I will save my people in the midst of Jerusalem and I will be to them a God of truth and justice.

Sequence: [this long hymn is not translated here: it evokes the power of God and recalls Old Testament figures pardoned their sins after repentance. It ends with an appeal to Mary to intercede with her son.]

The Gospel (Luke 4.38-44): In that time Jesus rising up out of the synagogue, went into Simon's house. And Simon's wife's mother was taken with a great fever: and they besought him for her. And standing over her, he commanded the fever: and it left her. And immediately rising, she ministered to them. And when the sun was down, all they that had any sick with divers diseases brought them to him. But he, laying his hands on every one of them, healed them. And devils went out from many, crying out and saying: Thou art the son of God. And rebuking them he suffered them not to speak; for they knew that he was Christ. And when it was day, going out he went into a desert place: and the multitudes sought him, and came unto him. And they stayed him that he should not depart from them. To whom he said: To other cities also must I preach the kingdom of God: for therefore am I sent. And he was preaching in the synagogues of Galilee.

Offertory: The priest stood between the living and the dead, with a gold censer in his hand, and offering the sacrifice of incense he appeased the anger of the Lord, and the plague ceased from the house and people of Israel.

Secret: We beseech you, O Lord, let the operation of your present sacrifice rescue the people, and powerfully release us from all faults and fears, and completely protect and defend us from threatened damnation.

Communion: A crowd of the sick, and those troubled by unclean spirits came to Jesus, for power came out of him and healed them all.

Post communion: Hear us, O God our salvation, and at the intercession of Mary, blessed mother of God, free your people from the terrors
of your anger and in mercy let them be secure in your bounty.

39. A prayer against pestilence to the Virgin Mary

This popular prayer (known by its Latin opening as *Stella Celi Extirpavit*) is
given here in two forms. The first is a prose translation of the Latin prayer as
it appears in the late- medieval Hours of the Blessed Virgin Mary. The second
is one of two English reworkings of the prayer by the fifteenth-century poet
John Lydgate. Lydgate's spelling and punctuation have been modernised, but
no attempt has been made to translate his verse into modern English or to
preserve the rhythms of the original.

(a) in prose: C. Wordsworth (ed), *Horae Eboracensis: the prymer or hours of the
Blessed Virgin Mary*, Surtees Society CXXXII, 1920 for 1919, p. 69.

Star of Heaven, who nourished the Lord and rooted up the plague of
death which our first parents planted; may that star now deign to
counter the constellations whose strife brings the people the ulcers of
a terrible death. O glorious star of the sea, save us from the plague.
Hear us: for your Son who honours you denies you nothing. Jesus, save
us, for whom the Virgin Mother prays to you.

(b) in verse: H.N. MacCracken (ed), *The Minor Poems of John Lydgate* I, Early
English Text Society, extra series CVII, 1911, pp. 295-6.

O blessed queen, above the starred heaven
Which of the sea art called chief lodestar,
Thy dwelling is above the stars seven,
Where ever is joy, and peace without war,
Cast down on us thy look, that art so far
From all mischief, be thou our chief defence,
In our most trouble thy succour let be near
And be our shield from stroke of pestilence.

In paradise with joy and all pleasance
Adam was put, to have lived without end,
But through his sin befell him great mischance
Brought in first death through tempting of the fiend,
But thou lady that art so good and kind
To thee be praise, with joy and reverence,
Thou broughtest life, to me and all mankind
And puttest away eternal pestilence.

Thou glorious star this world to illumine,
Thy name to praise I have no sufficiency,
On us sinners thy mercy let down shine,
Of infect airs oppress all their utterance
Us to infect, that they have no puissance;
From their battle be thou our chief defence,
That their malice to us do no grievance
Of infecting or stroke of pestilence.

Thou resplendent star, of stars most sovereign,
Grant me these three, most excellent princess:
The first is this, I pray thee not disdain,
To have length of life not mixed with sickness;
Of wordly goods grant me also largesse,
Without strife, to God's reverence;
The third is that my soul, without distress,
May come to the bliss where dreaded is no pestilence.

40. A prayer made to St Sebastian against the mortality which
flourished in 1349

This popular verse invocation of St Sebastian appears in late-medieval *Horae*
or Primers, but this text has been taken from the chronicle of Gilles li Muisis,
and the heading above is li Muisis' own.

J-J. de Smet (ed), *Recueil des Chroniques des Flandre* II, Brussels, 1841, pp.
385-6.

O St Sebastian, guard and defend me, morning and evening, every
minute of every hour, while I am still of sound mind; and, Martyr,
diminish the strength of that vile illness called an epidemic which is
threatening me. Protect and keep me and all my friends from this
plague. We put our trust in God and St Mary, and in you, O holy
Martyr. You, citizen of Milan,[8] could, through God's power, halt this
pestilence if you chose. For it is known to many that you have that
merit: to Zoe, whom you miraculously healed and restored to health,
and to Nicostratus her husband. You comforted martyrs in their time
of trial, and promised them the eternal life which is the reward of
martyrs.[9] O martyr Sebastian! Be with us always, and by your merits

8 St Sebastian himself was born in Narbonne, but his parents came from Milan.
9 According to his *Life* the saint encouraged the martyrs Marcus and Marcellian
   when they were wavering in their resolution.

keep us safe and sound and protected from plague. Commend us to the Trinity and to the Virgin Mary, so that when we die we may have our reward: to behold God in the company of martyrs.

41. The sins of the times

The title by which this anonymous poem is usually known, 'On the Pestilence', was supplied by its editor, Thomas Wright; the original (Cambridge University Library MS Ee.vi.29 fo.31) is untitled. There is no evidence to suggest which of the fourteenth-century plagues the author has in mind in stanza 1.

Thomas Wright (ed), *Political Poems and Songs* I, Rolls Series, 1859, pp. 279-81.

See how England mourns, drenched in tears. The people, stained by sin, quake with grief. Plague is killing men and beasts. Why? Because vices rule unchallenged here.

Alas! The whole world is now given over to spite. Where can a kind heart be found among the people? No one thinks on the crucified Christ, and therefore the people perish as a token of vengeance.

Peace and patience are thoroughly plundered; love and justice are not at home. Men cuddle up to errors and vices; children die for the sins of their fathers.

The sloth of the shepherds leaves the flocks straying. The trusting are tricked by the cunning of traders; fraud and avarice go hand in hand like sisters; the poor suffer through the depravity of the rich.

Nourished by simony, Simon Magus flourishes.[10] The balance is crooked, truth has departed; the flock of Christ is scattered, the wolf rages; and plague is poured out, engulfing the lambs.

Rulers are moved by favour not wisdom; power thrusts the unworthy into jobs; the mercy of kings is governed by favourites; patrons are swayed by love and lucre.

The brave warriors of Christ have now retreated; the satellites of

---

10 Simon Magus was a sorcerer of Samaria converted to Christianity by the Apostle Philip. He then offered money to be given the power (enjoyed by the Apostles themselves) of transmitting the Holy Ghost by the laying on of hands, and was rebuked by Peter for thinking that the gifts of God could be purchased for cash [Acts 8]. He therefore gave his name to simony, the sin of buying spiritual office. He also became the medieval stereotype of the fraudulent magician, a side of his career amplified by the apocryphal Acts of the Apostles: V. I. J. Flint, *The Rise of Magic in early medieval Europe*, Oxford, 1991, pp. 338-44.

Satan have overturned the temple. They have lost the wounded and sickly sheep. Cuckoos intrude into the monastic nest.

Noble fathers once put the plague to flight and the firm in faith healed the sick. Their holy life shone as a bright example and by their praiseworthy deeds they showed themselves soldiers of Christ.

Such men dressed in rough garments, but few do so these days; instead they wear soft fabrics. They were distinguished by moral excellence, but the youth of today are learned only in squalid rites.

Alas! rectors and vicars have changed their ways, they're hirelings now, not true shepherds, and their works are motivated by the desire for money. Such workers deserve to come to grief.

Such men prefer furs to hair shirts; they stuff their bellies with dainties and then abandon themselves to limitless depravity. Buttressed by riches, they live contrary to right.

While chapels are lavishly rebuilt the Church – the Bride of Christ – is stripped naked. Untended, the vine is blighted by sin, and usurers dig it up like rooting pigs.

The priests of God are unchaste; their deeds not matching their name. They should be teaching and administering the sacraments, but they behave in ways inappropriate to their order.

Their names should be written with blood in heaven, but are to be read instead in the records of this world. Old sins should be purged with fire, but theirs weigh them down and now rule them.

Alas! Love and charity have grown cold in kingdoms. It is spite and harshness which blaze up in the people. Truth and faith are lukewarm in laymen and clerics alike. Nobility and renown are asleep in this realm.

Women are no longer bound by the restraints of their sex; the subtlety of merchants shifts into fraud; the guile of brothers turns the world topsy turvy. Man, if truth now reigns in you, rejoice.

42. The failings of the clergy

Heinrich von Herford, in Westphalia, was a Dominican, who died in the friary at Minden on 9 October 1370, although his chronicle ends considerably earlier, in 1355. His attack on the greed and ambition of the clergy, printed here, leads immediately into a list of natural and man-made calamities, beginning with the earthquake of January 1348. For his detailed account of the flagellants see below, 52.

A. Potthast (ed), *Liber de Rebus Memorabilioribus sive Chronicon Henrici de
Hervordia*, Göttingen, 1859, pp. 268-9.

At this time violent disagreements, rebellions, conspiracies, plots
and intrigues sprang up among both secular and regular clergy
everywhere, just as the apostle foretold in 2 Timothy 3 and 2
Corinthians 12.[11] At the same time there were also other disturbances, of young against old, ignoble against noble, and an unusual
degree of unrest (whether general or specific) in many cities, monasteries and congregations. The heresy of simony also grew so strong
among the clergy, and overwhelmed them so completely, that everyone, of whatever degree (great, middling or humble) and of whatever status (secular or regular) in some fashion openly bought and
sold spiritualities of all sorts. They did not blush for shame, they
were not reproved or criticised by anyone, let alone punished, so
that it might seem as if the Lord, far from expelling the buyers and
sellers from the temple, had made them at home there, or as if
simony was now to be judged not heretical but ecclesiastical, catholic and holy. They traded prebends, benefices, and all other ecclesiastical dignities, parish churches, chapels, vicarages and altars for
money, women and sometimes for concubines; they staked them, lost
and won them, on a game of dice.

Then there were many disturbances over contested kingdoms, princi-
palities, archbishoprics, bishoprics, prebends and other things of that
kind, such as between the Emperor Lewis, Charles King of Bohemia
and Count Gunther of Schwarzburg over who was to be King of the
Romans;[12] between John, King of France and Edward, King of
England over the kingdom of France; and between rival claimants for

11 Both these biblical citations have apocalyptic overtones.

2 Timothy 3.1-5: 'Know also this, that in the last days shall come dangerous times.
Men shall be lovers of themselves, covetous, haughty, proud, blasphemers,
disobedient to parents, ungrateful, wicked, without affection, without peace,
slanderers, incontinent, unmerciful, without kindness, traitors, stubborn, puffed up,
and lovers of pleasures more than of God: having an appearance indeed of godliness,
but denying the power thereof'.

2 Corinthians 12.20: 'For I fear lest perhaps, when I come, I shall not find you such
as I would, and that I shall be found by you as you would not. Lest perhaps
contentions, envyings, detractions, whisperings, swellings, seditions be among you'.

12 In July 1346 Pope Clement VI deposed the Emperor Lewis IV and called upon the
imperial Electors to chose a new king of the Romans. A group of Electors chose
Charles of Moravia, the effective ruler of Bohemia, and the two men were at war
when Lewis died in October 1347. His supporters adopted Count Gunther of
Schwarzburg as their candidate in 1349.

the archbishopric of Mainz and for Bremen, Minden, Hildesheim, Halberstadt, Worms, Schleswig and many others. Prebends, dignities and inordinate numbers of lesser posts were neglected.

Then each religious order was wrenched asunder by its members, as the birth of vipers tears apart the maternal womb.[13] Every office and appointment among them could only be secured by money, or favouritism, or some other useful gift. Just as once prebends and dignities of that sort were sought and obtained from prelates or in the Roman Curia, so the offices of abbot, prior, warden, master, lector, definitor, and everything else, however petty, was bought, occupied and held by whoever possessed the necessary money (by theft or some other means), regardless of whether they were foul tempered, boorish, illiterate, under age, inexperienced, stupid, or lacking in any other way whatsoever. And in these days distinguished people cannot easily be found (as was once the case) among the secular and regular clergy. Look at all these abbots, priors, wardens, masters, lectors, provosts and canons, and groan! Look at their life, the example they give, their career and their doctrine, and at the risks to their people, and tremble! And you too, Lord, father of mercies, look down and have mercy, for we have sinned against you.

In the 31st year of Emperor Lewis, around the feast of the Conversion of St Paul [25 January] there was an earthquake throughout Carinthia and Carniola which was so severe that everyone feared for their lives. There were repeated shocks, and on one night the earth shook 20 times. Sixteen cities were destroyed and their inhabitants killed. One city, called Cencenighe, was entirely destroyed along with the Franciscan friary there and not one man escaped. And in many places it is hard to belive that anyone ever lived there. Thirty-six mountain fortresses and their inhabitants were destroyed and it has been calculated that more than 40,000 men were swallowed up or over-whelmed. Two very high mountains, with a highway between them, were hurled together, so that there can never be a road there again. This information comes from a letter of the house of Friesach to the provincial prior of Germany. It says in the same letter that in this year fire falling from heaven consumed the land of the Turks for 16 days; that for a few days it rained toads and snakes, by which many men were killed; that a pestilence has gathered strength in many parts of

13 It was believed that when young vipers were ready to be born, they tore their way out of their mother's side and so killed her — hence the proverbial ingratitude of vipers.

the world; that not one man in ten escaped in Marseilles; that all the Franciscans there have died; that beyond Rome the city of Messina has been largely deserted because of the pestilence. And a knight coming from that place said that he did not find five men alive there. All these things from the same letter.

43. Divine disapproval of tournaments

This account by Henry Knighton immediately precedes his description of the plague [21] and readers were presumably expected to see a causal connection.

J. R. Lumby (ed), *Chronicon Henrici Knighton vel Cnitthon monachi Leycestrensis,* 2 vols, Rolls Series, 1889-95, II, pp. 57-8.

In those days a murmuring and great complaint arose among the people, because whenever and wherever tournaments were held a troop of ladies would turn up dressed in a variety of extraordinary male clothing, as if taking part in a play. There were sometimes as many as forty or fifty of them, representing the showiest and most beautiful (but not the most virtuous) women of the whole realm. They were dressed in particoloured tunics with short hoods and liripipes like strings wound around the head,[14] and wore belts thickly studded with gold and silver slung across their hips, below the navel, with knives called daggers in pouches suspended from them. Dressed thus, and mounted on chargers or on other horses with elaborate trappings, they rode to the tournament ground. In this way they spent and wasted their goods, and (according to the common report) abused their bodies in wantonness and scurrilous licentiousness. They neither feared God nor blushed at the criticism of the people, but took the marriage bond lightly and were deaf to the demands of modesty. Nor, in following these pursuits, did they remember how much favour and outstanding support God, the liberal giver of all good things, had shown the English army against all their enemies, and with what special backing he had carried them to triumphant victories in every place.[15] But God, present in these things as in everything, supplied a marvellous remedy to prevent their frivolity; for at the times and places appointed for these vanities he sent down heavy rain, with thunder and flashing lightning, and tempestuous winds, and so scattered them.

14 Liripipes: the long 'tails' of hoods.
15 A reference to the Crécy campaign (1346) and the siege of Calais (1346-47).

44. Indecent clothing as a cause of the 1348-49 epidemic

This comes from the continuation of the Westminster chronicle covering the period 1325-45 and written by an anonymous monk of the abbey. From 1345 the continuation is the work of John of Reading [20, 25h, 45b].

James Tait (ed), *Chronica Johannis de Reading et Anonymi Cantuariensis 1346-1367*, Manchester, 1914, pp. 88-9.

[1344] There were few other good things worth noting this year. Ever since the arrival of the Hainaulters about eighteen years ago the English have been madly following outlandish ways, changing their grotesque fashions of clothing yearly.[16] They have abandoned the old, decent style of long, full garments for clothes which are short, tight, impractical, slashed, every part laced, strapped or buttoned up, with the sleeves of the gowns and the tippets of the hoods hanging down to absurd lengths, so that, if the truth be told, their clothes and footwear make them look more like torturers, or even demons, than men. Clerics and other religious adopted the same fashions, and should be considered not regulars but irregulars. Women flowed with the tides of fashion in this and other things even more eagerly, wearing clothes that were so tight that they wore a fox tail hanging down inside their skirts at the back, to hide their arses. The sin of pride manifested in this way must surely bring down misfortune in the future.

45. Indecent clothing as a cause of later outbreaks

(a) F. S. Haydon (ed), *Eulogium Historiarum sive Temporis*, 3 vols, Rolls Series, 1858-63, III pp. 230-1.

In the same year [1362] and in the previous year, the whole of England was thrown into madness and excitement by a rage for bodily adornments. The fashion was firstly for full doublets, cut short to the loins; and for a long garment reaching to the ankles, not opening in the front, as is proper for men, but laced up the side to the armhole in the style of women's clothes, so that from the back their wearers look more like women than men. This garment has an apt name, being called

16 The Hainaulters were the servants and associates of Edward III's queen, Philippa of Hainault. The marriage took place in January 1328, but the couple had been betrothed earlier, before the 1326 invasion of Edward's mother Isabella and her lover, Roger Mortimer, which deposed Edward II. The cost of the mercenaries from Hainault who provided the military muscle for the invasion was much resented, and perhaps explains the hostile tone of this passage, since Philippa herself seems to have been a popular figure.

gown in the vernacular, and well called, since it is said that 'gown' derives from *gounyg*, which ought properly to be pronounced *wounyg*, that is to say, 'wide open to mockery'.[17] They also have little hoods, tightly buttoned under the chin in the fashion of women, and sewn around with gold and silver thread and precious stones, the liripipe ankle-length and slashed like a jester's clothes.

They have also a garment of silk, called a *paltok* in the common tongue, a term which ought properly to be applied to ecclesiastical rather than to secular wear; of which it is said in the Book of Kings that Solomon in all his life never used such things.[18] They also have particoloured and striped hose, which they tie with laces to their paltocks, and which are called *harlottes*, and thus one 'harlot' serves another, as they go about with their loins uncovered.[19] They own immensely valuable belts studded with gold and silver: wealthy men have belts worth 20 marks; the middling sort, such as esquires and freeholders, own belts priced between £1–£5, even when they do not have 20 pence to rub together.

17 The word 'gown' is usually derived via Old French *goune* from medieval Latin *gunna*, a cloak, although the origins of the word are obscure. But the writer here is combining amateur etymology with some conscious word-play.

   As a result of borrowing words, English speakers were familiar with alternative forms with initial g– and w–, usually from Central French or Norman French, doublets such as guarantee/warranty, guard/ward. So it was easy for the writer to connect *gounyg* and *wounyg*. *Gounyg* is probably from the same root as *gounie*, a goon or simpleton, while *wounyg* is related to Old English *wanhoga*, an idiot, and *wohness*, crookedness or perversity.

   I owe this note to the kindness of Gerard M-F Hill.

18 It is not clear what passage the author has in mind here. The immediate reference may be to 3 Kings 10.24–25: 'And all the earth desired to see Solomon's face .... And everyone brought him presents, garments and armour....' But there is surely also an echo of Matthew 6.29 or Luke 12.27: 'But I say to you, not even Solomon in all his glory was clothed like one of these'. 'These' are the lilies of the field, and the point is that they are beautifully 'clothed' without working.

   The author's comment that the term is more fittingly applied to ecclesiastical than to secular wear cannot literally mean that the garment ought to be worn by priests rather than laymen – although this is how it is often interpreted. The explicit description of the garment in 45b makes it clear that it was far too immodest for clerical wear. The most likely explanation of the author's comment is that the term 'paltock' originally referred to an item of ecclesiastical clothing (probably a cassock or cloak) and had been mockingly applied by irreverent laity to a strikingly indecent garment – something hardly likely to amuse a clerical writer.

19 The implication of this rather cryptic comment is that the combination of short doublet (the paltock) and long hose left the genitalia inadequately covered and hence was an invitation to lechery. The next passage [45b] develops this theme. All three terms used there for the long hose have strong overtones of sexual laxity: harlots, *gadelinges* (gadabouts) and *lorels* (rogues).

They also possess shoes with pointed toes as long as a finger, which are called *crakowes*. These are more like devils' talons than apparel for men, and their wearers look more like minstrels and jesters than barons, like actors rather than knights, buffoons rather than esquires. In hall they are lions, hares on the battlefield; slow in giving gifts, they are quick to accept them; eager for spectacle, they are bored by prayers. Because the people wantonly squander the gifts of God on rage, pride, lechery and greed – and all the rest of the deadly sins – it is only to be expected that the Lord's vengeance will follow. Wherefore we pray for the mercy and pardon of God for past offences, and that we should not fall in the future but continue in grace.

(b) John of Reading, in *Chronica Johannis de Reading et Anonymi Cantuariensis* pp. 166-8.

[1365] Many serious things were prophesied because of the triple planetary conjunction: firstly, on 4 August this year, the conjunction of Mars and Jupiter in the twentieth degree of Libra; secondly the mean conjunction of Mars and Saturn on the 19th of the same month in the thirtieth degree of Libra; and thirdly the great conjunction of Jupiter and Saturn in the eighth degree of Scorpio on 30 October, something which has not happened for 200 years. But the time went by, and the days passed, thank God, without harm to the English – unless one counts harm to their animals. For during haymaking heavy rain destroyed the hay and the standing corn, and at the same time there were battles of sparrows in various places, which left countless bodies in the fields. An unexpected pestilence followed, in which many people went to bed healthy and died suddenly. Pustules, called *pokkes* in English, infected and killed men and various kinds of animals. The west wind, which for the past three years has been dreadfully destructive, did terrible damage to the monastery of Reading and its neighbourhood, and the devil appeared there in the shape of a deformed man.

And no wonder, given the empty headedness of the English, who remained wedded to a crazy range of outlandish clothing without realising the evil which would come of it. They began to wear useless little hoods, laced and buttoned so tightly at the throat that they only covered the shoulders, and which had tippets like cords. In addition they wore *paltoks*, extremely short garments, some of wool and others padded and quilted, which failed to conceal their arses or their private parts; they also wore very long legged hose called *harlotes, gadelinges* or *lorels*, tied to these short garments with laces; also shoes with long toes, and long knives hanging between their thighs; and caps of cloth twisted back into the shape of hose or sleeves. These misshapen and tight clothes did not allow them to kneel to God or to the saints, to their lords or to each other, to serve or do reverence without great discomfort, and were also highly dangerous in battle.

Infected by malice, cunning, deceit and evil, perverting every convention, decency and standard in their deeds, gestures and words, men considered that to deflower virgins and violate the chastity of wives and widows was doing them a favour, not an injury. Men did not have sexual intercourse with their wives, or married women with their husbands, but preferred to get bastards on strangers.

46. The disobedience of children

Reflections on the injunction to 'Honour thy parents' from an English treatise on the Ten Commandments. The text can be dated to the early 1360s by its reference to the death of children in the current pestilence. I have modernised the spelling and syntax, and have used the word 'honour' in place of 'worship' in the original – a word which now has rather different connotations.

British Library, Harleian Manuscript 2398, fos. 93-4.

He honours his father as he should who helps him in both his bodily and spiritual need, and so you should honour your father with bodily help and also help him spiritually, for he has need thereof. So the honour of father and mother stands principally in action. If your father and mother come to want and mischief by age or misfortune you are bound to help them both by service with your body and help with your possessions; and if they are in a state of sin or have need of spiritual teaching and comfort, you are obliged, if you can, to teach and comfort them. If you cannot, you are obliged to do what you can to get others to help them. And if they are dead, you are obliged to pray night and day to God to deliver them from pain. This is the reverence and honour in action that the child should do to the father and mother, and this lesson should be taught by every bodily father and mother, and spiritual father and also by god fathers and mothers to their children; and if this lesson had been taught and kept in England I am sure that the land would have stood in more prosperity than it has stood for many a day, and it may be that it is in vengeance of this sin of dishonouring and despising fathers and mothers that God is slaying children by pestilence, as you see daily. For in the old law children who were rebellious and disobedient to their fathers and mothers were punished by death, as the fifth book of holy writ testifies as follows: 'If a man has a son who is rebellious or wicked, and pays no heed to the commands of his father and mother and, when constrained, still refuses to obey, they shall take him and lead him to the elders of the city and to the gate of judgement, and then they shall say to them, 'This our son is wicked and rebellious and despises our teaching, and indulges in gluttony, lechery and feasting'. Then he shall be stoned to death so that all the people, hearing of the punishment, shall be afraid to rebel against father or mother.'[20] And though God no longer wills that this punishment of bodily death be executed as it was in those days for such trespasses, yet the punishment is no less, but rather harder and longer lasting; for unless such rebellious and disobedient children amend during their life, God will smite them with the sword of vengeance in the hour of their death, putting their souls into the pains of hell, and on the last day of judgement he shall put both body and soul into the everlasting pains of hell. Therefore obey this commandment and follow the noble teacher Paul, who says: 'Children, be obedient to your father and mother, for it is right to honour your father. That is the first commandment, so that it shall go well with you and that you shall be long living upon the earth' [Ephesians 6.1-3].

47. The Sermon of Reason

William Langland, *Piers the Plowman*, passus V, lines 1-62.

The king and his knights to the church went
To hear the day's matins and mass after.
Then woke I from my sleeping and was sad to think
That I had not slept sounder and seen more.
But I had not gone a furlong before faintness seized me
So I could go no further on foot for lack of sleep;
I sat softly down and said my Creed
And pattering my Pater noster sent me to sleep.
    And then I saw much more than I told before
For I saw the field full of folk, that I spoke of before,
And how Reason prepared himself to preach to the realm
And with a cross before the king began thus to teach.
    He proved that these pestilences were purely for sin

---

20 A paraphrase of Deuteronomy 21.18-21.

And the southwest wind last Saturday evening
Was evidently sent for pride and nothing else.[21]
Pear trees and plum trees were blown to the earth
As a sign to you men that you should do better.
Beeches and broad oaks were blown to the ground,
Turning their roots upwards in token of terror,
That deadly sin at Domesday shall undo them all.
Of this matter I might go on a long while
But I shall say what I saw, with God's help.
How plainly before the people Reason began to preach.
He bade Waster go work at what he did best
And earn what he'd wasted with some manner of craft.
And prayed Peronelle to put by her finery
And keep it in her box, to be sold as necessary.
Tom Stowe he taught to take two staves
And fetch Felicity home from gadding about.[22]
He warned Watt his wife was at fault –
Her hat was worth half a mark, his hood not worth fourpence.
And bade Bat cut a bough or two
And beat Betty therewith, if she wouldn't work.
And then he charged chapmen to chastise their children
'Don't let wealth spoil them while they are young
Nor for fear of the pestilence indulge them beyond reason.
My father and mother both told me
That the dearer the child the more teaching it needs.
And Solomon said the same, in his book of Wisdom:[23]
Qui parcit virge odit filium,
Which is in English, if you want to know:
Who spares the rod, spoils the child.'
And then he prayed prelates and priests alike,
'What you preach to the people, prove on yourselves,
Follow it in your deeds, it shall draw you to good,
If you live as you teach us, we'll believe you the better.'
Then he counselled religious to live by their rule:

21 For the great wind on the night of 15 January 1362 see 25e.

22 A free translation of a cryptic sentence usually taken to mean that Tom should fetch
Felicity home rather than risk her suffering the punishment of women, that is, the
ducking stool. Since Tom had to fetch her *home* her fault was evidently gadding
about, something which many contemporary moralists thought a particular failing
of women.

23 Wisdom 13.24.

'Lest the king and the council cut back your provisions
And administer your lands until you be ruled better.'
Then he counselled the king the Commons to love:
'They're your treasure in treason, a remedy in need'.
And then he prayed the pope to pity holy church
And before dispensing grace to govern himself first.
'And you who uphold the law, be covetous of truth
Rather than gold or gifts, if you wish to please God.
For whoever denies truth, as is said in the gospel,
God knows him not, nor do the saints in Heaven:
    Amen dico vobis, nescio vos.[24]
And you that seek St James and the saints of Rome,
Seek St Truth, for he may save you all
Qui cum patre et filio.[25] May good attend
Those who follow my sermon.'

48. The sins of the English

This and the following text come from sermons preached by the Bishop of
Rochester, Thomas Brinton, in 1375. Brinton, a Benedictine monk, was one of
the great preachers of his day and was not afraid to berate his contemporaries
– his motto was *Veritas liberabit* [the truth will deliver us]. Most of his
sermons were probably preached in English and the surviving Latin texts are,
in effect, Brinton's notes, so that the slightly stilted language is not a fair
reflection of his oratory.

This extract is from a sermon preached on 21 January 1375. This was before
the major outbreak of plague that year, but plague is one of the afflictions
which Brinton lists as the due punishment for the sins of contemporaries. His
text is 'Serving the Lord' [Romans 12.11], and the sermon is an extended
discussion of temporal and spiritual lordship and service. The first third, not
printed here, discusses the nature of temporal dominion. Brinton then turns to
the necessity of serving God.

Sister Mary Aquinas Devlin (ed), *The Sermons of Thomas Brinton*, 2 vols,
Camden Society, third series LXXXV-VI, 1954, I no 48.

Firstly, since the Lord is to be served holily, it is necessary that the
heart be prepared for his service with all diligence. As, indeed, you

---

24 Amen I say to you, I know you not. The reference is to Matthew 25.12: the
bridegroom's response to the foolish virgins.

25 Who, with the father and son. Medieval preachers ended by invoking the Trinity
and this identifies 'St Truth' in the previous line with the Holy Spirit, the third
person of the Trinity.

would prepare a heart for a lord's dinner, firstly impurites are drawn out of it, then it is washed, and then finally it is cooked or assayed over a clean fire – just so, spiritually, impurities are drawn from the human heart when the sin committed, with its attendant circumstances, is thoroughly examined: who has sinned, what is their age and social status, are they laymen or clerics, how knowledgeable are they, what sex are they, when and where was the sin committed, how often, is the sin notorious or a cause of scandal, in what manner and with whose help was it performed? Afterwards the heart is washed by full and true confession and an abundance of tears. Next it is assayed by the divine fire of love, or by thinking deeply on the passion of Christ. And thus a sacrifice is offered to God of the whole heart, and service tendered through proper reparation, as Scripture says: 'Serve the Lord with all your heart' [1 Kings 12.20].

And I say this as a warning to those who in making ready their bodies take great pains to acquire costly and well-made garments, but who are amazingly careless in making ready their heart or soul. Truly it seems acceptable to perform good deeds in this mortal life to acquire grace more quickly, or multiply worldly wealth, or to suffer less want, but not to earn eternal glory, and they do not please God or his saints by this kind of service. A story to illustrate this. There was a man who served the Virgin devotedly in vigils, fasting and prayers, but did not keep his heart and senses from defilement. One night, when he was dying for a drink and invoked the help of the Virgin, she appeared to him and offered him a delightful drink in a filthy cup. He said to her, 'Most sweet lady, I cannot drink from such a foul cup'. And she answered, 'As much as you now take physical pleasure in drinking, so much do I derive spiritual pleasure from the devoted service done for me – but because I must drink your devotions from a foul cup, that is from a filthy heart, your service is abhorrent to me until you cleanse your heart'. Dearly beloved, the Lord Jesus seeks nothing from you in return for all the great benefits you enjoy and his bitter pain except the cleansing of your heart. I refer you to what I said before: 'Prepare your hearts unto the Lord, and serve him only' [1 Kings 7.3]. And so much for the first point.

Secondly I said that the Lord is to be served justly. For we deserve justly of the Lord when we justly observe his commandments and rules, in other words when we do not hurt our neighbour, whether in his possessions (by theft, rapine, exactions or extortion), in his person (by beating, wounding or even killing him), in his soul (by giving bad advice or leading him astray) or in his reputation (by abusing or slandering him). We ought instead to love our neighbours as ourselves and as far as possible defend them by the weapons of justice. As the apostle says: 'In all things let us exhibit ourselves as the ministers of God, in much patience ... by the armour of justice' [2 Corinthians 6.4, 7].

Slanderers and false merchants violate and contravene this rule of justice. To take slanderers first: if they should see a man and woman of good standing, perhaps talking together, they immediately clamour in everybody's ears that they have sinned together, and by reason of this clamour the couple acquire a bad name throughout the whole neighbourhood. They compel the two people, however innocent, to be cited in the church courts as though they were guilty in the matter. But such slanderers should beware of two things. Firstly of the Council of Exeter, which ordered the excommunication of all those who, motivated by money, fear or favour, accuse someone of good reputation of a crime, with the result that the person is summoned to purgation or penalised in other ways. Secondly they should beware of the pains of hell if they do not satisfy as they ought those whom they defamed and slandered. For the slanderer or tale-spreader is not only bound to restore their good name as far as possible, but to provide recompense for the damage suffered from the infamy, and sin is not remitted unless what was lost is restored.

False merchants, secondly, infringe the rule of justice. Throughout the whole profession such great falsehood is practised in measures, charging interest, weights, scales, adulteration, lies and false oaths, that each studies to deceive the next man, whom they ought rather to serve in mutual love, as the apostle says: 'By charity of the spirit serve one another' [Galatians 5.13]. Merchants who outwit their brothers in business should beware, however, for of all these matters 'God is the Judge' [2 Timothy 4.1]. And so much for the second point.

I said thirdly that God is to be served with delight, as the Psalmist says: 'Delight in the Lord: and he will give thee the requests of thy heart' [Ps 36.4]. What more delightful thing can be imagined than to serve the Lord with delight, who sees the intention of service to him as an accomplished fact. The servants of earthly lords certainly work with more delight when they can see that their lord is present. But as Scripture says: 'The eyes of the Lord in every place behold the good and the evil' [Proverbs 15.3]. Therefore we ought to fear his presence and respect him everywhere. Happy therefore the servant in life, to whom in death Christ says 'Good and faithful servant ... Enter thou into the joy of thy Lord' [Matthew 25.21]. What more delightful than to serve the Lord whom the angels serve? In sign of which, when John in the Book of Revelation saw the angel and wished to fall down and worship him, the angel forbade him, saying 'See thou do it not, I am thy fellow servant' [Apoc. 19.10]. What more delightful than to serve the Lord, when to serve him is to reign? Earthly lords hardly give their servants their due and agreed wages. Indeed it frequently happens that lords are false to the command of God, witholding wages, and servants become thieves, appropriating the lord's goods for their own ends. But Christ the Lord rewards his servants beyond their deserts, for, as the Psalmist says: 'The Lord will give grace and glory' [Ps 83.12].

The earlier that service is offered to the Lord – in the morning of the day or of a man's life – the more pleasing it is to him. The Bestiary tells us that because the lark, wakeful early in the morning, serves God with singing, it will find food for that day, whatever tempest may lash down on any part of the earth. If the Lord of all things thus generously rewards and feeds a bird for praising him in the morning, how much easier is it to belive that if one of us – we who have been born from the womb of woman to serve God, as the prophet says: 'Forming me from the womb to be his servant' [Isaiah 49.5] – has served God in the morning with appropriate vigils, prayers and especially attendance at mass, he will be so directed by the Lord that he shall lack nothing which is necessary to sustain life. Nor is this surprising, for, according to teachers, hearing mass devoutly confers the following privileges: first, the things necessary for sustenance that day; secondly, forgiveness of idle words and oaths; thirdly that he will not go blind that day; fourthly that he will not die unexpectedly; fifthly, that while they are listening to the mass people grow no older; sixthly, the steps to and from mass are numbered by the angels. For such reasons it could be said by the apostle: 'Being made free from sin and become servants to God, you have your fruit unto sanctification' [Romans 6.22].

And I say this by way of warning to those who, when they ought to be serving God in the morning with delight and in the company of the angels, are instead drowsy, lazy and sluggish. Rather than serving sloth they ought to consider no time well spent unless it is in the worship of God. For in truth, if the earth does not yield its fruits in abundance, or if misfortunes, pestilences and wars befall the kingdom of England, this ought to be blamed on our sloth, for two reasons. Firstly, because the earth is inferior to man, it serves him, and because man is inferior to God, he serves him – it therefore seems that the earth and the other elements ought to serve man exactly in proportion to the service which man gives God: if well, well; if badly, badly. But men and most young people, being slothful, have withdrawn the service which they owe to God, and as a result God justly allows the earth and the other elements to become not a source of profit but of loss to their superior, man. The second reason is that where there is sloth, there is every other evil as well: theft, rape, greed, lechery, incest and adultery. There is no nation under heaven as ill-famed as the English, as is sufficiently proved in the letter which Boniface, pope and martyr, wrote to the king of the English: 'If the English race, as it has been reported, shall take to adultery, scorning legitimate marriage, then, because its life is foul, its people will not be strong in war or firm in faith, not honourable in the eyes of the world nor loved of God, but they will beget degenerate, leprous children'.[26]

Let us look at what is happening now. We are not strong or fortunate in war. We are not stable in faith. We are not honourable in the eyes of the world – on the contrary, we are of all men the falsest, and in consequence are not loved by God. It is undoubtedly for that reason that there exists in the kingdom of England so marked a diminution of fruitfulness, so cruel a pestilence, so much injustice, so many illegitimate children – for there is on every side so much lechery and adultery that few men are contented with their own wives, but each man lusts after the wife of his neighbour, or keeps a stinking concubine in addition to his wife, however beautiful and honest she might be; behaviour which merits a horrible and wretched death. Take the example of a certain English nobleman who, when it was announced to him during a massacre of the nobility that he was to die a shameful death later that day, fell to the ground and cried out, 'Woe is me that I never loved my wife', so acknowledging that it was adultery which was the cause of his death.

Dearly beloved, do not be like this, but consider, you lazy ones, how sloth and voluptuousness are the weapons with which the devil captures souls. Certainly it was idleness, due to an abundance of food, which led to the overthrow of Sodom and Gomorrah. Therefore be watchful and serve your Lord Christ cheerfully in honest toil and work, considering deeply that, according to Anselm, all the time

26 A paraphrase of part of a letter written from St Boniface to King Ethelbald of Mercia in 746-7: E. Emerton, *The Letters of St Boniface*, Columbia, 1940, p. 128. Boniface was martyred in 754. Brinton is wrong in describing him as a pope; he may have muddled him with Pope Boniface V, whose pastoral letter to King Edgar is recorded by Bede.

granted to you ought to be spent in this way. Consider also, you adulterers, the privileges and dignities of the order of matrimony. Firstly, the authority by which it was instituted. For whereas various holy men instituted the religious orders, God himself instituted the order of matrimony. If, therefore, an apostate or an offender against the Rule of St Benedict or that of St Augustine is considered blameworthy, how much more blameworthy is an offender against the order of God himself? Secondly, the place where it was instituted, for all the other orders were instituted outside Paradise, but this within it. Thirdly, that God preserved the order of matrimony at the time of the Flood. Fourthly, that God honoured the order of matrimony when, in the presence of his mother and disciples, he blessed the nuptials by the miracle of turning water into wine, as is described in the gospel for today. Fifthly, the excellence of the blessing which it is customary to give in the nuptials, but which is not repeated in subsequent marriages, for flesh once blessed transmits its virtue to unblessed flesh, just as consecrated oil absorbs unconsecrated oil and makes it holy. Sixthly, the virtue inherent in marriage makes that act venial which, outside marriage, is a horrible and mortal sin.[27] Seventhly, the virtue of marriage defends man in the direction from which the devil most often attacks. Consider these matters, you lechers and particularly you adulterers, who have previously been living dangerously and serving your body in filthiness, and henceforward, as the Psalmist says, 'Serve the Lord in gladness' [Ps 99.2]. And so much for the third point.

Fourthly and lastly I said that the Lord is to be served with constancy. For if the Lord cares for us so greatly that he ensures that the least hair of our head does not perish, it is only right that we should serve him so constantly that we do not lose a single moment from his service. For the man who rules himself reasonably and follows a regimen in eating, drinking, waking and sleeping, and does this without mortal sin, is constantly and continually serving God. And the man who, in worshipping God 'shall have persevered to the end, he shall be saved' [Matthew 10.22]. And this is directed against the many sons of the nobility who, when they are young and under the guidance of a master, arise in the morning and serve God at matins, vespers and at mass, recite the litany, and have a conscience in such matters, but who, when they have taken their full lordship upon them, lie in bed

27 i.e. the sexual act. Note that Brinton does not see sexual intercourse within marriage as entirely without sin, but the sin is venial, not mortal – in other words did not bring the risk of damnation and did not have to be confessed before receiving the Eucharist.

until terce[28] and skimp divine service, in spite of the fact that they are the more bound to serve God because they have received so much from him. The Psalmist says: 'When the people assemble together, and kings, to serve the Lord' [Ps 101.23].

This is also directed against the many churchmen who, when they are poor and without a benefice, celebrate mass daily, take no heed to the world, mortify the flesh, and with all diligence execute and observe the commands of God, but who, when they have been advanced to a rich living, scarcely ever hear mass, let alone say it, esteem the world, are slaves to the flesh, busy themselves about saying prayers for the souls of the great rather than looking after their benefices, and allow their duties to be performed by hirelings. Such men are not paying attention to what is figured by the sons of Levi, whom God separated from the people and ordered to serve him, so that they can say with the apostle, 'They and I are ministers of Christ'.[29] Not thus did the most glorious virgin Agnes, whose feast we are celebrating today, behave, but, as the narratives and stories of her life declare, she served the Lord in holiness and justice, with delight and constancy, considering Scripture: 'At first light, let us serve the Lord in holiness (that is the first point), and justice (the second point), before his face (the third point) for all the days of our life (the fourth point)'.

Therefore may the son of God and man, our lord Jesus Christ 'who did not come to be ministered unto, but to minister' [Matthew 20.28] and who also said to his father, 'Father, I will that where I am, there also may my servant be',[30] make you serve so worthily that you may come to rule with him for ever.

49. Be Watchful

This sermon is related to the Archbishop of Canterbury's letter of July 1375 [37] and was probably preached that month. Brinton takes as his text 'Be watchful' [1 Peter 5.8] and the sermon is structured around four reasons why it behoves contemporaries to be watchful, the first two of which (accounting for about three quarters of the sermon) are printed here.

28 Terce is the third hour of the liturgical day, which started at dawn (prime). Its exact time therefore varied, but was around 9 a.m.

29 An abridgement of 2 Corinthians 11.23, which alters the sense of the text. The original reads: 'They are ministers of Christ (I speak as one less wise); I am more....'

30 A paraphrase of John 17.24, reworded to clarify its relevance to Brinton's theme of service. The original reads: 'Father, I will that where I am, they also whom thou hast given me may be with me'.

Sermons of Thomas Brinton, II no. 70.

Since according to the apostle 'It is proper, first of all, that supplications, prayers, intercessions and thanksgivings be made for the king
and for all that are in high station, that they may have a quiet life'[31] and
the lord king in his letters has requested the same for our expedition,
I do not know of any words more useful and health-giving to put
before you at the beginning of a sermon than those of the saviour:
'Take heed, watch and pray' [Mark 13.33]. Take heed prudently,
watch diligently and pray wisely etc.

At the present time four things specially lead us to watch with all
diligence: first, the archbishop's pastoral injunction; the imminent
danger of pestilence; the malicious attack of our enemy; and the reason
explicitly given by Christ. Concerning the first, nature provides an
example. Cranes are so prudent that they share out the night watches
among themselves, and the one who is on watch holds a stone in its
claw, so that if it happens to fall asleep through weariness, the others,
alerted by the fall of the stone, will be safe from dangers. To the point.
By the cranes taking turns to watch, I take to be meant the shepherds
of souls and the prelates, who ought to watch studiously to benefit the
holy church of God. They ought to hold a stone in one foot, that is, to
think assiduously about the burden of their cure of souls, for if a sheep
from their flock perish through their negligence, they do not pay
money in reparation, but pay a soul for a soul. 'Keep this man, for if he
shall slip away, thy life shall be for his life' [3 Kings 20.39].

The form of this vigil is shown in Luke 2, where it is figured: 'There
were in the same country shepherds watching etc' [Luke 2.8]. In this
passage the authority touches on three things. Firstly, the office was
that of a shepherd – *there were shepherds* – not a hireling, to whom the
sheep were of no concern [John 10.12]. It does not say that they were
thieves and robbers who entered not by the door but by some other
way: some, like deceitful men, by fraud; some, like ungovernable
gentlefolk, by power; some, like the ambitious, by worldly wisdom –
but they were shepherds, nurturing their flocks with the word of
instruction, the example of social intercourse, and (if they have the
resources) the succour of material help. Secondly, the authority
touches the place: *in the same country*. It does not say in a distant place
where they would not be able to exercise the pastoral office effectively.
Nor does it say in the courts of princes and great men, since courtier-
prelates do not generally visit their sheep but just send the shearers.

31 A paraphrase of 1 Timothy 2.1-2.

Thirdly, it touches the zealous duty: *watching*, for it is permissible for everyone to be summoned to the vigil, as Christ says: 'What I say to one, I say to all, watch' [Mark 13.37]. For Christ had found the disciples sleeping, and he chided Peter especially, saying, 'Simon, sleepest thou? Couldst thou not watch with me one hour?' [Mark 14.37]. To conclude this point, note how the apostle expresses it: 'But be thou vigilant: labour in all things: do the work of an evangelist', by announcing the whole truth; 'fulfill thy ministry' by demonstrating continuing holiness [2 Timothy 4.5]. And so much for the first point.

The second point is that imminent danger of death stirs us to watch. Living as we do in an earthly home weakened on all sides, whose walls are easily undermined by thieves coming to rob, it is obviously essential to watch with all vigilance. To the point. The house of the soul, that is to say the body, is weak mud and of the earth, because it is created of earth, returns to earth and is finally put under the earth. The thief wishing to undermine the house is death, who comes without warning, against whose coming we should watch carefully, as the Saviour showed in these words: 'If the householder knew at what hour the thief would come, he would surely watch and would not suffer his house to be broken open' [Luke 12.39]. On which Gregory says: 'The head of the family is our soul, who instructs and rules the body and all its functions like a father. If he were to know of the coming of the thief – that is, sudden death – he would not let him break into his house etc.' For if our soul were to contemplate unremittingly the day of death it would be shaken out of all its sluggishness. Not thus do the voluptuous watch amidst their delights; not thus do the lecherous watch amidst their foulness; not thus do the ambitious watch while amassing riches; not thus do hypocrites watch, too busy singing people's praises; not thus do the pleasure-seekers watch amidst their hunting parties, dances, wrestling matches and other frivolities. But the chosen of God ought to watch thus, in their works of mercy, penance and devotion, lest death should catch them sleeping in sin: 'Do penance. If then thou shalt not watch, I will come to thee as a thief' [Apocalypse 3.3].

Even so have the pestilence and other misfortunes come to pass in these days. Let those who ascribe such things to planets and constellations rather than to sin say what sort of planet reigned at the time of Noah, when God drowned the whole world except for eight souls, unless the planet of malice and sin. 'Since the wickedness of men was great on the earth, and all the thought of their heart was bent upon evil' [Genesis 6.5] God himself, the best astrologer, said, 'The earth is filled with iniquity, therefore I will destroy them with the earth' [Genesis 6.13]. Or what sort of planet, unless that of sin, reigned at the burning of the Sodomites? As the Lord says to Abraham, 'The cry of the Sodomites has come to me and their sin has increased. I shall go down etc'.[32] Or what sort of planet reigned at the time of David, when thousands of men were killed by plague, unless the planet of sin, for David had counted the people [2 Kings 24]. Therefore the law says [canon 16, qu. 6] 'Let them be turned back', for it is because of the evil deeds of men that the world is afflicted with famine and pestilence, as (to conclude this part of the argument) God said: 'I have watched over you, to afflict you' [Jeremiah 31.28].

Today the corruption of lechery and the imagining of evil are greater than in the days of Noah, for a thousand ways of sinning which were unknown then have been discovered now, and the sin of the Sodomites prevails beyond measure, and today the cruelty of lords is greater than in the time of David. And therefore, let us not blame the flails of God on the planets or the elements but rather on our sins, saying, as in Genesis, 'We deserve to suffer these things, because we have sinned' [Genesis 42.21]. For if sin has no dominion over us, neither Hell nor Purgatory can harm us, for as Gregory says: 'Adversity will do no harm, if iniquity has no dominion'. But you say, 'If sin is the occasion of these misfortunes, then by the just judgement of God notorious sinners should die, but not children or the just, who, by comparison, have not sinned'. In reply I say that children die not because of their own sins, but the sins of their parents. Take the example of the son of Bersabea, or the example of the deaths of children who would have followed the sins of their parents had they lived and whom God mercifully took, so that by the death of the body they avoided the eternal punishment which they would have earned had they lived. This is proved in the law [cause 1, questio 4, c.11] *The Church.* You can be sure that the children would have wished to follow the sins of their parents, and then God does them no injury, for death is a release from prison, an end of exile and toil, an escape from all danger, a breaking of chains, a return to the homeland, a going forth to glory.

Or say that God punishes the innocent to chastise us, the most evil and guilty. For in the manner of an archer, God, 'who has bent his bow and made it ready' [Ps 7.13] sometimes shoots the arrow of death beyond the target (that is, the sinner), by hitting a father, mother or other elderly person; sometimes this side of the target, by hitting a son or

32 A paraphrase of Genesis 18.20-21.

daughter or other young person; sometimes to the left hand side, by
hitting a neighbour; sometimes to the right hand side of the target, by
hitting a brother or sister. But he strikes the target when he snatches
the sinner sleeping in his sin by means of dreadful death. Take the
example of King William Rufus. Anselm saw in a dream how all the
English saints were making serious complaints against the king,
because he had plundered many churches in England and extorted
50,000 marks from the church of Lincoln. And the Lord said, 'Let
Alban the protomartyr of England draw near', and he handed a
flaming arrow to him, saying, 'Behold, the death of this man you are
complaining about'. When Alban had received it, he handed it over to
the avenger of the sins of a worthless spirit. As it flew through the air
in the form of a comet, Anselm, in the spirit, understood that the king
had died that night, hit by the arrow. And early the next morning,
when he had celebrated mass, he made preparations to return to his
church. And when he reached England he heard of the way in which
King William had been killed by an arrow while hunting in the New
Forest. And no wonder, when divine correction is so watchful to wield
the rod, as Jeremiah heard [Jeremiah 1].

But someone asks, 'Given that sin is the primary cause of the pestilence,
what remedies are available to stay the divine hand?' I reply that the
best remedy is the confession of sins. For how should the prayers of
the people halt the flail of the Lord when the third part of those people
is in a state of mortal sin? Scripture says: 'Confess your sins one to
another' and continues, 'Pray one for another, that you may be saved'
[James 5.16]. Concerning vigilance (that is, confession) it is written:
'Arise in the night in the beginning of your watches: pour out thy heart
like water' [Lamentations 2.19]. That is to say, you who have slept the
sleep of sin for a long time, *arise* from the sleep of sloth and
uncaringness, and go keenly to work; change the filth of corruption
and concupiscence to cleanliness, and presumption and pride to
humility. It goes on, *in the beginning of your watches,* which is to say that
just as the peacock (so the Bestiaries tell us) awakes and cries after his
first sleep because he believes that he has lost his beauty, so should
you, a sinner, seeing beside you the grace which you have lost, within
you the misery which you have incurred, against you the sentence
which you await and below you the punishment towards which you are
hastening. Like another Philothea you ought to watch in the morning
and cry to the Lord with all your heart to restore to you the grace
which you have lost, saying to the Lord: 'My soul hath desired you in

the night: yea, and with my spirit within me in the morning early I will watch to thee' [Isaiah 26.9].

Then it goes on *pour out thy heart like water.* He does not say like oil, which leaves a greasiness behind it; or like honey, which leaves a sweetness behind it; or like wine, which leaves a scent behind it; or like milk, which leaves a whiteness and a scent behind it; but like water, which is poured out so thoroughly that not a trace is left behind. Thus in confession the depths of the human heart are set forth, so that nothing of error should remain in the soul – no substance, odour, sweetness or colour. As Chrysostom has it: confession is the safety of souls, the recovery of grace, the remission of sin, the conquering of demons, the blocking of the gates of hell and the opening of the kingdom of heaven. Three things – fire, thieves and water – arouse men from sleep and urge them to bodily vigilance, and this is true spiritually, for there is hardly a day when the fires of depraved desires do not approach the house of conscience, hardly a day when thoughts of evil do not invade the heart of man, and in addition a hellish robber lies constantly in wait to devour us. You are placed in so many dangers by these things 'Watch ye: and pray that ye enter not into temptation' [Matthew 26.41].

50. Pilgrimage to Merevale, 1361

Robert de Stretton, Bishop of Coventry and Lichfield, to Thomas of Leicester, a monk of Merevale, 30 June 1361, arranging for absolution to be granted to pilgrims dying at the abbey. Although the plague is not explicitly mentioned, there is little doubt that it was one of the spurs to the pilgrimage. Two days after this letter was written the bishop ordered penitential processions to avert the plague which, although it had not yet entered his diocese, had 'emptied' other parts of the kingdom.

Lichfield Record Office, B/A/1/5ii fo. 43v.

We see it as our pastoral duty to extend our patronage in matters which concern the health of souls. We have been told that a great multitude of the faithful, for the expiation of their offences, pour almost daily to the chapel built beside the gateway of your monastery, which is dedicated to the praise and honour of the most glorious Virgin Mary, the Mother of God, and we have further gathered, by the testimony of people worthy of credence, that it often happens that many of our subjects, both men and women, travelling there away from home, are brought to the point of death by the crush of people or by falling sick of the various illnesses prevalent in these days.

We wish to make provision for the spiritual health of these people and accordingly (having complete faith in your circumspection and the sedulous affection which you are known to have towards the health of men's souls) we give you full and unlimited power to absolve those of our subjects who, while on pilgrimage to the aforesaid chapel, find themselves at the point of death and wish to make formal confession to you, and to impose a salutary penance upon them according to the nature of their fault. This power is also to extend to cases normally reserved to us, and is to last as long as we decide.

51. A wholesome medicine against the plague

This is from a fifteenth-century Italian book of medical remedies. Its message is that those afflicted by plague should not concern themselves with medicine for the body, but should make a good death. The 'medicines' it describes are the last rites administered to the dying: confession, the receiving of the *viaticum* and final unction (the anointing of the body with holy oil).

Wellcome Institute for the History of Medicine, London: Western MS 668 fos. 97v-98.

The advice of the reverend father Dom Theophilus of Milan, of the order of St Benedict, against the plague; also a most wholesome medicine against all infirmities. Note it well.

Whenever anyone is struck down by the plague they should immediately provide themselves with a medicine like this. Let him first gather as much as he can of bitter loathing towards the sins committed by him, and the same quantity of true contrition of heart, and mix the two into an ointment with the water of tears. Then let him make a vomit of frank and honest confession, by which he shall be purged of the pestilential poison of sin, and the boil of his vices shall be totally liquified and melt away. Then the spirit, formerly weighed down by the plague of sin, will be left all light and full of blessed joy. Afterwards let him take the most delightful and precious medicine: the body of our lord and saviour Jesus Christ. And finally let him have himself anointed on the seat of his bodily senses with holy oil. And in a little while he will pass from transient life to the incorruptible country of eternal life, safe from plague and all other infirmities.

Compared with this all other remedies of doctors are futile and profit little against the plague, which God keeps for the chastisement of sin and which is without remedy save through him and his power.

52. The flagellants

Almost every European chronicler described the penitential movement which swept across continental Europe. This account is one of the fullest, and it continues with a detailed analysis (not printed here) of the configuration of the heavens at the beginning of the astrological year (3 a.m. on 12 March 1349, when the sun entered Aries) to demonstrate that the movement and its characteristics were prefigured in the stars. For instance, the conjunction of Mars and Mercury foretold blows and the shedding of blood; while the fact that Scorpio (associated with deceitfulness) occupied the mid heaven forecast the movement's numberless lies.

A. Potthast (ed), *Chronicon Henrici de Hervordia*, Göttingen, 1859, pp. 280-4.

In 1348 a race without a head[33] aroused universal wonder by their sudden appearance in huge numbers. They suddenly sprang up in all parts of Germany, calling themselves cross bearers or flagellants. They were said, as if in confirmation of the prophecy, to be without a head either because they literally had no head – that is to say no one to organise and lead them – or because they had no head in the sense of having no brain and no judgement; they were fools, laying claim to a form of piety but, as will appear, spoiling everything when their stupidities began to ferment. They were called cross bearers either because they followed a cross carried before them on their travels, or because they prostrated themselves in the form of a cross during their processions, or because they identified themselves with a cross stitched to their clothes. They were called flagellants because of the whips [*flagella*] which they used in performing public penance. Each whip consisted of a stick with three knotted thongs hanging from the end. Two pieces of needle-sharp metal were run through the centre of the knots from both sides, forming a cross, the ends of which extended beyond the knots for the length of a grain of wheat or less. Using these whips they beat and whipped their bare skin until their bodies were bruised and swollen and blood rained down, spattering the walls nearby. I have seen, when they whipped themselves, how sometimes those bits of metal penetrated the flesh so deeply that it took more than two attempts to pull them out.

Flocking together from every region, perhaps even from every city, they overran the whole land. In open country they straggled along

---

33 The race without a head is a reference to the 'Cedar of Lebanon' prophecy; see 23. The prevalence of the prophecy meant that the phrase occurs in various contexts at this time. The English chronicler Knighton, for instance, uses it of the French invaders of Gascony in 1348: *Chronicon* II p. 57.

behind the cross in no particular order, but when they came to cities, towns and villages they formed themselves into a procession, with hoods or hats pulled down over their foreheads, and sad and downcast eyes, they went through the streets singing a sweet hymn. In this fashion they entered the church and shut themselves in while they stripped off their clothes and left them with a guard. They covered themselves from the navel down with a pleated linen cloth like the women's undergarment which we call a kirtle, the upper part of the body remaining bare. Then they took the whips in their hands. When that was done, the north door of the church, if it had one, was opened.[34] The eldest came out of the church first and threw himself to the ground immediately to the east of the door, beside the path. After him, the second lay down on the west side, then the third next to the first, the fourth next to the second and so on. Some lay with right hand raised, as though taking an oath, others lay on their belly or back, or on their right or left side, representing in this way the sins for which they were performing penance.

After this, one of them would strike the first with a whip, saying, 'May God grant you remission of all your sins. Arise'. And he would get up, and do the same to the second, and all the others in turn did the same. When they were all on their feet, and arranged two by two in procession, two of them in the middle of the column would begin singing a hymn in a high voice, with a sweet melody. They sang one verse and then the others took it up and repeated it after them, and then the singers sang the second verse and so on until the end. But whenever they came to the part of the hymn which mentioned the passion of Christ they all suddenly threw themselves down prostrate on the ground, regardless of where they were, and whether the ground was clean or filthy, whether there were thorns or thistles or nettles or stones. And they did not lower themselves gradually to their knees or steadying themselves in some other way, but dropped like logs, flat on their belly and face, with arms outstretched, and, lying there like crosses, would pray. A man would need a heart of stone to watch this without tears. At a sign given by one of them they would rise and

---

34 Because the north side of the church is the dark side in the northern hemisphere it acquired negative connotations. Burial there was often reserved for those whose state of grace was compromised; suicides, victims of violence or still-born babies. If a northern door existed at all it was rarely used, although in some places it was opened at baptism, a practice popularly believed to create an escape route for the devils cast out by the sacrament. In preferring the north door the flagellants were thus making a statement about their own unworthiness.

resume their procession as before. And usually they sing the hymn three times, and prostrate themselves, as described, three times. And then, when they have returned to the same door by which they left the church, they re-enter and resume their clothes, taking off the linen cloths. As they leave the church they ask for nothing, requesting neither food nor lodging, but accepting with gratitude the many offerings freely made to them.

However, just as annoying tares and persistent burrs often grow among the corn, so the ignorant and stupid, not content with penitential whippings, annoyingly and persistently took upon themselves the job of preaching. They did not think or speak of the clergy and the sacraments of the church with proper reverence, but rather with contempt; spat back rebukes and criticism, and despised persuasion. When they met up with two Dominicans in a field they were so infuriated by their exhortations that they tried to kill them, and although the more nimble managed to make his escape they stoned the other, and left his body under a pile of stones on the outskirts of Meissen. And they did similar things in many other places.

If somebody said to them, 'Why are you preaching, because you have not been sent, as the apostle says: "How shall they preach, unless they be sent?",[35] and why do you teach what, because you are illiterate, you cannot understand?' they would reply, as if clinching the argument, 'And who sent you, and how do you know that you are consecrating the body of Christ, and that the gospel you are teaching is the truth?' If somebody answers them (as that Dominican answered them) that we have received these things from our Saviour, who consecrated his body and ordered his disciples to do likewise, thereby instituting the form of consecration which has come down to us through them, and that we have been sent by the church and that the gospel that we preach teaches the truth and cannot err, for it is guided by the Holy Spirit; they say that they have been instructed and sent directly by the Lord and by the spirit of God, according to Isaiah 48.16: 'The Lord has sent me and his spirit'.

But Pope Innocent III said this about heretics: 'Since the order of teachers is almost pre-eminent in the church, no one ought to usurp the office of preacher casually. For according to the apostle, how can they preach unless they are sent?' If someone should reply that such things should be sent invisibly by God, rather than visibly by man, for

---

35 Romans 10.15.

an invisible sending is of higher dignity than a visible, and divine things far better than human; it can reasonably be answered that since an inward sending is invisible, it is not enough for anyone just to say that he has been sent by God, as a heretic would claim, but it is necessary that he should demonstrate his invisible sending by working a miracle or the testimony of scripture. Thus when God chose to send Moses to the children of Israel in Egypt, he gave him a sign so that they would believe that he had been sent by God, and turned his staff into a snake and back again. On the other hand, John the Baptist pointed to scripture as witness of his special sending, saying: 'I am the voice of one crying in the wilderness, make straight the way of the Lord, as said the prophet Isaias' [John 1.23].

However the flagellants ignored and scorned the sentence of excommunication pronounced against them by bishops. They took no notice of the papal order against them – until princes, nobles and the more powerful citizens started to keep them at a distance. The people of Osnabrück never let them in, although their wives and other women clamoured for them. Afterwards they disappeared as suddenly as they had come, as apparitions or ghosts are routed by mockery. Horace puts it well towards the end of his letters: 'Do you laugh at nocturnal ghosts or Thessalian portents?'[36]

53. The flagellants in England

(a) Robert of Avesbury: E. M. Thompson (ed), *Robertus de Avesbury de Gestis Mirabilibus Regis Edwardi Tertii*, Rolls Series, 1889, pp. 407-8. The description follows immediately upon the account of the plague printed above [14].

In that same year of 1349, about Michaelmas [29 September], more than 120 men, for the most part from Zeeland or Holland, arrived in London from Flanders. These went barefoot in procession twice a day in the sight of the people, sometimes in St Paul's church and sometimes elsewhere in the city, their bodies naked except for a linen cloth from loins to ankle. Each wore a hood painted with a red cross at front and back and carried in his right hand a whip with three thongs. Each thong had a knot in it, with something sharp, like a needle, stuck through the middle of the knot so that it stuck out on each side, and as they walked one after the other they struck

---

36 Horace, Epistles II.2. Thessaly (N.E. Greece) was regarded by classical authors as a country of witches, who had a reputation for wonder-working.

themselves with these whips on their naked, bloody bodies; four of
them singing in their own tongue and the rest answering in the
manner of the Christian litany. Three times in each procession they
would all prostrate themselves on the ground, with their arms
outstretched in the shape of a cross. Still singing, and beginning with
the man at the end, each in turn would step over the others, lashing the
man beneath him once with his whip, until all of those lying down had
gone through the same ritual. Then each one put on his usual clothes
and, always with their hoods on their heads and carrying their whips,
they departed to their lodgings. It was said that they performed a
similar penance every night.

(b) Thomas Walsingham: H. T. Riley (ed), *Historia Anglicana 1272-1422*, 2
vols, Rolls Series, 1863-64, I p. 275.

[1350] In this year penitents arrived in England – noble men of
foreign birth, who lashed themselves viciously on their naked bodies
until the blood flowed, now weeping, now singing. However, it was
said that they were doing these things ill advisedly, in that they did
not have permission from the apostolic see.

54. Rumours of Antichrist

A note of rumours current around Rome in 1349, sent by William of Blofield
(Norfolk) to a Dominican friar at Norwich. Blofield was a brother of the
Carmelite friary at Cambridge and was, it seems, distinctly doubtful about the
validity of the rumours he was passing on.

Robert E. Lerner, 'The Black Death and Western European Eschatological
Mentalities', *American Historical Review* LXXXVI, 1981, p. 552.

The rumours noted below were written in 1349 by Brother William of
Blofield in England to a brother of the Dominican friary at Norwich.
There are various prophets in the regions around Rome, whose
identity is still secret, who have been making up stories like this for
years. They say that this very year, 1349, Antichrist is aged ten, and
is a most beautiful child, so well educated in all branches of knowledge
that no one now living can equal him. And they also say that there is
another boy, now aged twelve and living beyond the land of the
Tartars, who has been brought up as a Christian and that this is he
who will destroy the Saracens and become the greatest man in
Christendom, but his power will be quickly brought to an end by the
coming of Antichrist.

These prophets also say, among a great deal else, that the present pope will come to a violent end, and that after his death there will be more revolutions in the world than there have ever been before. But after that another pope will arise, a good and just man, who will appoint God-fearing cardinals, and there will be almost total peace in his time. And after him there will be no other pope, but Antichrist will come and reveal himself.

55. Millenarianism in Germany

Johann von Winterthur was a Franciscan friar, who composed an account of the events of his own times, ending in 1348 with the Black Death. Many contemporary writers discuss the plague in implicitly apocalyptic terms, but Winterthur is unusual in describing (and carefully refuting) the millenarian fantasies triggered by the plague.

Die Chronik Johanns von Winterthur, Monumenta Germaniae Historica: scriptores rerum Germanicarum, new series III, Berlin, 1924, pp. 280-2.

In these times it was freely spread abroad among men of various races, indeed of every race, that the Emperor Frederick II (with whom I began the second part of this work) would return in the full might of his power to reform the corrupt church completely. The men who believed this also added that it was inevitable that he would return, even if he had been cut into a thousand pieces, or burnt to ashes,[37] because it had been foretold that this would happen and it could not possibly be otherwise. According to this claim, once raised up and restored to the peak of his power, he will marry rich men to poor girls and women, and *vice versa*; marry off nuns and members of secular sisterhoods; find wives for monks; restore the goods taken from wards, orphans, widows and from everyone who has been despoiled; and give justice to all. He will persecute the clergy so savagely that they will hide their tonsures with cattle dung, if they have no other covering, so that they do not appear tonsured. He will drive out the regular clergy, especially the Franciscans, who by announcing the papal proceedings against him, drove him from power.[38] After resuming a power more

37 Frederick II (d.1250) had already been identified as the Emperor of the Last Days in his own lifetime. Within a generation of his death a pseudo-Frederick, who claimed to be the resurrected emperor, had appeared. He was captured and burnt at the stake, and von Winterthur's reference to people believing in Frederick's resurrection even if he had been burnt to ashes is a reference to this episode: N. Cohn, *The Pursuit of the Millenium*, London, 1970, chapter 6.

38 Frederick was excommunicated by the pope, who used the friars to spread the news throughout Italy.

just and a rule more glorious than before, he will cross the seas with a large army and will resign his power on the Mount of Olives or at the dry tree.

I do not cease to be amazed by this false belief; that anyone could hope for or believe in the revival of a man dead 80 years, who was emperor for 30 years. The men who hold this false belief have been deceived just like the Jews, who believe that King David will be raised up by the Lord to reign again over Israel as he did in the past. They believe it on the basis that the Lord, speaking through the prophets, said: 'I will raise up my faithful servant David'.[39] For Ezechiel says: 'One king shall be king over them all' [37.22] and a little later it continues: 'and my servant David shall be king over them' [37.24]. And Jeremiah says: 'And they shall serve the Lord their God and David their king, whom I will raise up to them' [30.9]. But these and other similar authorities are to be understood as referring to Christ or to another of the race of David, as in Jeremiah: 'Behold the days come, saith the Lord and I will raise up to David a just branch. And a king shall reign' [23.5] – not David in person, but his branch; that is, someone of his race: Christ.

I do not deny that the dead will arise, be brought back to life and raised up, as Isaiah says: 'Thy dead men shall live, thy slain shall rise again. Awake, and give praise, ye that dwell in the dust' [26.19] and Daniel: 'And many of those that sleep in the dust of the earth shall awake: some unto life and others unto reproach' [12.2] and Ezechiel: 'I will open your graves and will bring you out of your sepulchres ... and will bring you into the land of Israel ... and they shall rest upon their own land' [37.12, 14]. These and similar authorities are to be understood as referring to the general resurrection in the future or to the several individual resurrections in the past. That anyone dead and burnt should arise again, to reign and dwell on the earth now as formerly, is contrary to the catholic faith and contradicted by scripture in many places, of which I shall touch on a few. Job says: 'Remember that my life is but wind: and my eyes shall not return to see good things. Nor shall the sight of man behold me .... He that shall go down to hell shall not come up. Nor shall he return any more into his house: neither shall his place know him any more' [7.7-10]. Solomon says: 'For the living know that they shall die, but the dead know nothing more. Neither have they a reward any more: for the memory of them is forgotten' [Ecclesiastes 9.5], and David: 'He shall go in the generations of his

---

39 Not a direct Biblical quotation, but a conflation of the three citations which follow.

fathers: and he shall never see light' [Ps 48.20] and elsewhere: 'For the spirit shall pass in him, and he shall not be: and he shall know his place no more' [Ps 102.16]. From these we may conclude that it is the height of madness and stupidity to believe that Frederick, once emperor and heretic, will be resurrected and rule the earth again.

IV: Scientific explanations

56. The report of the Paris medical faculty, October 1348

This is the most authoritative contemporary statement of the nature of the plague and therefore forms an appropriate introduction to this section. The full text consists of two parts: three chapters on the causes of the plague, and seven on remedies and regimen. Only the first part is printed here.

R. Hoeniger (ed), *Der Schwarze Tod*, Berlin, 1882, appendix III, pp. 152–6.

Seeing things which cannot be explained, even by the most gifted intellects, initially stirs the human mind to amazement; but after marvelling, the prudent soul next yields to its desire for understanding and, anxious for its own perfection, strives with all its might to discover the causes of the amazing events. For there is within the human mind an innate desire to seize on goodness and truth. As the Philosopher makes plain, all things seek for the good and want to understand.[1] To attain this end we have listened to the opinions of many modern experts on astrology and medicine about the causes of the epidemic which has prevailed since 1345. However, because their conclusions still leave room for considerable uncertainty, we, the masters of the faculty of medicine at Paris, inspired by the command of the most illustrious prince, our most serene lord, Philip, King of France, and by our desire to achieve something of public benefit, have decided to compile, with God's help, a brief compendium of the distant and immediate causes of the present universal epidemic (as far as these can be understood by the human intellect) and of wholesome remedies; drawing on the opinions of the most brilliant ancient philosophers and modern experts, astronomers as well as doctors of medicine. And if we cannot explain everything as we would wish, for a sure explanation and perfect understanding of these matters is not always to be had (as Pliny says in book II, chapter 39: 'some accidental causes of storms are still uncertain, or cannot be explained'), it is open to any diligent reader to make good the deficiency.

We shall divide the work into two parts, in the first of which we shall investigate the causes of this pestilence and whence they come, for

---

1 'The Philosopher' is Aristotle.

without knowledge of the causes no one can prescribe cures. In the second part we shall include methods of prevention and cure. There will be three chapters in the first part, for this epidemic arises from a double cause. One cause is distant and from above, and pertains to the heavens; the other is near and from below and pertains to the earth, and is dependent, causally and effectively, on the first cause. Therefore the first chapter will deal with the first cause, the second with the second cause, and the third with the prognostications and signs associated with both of them. There will be two treatises in the second part. The first will deal with medical means of prevention and cure and will be divided into four chapters: the first on the disposition of the air and its rectification; the second on exercise and baths; the third on food and drink; the fourth on sleeping and waking, emptiness and fullness of the stomach and on the emotions. The second treatise will have three chapters: the first on universal remedies; the second on specific remedies appropriate to different patients; the third on antidotes.

CHAPTER 1 OF THE FIRST PART: CONCERNING
THE UNIVERSAL AND DISTANT CAUSE

We say that the distant and first cause of this pestilence was and is the configuration of the heavens. In 1345, at one hour after noon on 20 March, there was a major conjunction of three planets in Aquarius. This conjunction, along with other earlier conjunctions and eclipses, by causing a deadly corruption of the air around us, signifies mortality and famine – and also other things about which we will not speak here because they are not relevant. Aristotle testifies that this is the case in his book *Concerning the causes of the properties of the elements*,[2] in which he says that mortality of races and the depopulation of kingdoms occur at the conjunction of Saturn and Jupiter, for great events then arise, their nature depending on the trigon in which the conjunction occurs. And this is found in ancient philosophers, and Albertus Magnus in his book, *Concerning the causes of the properties of the elements* (treatise 2, chapter 1) says that the conjunction of Mars and Jupiter causes a great pestilence in the air, especially when they come together in a hot, wet sign, as was the case in 1345.[3] For Jupiter, being wet and hot, draws up evil vapours from the earth and Mars, because it is immoderately

---

2 This work, although credited to Aristotle in the middle ages, was not by him. It was the subject of a commentary by Albertus Magnus (Albert the Great, d. 1280), which the medical faculty cites in the next sentence.

3 The houses of the zodiac are each associated with one of the elements, listed in 58. Aquarius is one of the air signs, and therefore hot and wet.

hot and dry, then ignites the vapours, and as a result there were lightnings, sparks, noxious vapours and fires throughout the air.

These effects were intensified because Mars – a malevolent planet, breeding anger and wars – was in the sign of Leo from 6 October 1347 until the end of May this year, along with the head of the dragon, and because all these things are hot they attracted many vapours; which is why the winter was not as cold as it should have been.[4] And Mars was also retrograde and therefore attracted many vapours from the earth and the sea which, when mixed with the air, corrupted its substance.[5] Mars was also looking upon Jupiter with a hostile aspect, that is to say quartile, and that caused an evil disposition or quality in the air, harmful and hateful to our nature.[6] This state of affairs generated strong winds (for according to Albertus in the first book of his *Meteora*, Jupiter has the property of raising powerful winds, particularly from the south) which gave rise to excess heat and moisture on the earth; although in fact it was the dampness which was most marked in our part of the world. And this is enough about the distant or universal cause for the moment.

CHAPTER 2 OF THE FIRST PART: CONCERNING
THE PARTICULAR AND NEAR CAUSE

Although major pestilential illnesses can be caused by the corruption of water or food, as happens at times of famine and infertility, yet we still regard illnesses proceeding from the corruption of the air as much more dangerous. This is because bad air is more noxious than food or drink in that it can penetrate quickly to the heart and lungs to do its damage. We believe that the present epidemic or plague has arisen

4 Leo is one of the fire signs – hot and dry – and therefore intensifies the hot/dry characteristics of Mars.

5 When observed from the earth against the background of the fixed stars, planets at times appear to loop backwards (to be retrograde) or to stand still. Mars makes a backward loop in some part of the sky once every 780 days.

6 As they move round the heavens, through the twelve houses of the zodiac, the planets' position relative to each other sometimes takes on particular significance, whether for good or bad. In these positions the planets are said to be looking at each other, and the positions are known as aspects. For instance, two planets in opposite houses of the zodiac (i.e. separated by 180° of the 360° circle) are said to be in opposition, and the aspect is malign. The other aspects are: trine (120° apart, benign), quartile (90° apart, malign) and sextile (60° apart, benign).

7 As the authors immediately make clear, they do not mean by this that the *nature* of the air changed, which would be impossible, but that it was corrupted by being mixed with bad vapours. John of Burgundy [62] makes the same point, but uses 'substance' in the opposite sense, to mean the unchanging, essential nature of an element, rather than (as here) its outward form.

from air corrupt in its substance, and not changed in its attributes.[7] By which we wish it be understood that air, being pure and clear by nature, can only become putrid or corrupt by being mixed with something else, that is to say, with evil vapours. What happened was that the many vapours which had been corrupted at the time of the conjunction were drawn up from the earth and water, and were then mixed with the air and spread abroad by frequent gusts of wind in the wild southerly gales, and because of these alien vapours which they carried the winds corrupted the air in its substance, and are still doing so. And this corrupted air, when breathed in, necessarily penetrates to the heart and corrupts the substance of the spirit there and rots the surrounding moisture, and the heat thus caused destroys the life force, and this is the immediate cause of the present epidemic.[8]

And moreover these winds, which have become so common here, have carried among us (and may perhaps continue to do so in future) bad, rotten and poisonous vapours from elsewhere: from swamps, lakes and chasms, for instance, and also (which is even more dangerous) from unburied or unburnt corpses – which might well have been a cause of the epidemic. Another possible cause of corruption, which needs to be borne in mind, is the escape of the rottenness trapped in the centre of the earth as a result of earthquakes – something which has indeed recently occurred. But the conjunctions could have been the universal and distant cause of all these harmful things, by which air and water have been corrupted.

CHAPTER 3: CONCERNING PROGNOSTICATION AND SIGNS

Unseasonable weather is a particular cause of illness. For the ancients, notably Hippocrates, are agreed that if the four seasons run awry, and do not keep their proper course, then plagues and mortal passions are engendered that year. Experience tells us that for some time the seasons have not succeeded each other in the proper way. Last winter was not as cold as it should have been, with a great deal of rain; the spring windy and latterly wet. Summer was late, not as hot as it should have been, and extremely wet – the weather very changeable from day to day, and hour to hour; the air often troubled, and then still again, looking as if it was going to rain but then not doing so. Autumn too was very rainy and misty. It is because the whole year here – or most

8 'Spirit' in these medical tracts has a very precise meaning. It was a substance created by the heart from inhaled air, and was envisaged as an extremely thin, light vapour, which was carried through the body by the arteries. It was, in a literal and immediate sense, the life force, and without it the body would die.

of it – was warm and wet that the air is pestilential. For it is a sign of pestilence for the air to be warm and wet at unseasonable times.

Wherefore we may fear a future pestilence here, which is particularly from the root beneath,[9] because it is subject to the evil impress of the heavens, especially since that conjunction was in a western sign. Therefore if next winter is very rainy and less cold than it ought to be, we should expect an epidemic round about late winter and spring – and if it occurs it will be long and dangerous, for usually unseasonable weather is of only brief duration, but when it lasts over many seasons, as has obviously been the case here, it stands to reason that its effects will be longer-lasting and more dangerous, unless ensuing seasons change their nature in the opposite way. Thus if the winter in the north turns out to be cold and dry, the plagues might be arrested.

We have not said that the future pestilence will be exceptionally dangerous, for we do not wish to give the impression that it will be as dangerous here as in southern or eastern regions. For the conjunctions and the other causes discussed above had a more immediate impact on those regions than on ours. However, in the judgement of astrologers (who follow Ptolemy on this) plagues are likely, although not inevitable, because so many exhalations and inflammations have been observed, such as a comet and shooting stars.[10] Also the sky has looked yellow and the air reddish because of the burnt vapours. There has also been much lightning and flashes and frequent thunder, and winds of such violence and strength that they have carried dust storms from the south. These things, and in particular the powerful earthquakes, have done universal harm and left a trail of corruption. There have been masses of dead fish, animals and other things along the sea shore, and in many places trees covered in dust, and some people claim to have seen a multitude of frogs and reptiles generated from the corrupt matter; and all these things seem to have come from the great corruption of the air and earth. All these things have been noted before as signs of plague by numerous wise men who are still remembered with respect and who experienced them themselves.

No wonder, therefore, that we fear that we are in for an epidemic. But it should be noted that in saying this we do not intend to exclude the possibility of illnesses arising from the character of the present year –

9 By the 'root beneath' the authors mean terrestrial causes as distinct from celestial ones. Exactly the same phrase is used by the translator of Bengt Knutsson [59].

10 No comet was seen before the first plague epidemic and the authors are presumably referring to the mysterious 'star' which appeared over Paris in August 1348 [7].

for as the aphorism of Hippocrates has it: a year of many fogs and damps is a year of many illnesses. On the other hand, the susceptibility of the body of the patient is the most immediate cause in the breeding of illnesses, and therefore no cause is likely to have an effect unless the patient is susceptible to its effects. We must therefore emphasise that although, because everyone has to breathe, everyone will be at risk from the corrupted air, not everyone will be made ill by it but only those, who will no doubt be numerous, who have a susceptibility to it; and very few indeed of those who do succumb will escape.

The bodies most likely to take the stamp of this pestilence are those which are hot and moist, for they are the most susceptible to putrefaction. The following are also more at risk: bodies bunged up with evil humours, because the unconsumed waste matter is not being expelled as it should; those following a bad life style, with too much exercise, sex and bathing; the thin and weak, and persistent worriers; babies, women and young people; and corpulent people with a ruddy complexion. However those with dry bodies, purged of waste matter, who adopt a sensible and suitable regimen, will succumb to the pestilence more slowly.

We must not overlook the fact that any pestilence proceeds from the divine will, and our advice can therefore only be to return humbly to God. But this does not mean forsaking doctors. For the Most High created earthly medicine, and although God alone cures the sick, he does so through the medicine which in his generosity he provided. Blessed be the glorious and high God, who does not refuse his help, but has clearly set out a way of being cured for those who fear him. And this is enough of the third chapter, and of the whole first part.

57. Simon de Covino, De Judicio Solis

Simon de Covino of Liège wrote On the Judgement of Sol at the Feasts of Saturn in 1350. It is a long allegorical poem of 1132 hexameters describing the planetary conjunctions and their consequences in terms of the classical deities. Thus Saturn holds a feast in his house (the zodiac sign of Aquarius) to which the other gods (planets) are invited. Covino supplied a prose prologue to the poem, setting out the contents and 'translating' the allegory, and it is that which is printed here.

Master Simon de Covino, De Judicio Solis in Conviviis Saturni, ed E. Littre, *Bibliothèque de l'école des Chartes* II, 1840-1, pp. 206-208.

In case the material in this little book should seem too burdensome, I here explain it in four parts. In the first I describe, in the manner and fashion of poets, how Saturn prepared a great feast in his own house and invited all the other gods. This description signifies how all the planets were in conjunction with Saturn in his own house of the Zodiac, that is Aquarius, in three months of 1345 – January, February and March. That is not to say that all the planets were in conjunction with Saturn at once, but one after the other on various days in those three months. My main intention is to describe the great conjunction of Jupiter and Saturn, which only happens in Aquarius every ninety years; a conjunction which, according to philosophers, signifies great and amazing upheavals. Aristotle in his book on the properties of the elements says that because of the conjunction of Saturn and Jupiter in Aquarius kingdoms have been emptied and the earth depopulated.

And when all the gods had come to this feast, and Jupiter had entered the house of Saturn, a great dispute arose between Saturn and Jupiter over the human race. And in this way I describe the hostility and contradiction of these two planets, both in complexion and in effect. For Saturn is excessively cold and dry, and as a result is a corrupter of human life. Jupiter is moderately warm and moist, and therefore can be said to be a friend of the human condition.

In the second part of this work, on the strife and conflict of these two planets, Sol is described as judge, and deservedly, for he is the king and prince of all the planets and the heart of the heavens, according to philosophers. For just as (according to Aristotle in his book on animals) the heart of man is in the centre of the human body, as if ruler and prince of all the other members, so Sol is in the centre of the planets.[11] In addition, since all the other heavenly bodies pour and shed on the world only transmitted rays, and would have no light at all if it were not for the Sun, as many philosophers assure us, it seems that all the other heavenly bodies have their influence and their virtues from Sol. From which it is obvious that all decisions on the workings of the celestial bodies are determined by the Sun. And everyone who has discussed these matters is in full agreement that all the planetary conjunctions in the ensuing year take their significance from the state of the heavens at Sol's entry into Aries.[12] For while in Aries, Sol is said

11 Covino is not implying a heliocentric universe. The orbits of the seven planets formed a series of concentric circles around the earth and the sun's orbit was the fourth, i.e. the central, one of the seven. Similarly, in schemes of the seven ages of man, where each of the planets was identified with one of the ages (the moon with infancy, Mercury with childhood and so on), the sun represented the prime of life: the high point on the arch of human development and decline.

12 The entry of the sun into Aries marked the beginning of the astrological year and

to be exalted and crowned like a king in majesty on his throne, and that was the place he occupied when he was created by God. And that this was the first position of the heavens is the opinion of Plato and of theologians, and Scripture agrees with them: 'Let the earth bring forth green plants' etc [Genesis 1.11]. For this reason I have made Sol the judge in the case brought between Saturn and Jupiter. And then I describe the seat of the judge, and the manner and form in which he was enthroned there. And in the presence of this king or judge of the heavens, Saturn puts forward reasons for the destruction of the human race and Jupiter puts forward a defence to them.

When both parties have presented their reasons, Mercury arises, as prosecutor in the heavenly court. For he is called Sol's knight, because he is never far from the Sun. And moreover from the time when Sol entered Aries in 1345 (after which Jupiter and Saturn were in conjunction) Mercury himself was in conjunction and unity with Sol in the first degree of Aries. And because that makes him partake of the influence and nature of the planet with which he is in conjunction, therefore I describe him as holding office in the court of his lord, the Sun. And because it is the common opinion that this mortality proceeded from God because of the sins of the human race, just as in the time of the Flood, therefore Mercury, as prosecutor in the court, proposes that the crimes of men are greater than they were at the time of the Flood, and brings celestial records, charters and documents to prove his case. And when Jupiter sees such great crimes proved against the human race then he turns in horror from mankind's cause and will abandon it completely, because he mainly represents faith, holiness and religion, and purity of mind and body. Therefore he will abandon the accused sinners to their just punishment, and he makes peace and concord with Saturn and aims to obey him in the matter. And this obedience signifies that Saturn is superior to Jupiter, partly because of their orbits, partly because of the house of Aquarius in which they have both been joined together.[13]

In the third part of this work the judgements of Sol begin. But first

---

the position of the planets at that moment was thus of particular importance for the rest of the year. In effect the year was 'born' then, and its horoscope could be read from the configuration of the heavens.

13 As the outermost of the planets, Saturn had the widest orbit, which was thought to give him great power – enhanced in 1345 because the conjunction was taking place in his mansion of Aquarius. Most astrologers also believed that in 1345 Saturn was the lord of the year: the planet which ruled affairs for that astrological year. Covino refers to the lord of the year in the next paragraph.

mention is made of how other matters had a bearing on the mortality, namely the change of the lord of the year and the many causes also signified by the conjunction of the said planets, as is afterwards set out in the words of the judge. And first Sol appointed the principal lord of the year and the other rulers over the regions of the world, who are called lords of the year. Afterwards Sol gives his judgement and condemns the human race to pestilential death. And afterwards he gives his judgements on all the other matters signified by the conjunction of the planets, according to the writings of Master Jean de Murs, Master Firmin de Beauval and Master Leo the Jew of Montpellier, and I have added nothing of my own to the judgement of Sol beyond putting it into verse.[14]

After he has passed judgement, Sol appoints Saturn, Jupiter and Mercury to put his judgements into effect. And this signifies that, although the decisions of the planets derive from Sol, as I explained above, nevertheless execution of the judgements on us seems rather to come from the conjunctions of the planets. And the great eclipse of the moon is immediately described, which preceded by two days the actual conjunction of Jupiter and Saturn, that is to say it occurred about a week or so after the entry of Sol into Aries – which is to say, after the judgement of Sol. And immediately afterwards there is described the actual and bodily conjunction of Saturn and Jupiter in Aquarius, which followed nine days or so after the entry of Sol into Aries.[15] And there the work treats of the nature and workings of poisonous pestilence, and its manner of bringing about death, which is to say through the means of Saturn and Juno. For Saturn himself causes thick, heavy clouds which smother Juno – which is to say the lower atmosphere – and the smothered air becomes corrupt and poisonous. And then there follows death-bearing pestilence.

In the fourth part I deal with the remedies given against pestilence. And the poem treats of the three fatal goddesses – Clotho, Lachesis and Atropos. Clotho, who holds the distaff of life, represents generation; Lachesis, who draws out the thread of life, represents the span of human life from birth to death; Atropos, who breaks the thread of life, signifies corruption and death. And therefore I treat of remedies in this

---

14 All three were eminent contemporary astrologers who wrote prognostications following the 1345 conjunction but before the plague. That of Jean de Murs is mentioned by Gilles li Muisis [6].

15 The sun entered Aries on 11 March and the lunar eclipse was on 18 March. Saturn and Jupiter began their conjunction on 20 March.

fashion, putting them poetically into the mouth of Lachesis, who represents the lengthening of life and the means whereby that can be achieved. And she seeks these remedies to prolong life in opposition to her sister, Atropos, who represents decay. And although doctors arm her with remedies to fight against her sister, those arms, that is the remedies of doctors, are of little worth to her. Instead, she is defeated in the first battle of the war, and flees, and her followers and the doctors fall dead, as really happened in Montpellier, where there was a very great supply of doctors, of whom scarcely one escaped. But I go on to show which of the doctors' weapons are of use in this mortality, and which are not, and how some have managed to stay alive and by what means they have been able to resist, grouping this section according to the root of the infection. And afterwards I treat of the illness's usual symptoms and discuss my own views of the remedies. And finally I describe the effects of this illness, not with poetic imagination, but using real examples from various places. And so ends the little book concerning the judgement of Sol at the feasts of Saturn.

58. The astrological causes of the plague, Geoffrey de Meaux

Geoffrey de Meaux was a astrologer who had been associated with the French court earlier in the fourteenth century. The astrological measurements given in this treatise, however, relate to Oxford, which suggests that it was composed (or at least rewritten) there. Unlike the three astrologers mentioned in 57 de Meaux wrote this commentary on the 1345 conjunction after the outbreak of plague, and accordingly stresses the malign role of Saturn and Mars rather than the possible contribution of Jupiter.

Bodleian Library, Oxford, MS Digby 176 fos. 26-9.

I have been asked by some of my friends to write something about the cause of this general pestilence, showing its natural cause, and why it affected so many countries, and why it affected some countries more than others, and why within those countries it affected some cities and towns more than others, and why in one town it affected one street, and even one house, more than another, and why it affected nobles and gentry less than other people, and how long it will last. And they asked that after explaining the cause I should discuss appropriate remedies, drawing on my own opinions and medical advice. In order to demonstrate the cause of all these things I shall begin with the basics, as set forth by the wise authors, philosophers and astrologers who have had things to say on such matters.

Ptolemy in chapter 4 of the third book of his *Quadripartitum* cites Plato
and Aristotle in support of the contention that God first created the
heavens and the stars, and endowed them with the power to rule all
earthly matters, and because of this it can be said that everything
which befalls us happens at the will of God; for it is God himself who
moves the heavens and whatever is within them, and it is through this
motion that there come all the chances of generation and corruption,
and all the other chances which lie outside our free will. Haly also cites
Ptolemy as saying in the prologue to the first book of the
Quadripartitum that the heavenly bodies confer on the inferior bodies
below them similar powers, if they are naturally disposed to receive
them.[16] He also says in the *Quadripartitum* that heavenly bodies can
bring about changes and events when they are turned towards us, and
that this is a natural power, like the power of adamant to attract iron
or scammony to purge yellow bile.[17] Friar Roger Bacon in his treatise
on the significance of places says that every point on the earth is at the
apex of a pyramid formed by the converging lines of various heavenly
powers; and this explains why you get plants of various species within
one tiny piece of ground, or find twins who differ in character and
behaviour, and in their aptitude for scholarship, languages or business.

Ptolemy divided the twelve signs of the Zodiac, through which all the
planets move, into four groups of three, which he called trigons or
triplicities, each of which is identified with one element. Thus the
trigon of Aries, Leo and Sagittarius is identified with fire, which is hot
and dry; the trigon of Taurus, Virgo and Capricorn with earth, which
is cold and dry; the trigon of Gemini, Libra and Aquarius with air,
which is hot and wet; and the trigon of Cancer, Scorpio and Pisces with
water, which is cold and wet. Ptolemy also divided the whole inhabited
world into four principal parts, each of which he identifies with one of
the trigons. Ptolemy also says that the conjunctions of the two highest
planets, that is Saturn and Jupiter, are of three types: major, minor and
mean. A major conjunction is one in which these two planets begin
their conjunction in the trigon of fire and remain in conjunction in the
other trigons in turn until they return to the trigon of fire, but another

16 Haly or Haly Abbas is the tenth-century Islamic scientist Ali ben Al-Abbas Al-
Magusi. Here and elsewhere I have retained the names by which Islamic writers
were known in the Latin west.

17 Adamant was originally the name given to an intensely hard crystal, now usually
taken to be the diamond. Most medieval writers, however, conflated it with the
magnet or lodestone, which is the sense in which the word is being used here.
Scammony is the English name of *convolvulus scammonia*, a powerful purgative.

sign from that in which they started, and this happens every 960 years. A mean conjunction is when these two highest planets begin their conjunction in one of the four triplicities and it lasts until they enter another, and this happens every 240 years. A minor conjunction is when they come together in any one trigon and this happens about every 20 years.

Now that the basics have been discussed, you can consider the reasons for such a great mortality in so many countries, and how the illness came through the influence of the stars. Ptolemy in chapter 4 of the second part of the *Quadripartitum* says: the important things are the strengths and powers of the hour, the conjunctions and oppositions, eclipses of the sun and moon, and the places the planets cross at that hour. Wherefore it has been, and is, known by all astrologers that in the year 1345 (taking the year to begin in January) there was a total eclipse of the moon, of long duration, on 18 March. At the longitude of Oxford it began an hour after the moon rose, and at the time the two planets were in conjunction in Aquarius, and Mars was with them in the same sign, within the light of Jupiter.

The sun is the lord, the director of all events, both general and specific, and the moon is second to him in dominion and power, and their effect is to intensify the effects of the planets acting with them. It is therefore in the natural course of events, and not to be wondered at, that such a great configuration should bring about major events on the earth, from the nature of the planets which drew to themselves the natures of the sun and moon. For when the sun is directly opposite the moon, as occurs in a total eclipse, then the power of each of them reaches the earth in a straight line, and the mingling of the influence of sun and moon with that of the superior planets creates a single celestial force which operates in conformity with the nature of the superior planets, which have drawn to themselves the powers of the sun and moon. The same thing happens in compound medicines: turbith naturally expels phlegm from the stomach and veins, and if it is mixed with ginger the mixture expels phlegm, and since ginger is not in itself an expellant it has taken on the nature of turbith. It is the same with the planets. On their own they cannot achieve anything great or universal, but when compounded with the sun and moon (at a time when these are aligned with each other and with the earth) they bend the nature of the two luminaries to their own nature, and thus with the power of the two luminaries are able to achieve great things which have a general and universal impact.

These natural causes affect the whole inhabited world between east and north. According to Ptolemy, Saturn, which was one of the partners in the conjunction, governs the whole eastern part of the inhabited world; Mars the whole western part; and Jupiter, besieged by both of them in the conjunction, rules the whole northern part. Thus the greater part of the earth was influenced, because of the place of the conjunction and because the planets involved rule parts of the world, as I have just described, and also because all the parts of the world where the eclipse was visible above the horizon shared in the effect of the configuration. Therefore this is why it affected so many provinces. And the reason why some were affected more than others is that a planet has no effect in a place over which it exerts no influence, as Ptolemy testifies in his *Centilogium*, and the superior planets in this conjunction had an influence over the places they rule and not elsewhere. And the reason why some towns and cities were affected more than others in the same provinces is as follows. Each city, town and home has fixed stars and planets ruling it, as Ptolemy testifies in the *Centilogium*. Therefore wherever the rulers of these places agree in power and effect with the planets and stars bringing the general mortality, those subject to them will have been made ready to receive that celestial influence upon their bodies.

It now remains to assign a reason why in one town it affected one street more than another, and also one house more than another. The answer is the same in both cases. Not all streets were affected in the same way, or both sides of one street, or neighbouring houses, because they do not have the same influences or rulers, and therefore the impact of the heavens cannot affect them all equally – for that action of which I speak is natural and operates according to the rules of nature. It cannot act in the same way in every case, but only has an effect insofar as the ground has been prepared for it.

It now remains to say why nobles and gentry were less affected than the rest of the population. It was and is known to all astrologers that at the time of this eclipse the three superior planets were in the sign of Aquarius, where the fixed stars are not of the first magnitude and, save for one which is in the south, far distant from us, are lesser stars which signify the common people, and therefore the effect of the illness which they brought touched those people more....

It now remains to say how long the effects of that configuration on 18 March 1345 will last. It is known to all astrologers that the duration of obscurity of the lunar eclipse when there was the conjunction of the three superior planets was three hours, 29 minutes and 54 seconds. That three hours and a half (roughly) when multiplied by 20, which is the number of years between these minor conjunctions of Saturn and Jupiter, make 70, which, divided by the 13 lunar months which make up the solar year, give 5 years and 5 lunar months, denoting the duration of the universal effect of that configuration of the two superior planets together with the lunar eclipse, as Ptolemy witnesses in the second book of the *Quadripartitum* where he says: the impact of a solar eclipse will last for as many years as there were hours of darkness, and in the case of a lunar eclipse for as many months as there were hours of darkness. And the commentator adds at that point that this calculation relates just to the eclipse; when it occurs with something else, such as a conjunction of Saturn and Jupiter, the duration of its effect will be proportionately lengthened.

You should understand, however, that I do not wish to imply that the mortality comes only from Saturn and Jupiter but rather through Mars, which was mixed with them at the time of the eclipse. And the condition which resulted from all of these will last according to the nature of the dominant planets in that configuration....

Now it remains to write about the best remedy to be taken against this celestial influence, and you should know, as Ptolemy says in the third chapter of the first book of the *Quadripartitum*, that not all the things which befall men through the heavenly bodies are inevitable – that is, cannot be avoided. Some of the works of the stars are inevitable in this sense, and cannot in the nature of things be avoided, but others are things which it is possible to avoid, so that one part of the events befalling men arose through the general and universal pestilence, and did not befall them because of their individual nature. For in that mortality the greater and stronger force throws down the weaker and lesser. And you ought to know that should someone's nativity be the opposite of the configuration bringing the mortality, the mortality would not touch him; but should his nativity be broadly similar to the configuration, it would be clear that he lacks the contrary forces by which he could resist it. For as doctors and students of natural science know, transmutation is easy between bodies which have matching qualities. And where a person's nativity does not fully correspond to the configuration and yet is not totally contrary to it either, the body can (given a good regimen and certain medicines which I will describe later) be preserved from this pestilence, but if he adopts a bad regimen then he can easily contract it.

Now the nature of the sun and moon is drawn, as I said earlier, to the nature of the dominant planets in the configuration, and those were Saturn and Mars; not Jupiter, although at the time of the eclipse he was exalted above Mars both in the eccentric and epicycle.[18] For Jupiter is of a temperate power, and the more easily overcome as a result; just as temperate medicines are easily overwhelmed when mixed with intemperate medicines, and become intemperate themselves.[19] Thus at the time of the eclipse, Jupiter was besieged by both the infortunes[20] and, mixed with them, took the nature of both of them, but rather more of Saturn than of Mars; because Saturn was stronger than Mars in that place, because he had more dignities ·in that place, and because he was exalted above them in both the eccentric and epicycle. Saturn thus obtained dominion, and Mars was his second, as Ptolemy testifies.

Because Saturn was dominant, he brings cold (greater than the sun could counter) to each country under his rule, and because of the sign in which the conjunction occurred men will experience the onset of lingering illnesses such as tuberculosis, catarrh, paralysis and gout; passions of the heart arising from unhappiness; and the deaths of those who have endured long weakness. And since the conjunction was in the air sign of Aquarius it signified great cold, heavy frosts, and thick clouds corrupting the air; and since this is a sign which represents the pouring out of water, the configuration signifies that rivers will burst their banks and the sea flood. And because of the persistently cold atmosphere bitter humours cannot be expelled from the sea as usual, and because of the persistent cold there will be few fish in the sea and those that there are will rot because of the cold, which traps vapours and humours in their bodies. For his part, Mars in that sign denotes strife among men, and sudden death which comes among all sorts of men, especially among children and adolescents, and illnesses entailing fevers and the spitting of blood, and also violent death and ulcers.

18 An eccentric is a planetary orbit which does not have the earth at its exact centre. An epicyle is a revolution by a planet as it goes along the course of its orbit.

19 A body is 'temperate' when the contraries of which it is composed are well balanced; 'intemperate' when there is a dramatic imbalance. The Paris medical faculty was making the same point when it described Mars as 'immoderately' hot and dry [56].

20 The infortunes were the two malevolent planets, Saturn and Mars, which were known in Latin as *infortuna maior* and *minor* (the greater and lesser infortune). Conversely, the beneficent planets Jupiter and Venus were *fortuna maior* and *minor* (the greater and lesser fortune).

59. The dangers of corrupted air

This account is taken from the treatise of Bengt Knutsson, a mid-fifteenth century bishop of Västerås, near Stockholm. Knutsson took over wholesale one of the most popular plague tracts of the fourteenth century, that of John Jacobus (Jean Jacmé), written *c.*1364. Jacobus was a royal and papal physician and Chancellor of Montpellier, and the various autobiographical references later in the work refer to him, not to Knutsson.

This extract represents a little over half the treatise; the last two sections (on the comforts of the heart and blood-letting) have been omitted. The text is taken from a fifteenth-century English translation of Knutsson. I have modernised the spelling and made a few grammatical changes for the sake of clarity, but have not attempted a complete modern 'translation'.

A Little Book for the Pestilence, Manchester, 1911, a facsimile of a printed English translation of Knutsson in the John Rylands Library, Manchester.

Here begins a little book which treats and rehearses many good things necessary for the infirmity and great sickness called the Pestilence, the which often infects us, made by the most expert doctor in physic the Bishop of Arusiens in the realm of Denmark.

At the reverence and worship of the blessed Trinity and of the glorious Virgin St Mary and for the conservation of the common weal, as well for them that be whole as for remedy of them that be sick, I the Bishop of Arusiens in the realm of Denmark, doctor of physic, will write by the most expert and famous doctors, authorities in physic, some things about the infirmity of pestilence which daily infects us and soon suffers us to depart out of this life.

First I will write the tokens of this infirmity.

Secondly the causes whereof it comes.

Thirdly the remedies for the same.

Fourthly comfort for the heart and the principal members of the body.

Fifthly when it shall be the season to let blood.

First as I said the tokens of this infirmity. Seven things ought to be noted here:

The first is when on a summer's day the weather often changes, so in the morning the weather appears rainy, afterwards it appears cloudy and finally windy from the south.

The second token is when in summer the days appear all dark and look like rain, and yet it does not rain. And if many days continue thus, great pestilence is to be dreaded.

The third token is when there is a great multitude of flies upon the earth, then it is sign that the air is venomous and infected.

The fourth token is when stars often seem to fall, then it is a token that the air is infected with much venomous vapour.

The fifth token is when a blazing star is seen in the sky, then it should fortune that soon after there will be great manslaughter in battle.

The sixth token is when there is great lightning and thunder, namely out of the south.

The seventh token is when great winds blow out of the south for they be foul and unclean.

Therefore when these tokens appear great pestilence is to be dreaded, unless God of his mercy will remove it.

The pestilence comes of three things. Sometimes it comes from the root beneath, at other times from the root above, so that we may feel sensibly how the change of air apppears to us, and sometimes it comes of both together: from the root above as well as from the root beneath – as when we see a siege or privy next to a chamber or any other particular thing which corrupts the air in substance and quality, which is a thing which may happen every day. And thereof comes the ague of pestilence. And many physicians are deceived about this, not suspecting this ague to be a pestilence. Sometimes it comes of dead carrion or the corruption of standing waters in ditches or sloughs or other corrupt places, and these things are sometimes universal and sometimes particular. By the root above is meant the heavenly bodies, by whom the spirit of life is corrupted in man or beast. In like wise, as Avicenna says in his fourth book, by the form of the air above the bodies beneath may be infected. For the inspissation above corrupts the air and so the spirits of man are corrupted.[21] This infirmity comes also from the root above or beneath: when the inspissation above corrupts the air or when the putrefaction or rotten carrion of the vile places beneath cause an infirmity in man. And such an infirmity is sometimes an ague, sometimes an apostume or a swelling and that is in many things. Also the inspissated air is sometimes venomous and corrupt, hurting

21 Inspissation is a thickening, specifically in this context the condensation of corrupt vapours to form thick, wet clouds.

the heart so that nature is grieved in many ways, but so that he does not perceive his harm. For the urine appears fair and shows good digestion, yet nevertheless the patient is likely to die.[22] Wherefore many physicians, seeing the urine of their patients, speak superficially and are deceived. Therefore it is necessary that every patient provide himself with a good and expert physician.

These things before written are the causes of pestilence; but about these things two questions are asked. The first is why, within one town, one man dies and another does not. Where men are dead in one house, in another house no one dies. The other question is whether pestilence sores are contagious. To the first question I say that it may happen for two causes: that is to say because of the thing that does or the thing that suffers. An example of that thing that does: the influence of the bodies above affects that place or that place more than this place or this place. And one patient is more disposed to die than another. Therefore it is to be noted that bodies inclined to be hot have open pores, whereas infected bodies have the pores stopped with many humours. Where bodies have open pores, as in the case of men who abuse themselves with women or often have baths, or men who are hot with labour or great anger, they are the more disposed to this great sickness.

To the second question I say that pestilence sores are contagious because of infectious humours, and the reek or smoke of such sores is venomous and corrupts the air. And therefore one should flee such persons as are infected. In pestilence time nobody should stand in a great press of people because some man among them may be infected. Therefore wise physicians visiting sick folk stand far from the patient, holding their face towards the door or window, and so should the servants of sick folk stand. Also it is good for a patient to change his chamber every day and often to have the windows open against the north and east and to spar the windows against the south. For the south wind has two causes of putrefaction. The first is it that makes a man, whether whole or sick, feeble in his body. The second cause is as it is written in Aphorisms chapter 3, the south wind grieves the body and hurts the heart because it opens man's pores and enters into the heart. Wherefore it is good for a whole man in time of pestilence when the wind is in the south to stay within the house all day, and if it shall

22 Medieval physicians used their patient's urine as one of their main diagnostic tools. The assumption that illness was caused by corrupt humours meant that the body's excreta were the obvious source of information about the state of the humours inside the body.

be necessary for a man go out, yet let him abide in his house until the sun be up in the east and passing southward.

Here after follow the remedies for the pestilence.

Now it is to be known by what remedies a man may preserve himself from the pestilence. First see the writings of Jeremiah the prophet that a man ought to forsake evil things and do good deeds and meekly confess his sins, for it is the highest remedy in time of pestilence: penance and confession to be preferred to all other medicines. Nevertheless I promise you verily it is a good remedy to void and change the infected place. But some may not profitably change their places. Therefore as much as they can they should eschew every cause of putrefaction and stinking, and namely every fleshly lust with women is to be eschewed. Also the southern wind, which is naturally infective. Therefore spar the windows against the south in like wise as it is said before, until the first hour after the middle of the day then open the windows against the north. Of the same cause every foul stench is to be eschewed, of stable, stinking fields, ways or streets, and namely of stinking dead carrion and most of stinking waters where in many places water is kept two days or two nights. Or else there be gutters of water cast under the earth which cause great stink and corruption. And of this cause some die in that house where such things happen, and in another house die none as is said afore. Likewise in that place where worts and cabbages putrefy it makes a noisome savour and stinking. For in likewise as by the sweet odour of balsam the heart and the spirits have recreation, so of evil savours they be made feeble. Wherefore keep your house that an infected air enter not in, for an infected air most causes putrefaction in places and houses where folk sleep. Therefore let your house be clean and make clear fire of wood flaming. Let your house be made with fumigation of herbs, that is to say with leaves of bay tree, juniper, *uberiorgani* [unidentified] it is in the apothecary shops, wormwood, rue, mugwort and of the wood of aloes which is best but it is dear. Such a fume taken by the mouth and ears opens the inward parts of the body. Also all great repletion is to be eschewed because full bodies be easily infected as Avicenna says in the fourth canon: they that charge their bodies to repletion shorten their life.

Also common baths are to be eschewed, for a little crust corrupts all the body.[23] Therefore the people as much as is possible is to be

---

23 A crust is a scab, and Knutsson is saying that just as a localised infection can spread to affect the whole body, so one man in a crowd can infect the rest. Public baths

eschewed, lest of infectious breath some man be infected. But when the multitude of people may not be eschewed, then use the remedies following. In the morning when you rise wash a little rue and one or two filbert nuts clean and eat them, and if that cannot be had then eat bread or toast sopped in vinegar, namely in troublous and cloudy weather. Also in the time of pestilence it is better to abide within the house for it is not wholesome to go into the city or town. Also let your house be sprinkled especially in summer with vinegar and roses and with the leaves of the vine. Also it is good to wash your hands oft times in the day with water and vinegar and wipe your face with your hands and smell to them. Also it is good always to savour sour things. In Montpellier I might not eschew the company of people for I went from house to house because of my poverty to cure sick folks, therefore bread or a sponge sopped in vinegar I took with me holding it in my mouth and nose because all sour things stop the way of humours and suffer no venomous things to enter into a man's body and so I escaped the pestilence, my fellows supposing that I should not live. These forsaid things I have proved by my self.

60. Earthquakes as the cause of plague

This is the final section of a treatise usually known, from its opening words, as *Is it from divine wrath that the mortality of these years proceeds.* It was probably produced in Germany in the generation after the 1348-49 outbreak. In the first part of the treatise, not printed here, the author considers various explanations of the plague, including the astrological one – which he rejects on the grounds that similar conjunctions occur frequently without being followed by plague, and that the configuration of the heavens should have an equal impact on all mankind, which the plague did not. He then turns to his preferred explanation: that the earthquakes of 1347 released poisonous fumes into the atmosphere.

Karl Sudhoff, 'Pestschriften aus den ersten 150 Jahren nach der Epidemie des 'schwarzen Todes' 1348: XI', *Archiv für Geschichte der Medizin* XI, 1918-19, pp. 47-51.

There is a fourth opinion, which I consider more likely than the others, which is that insofar as the mortality arose from natural causes its immediate cause was a corrupt and poisonous earthy exhalation, which

---

were notoriously used for sexual assignations and were regarded by contemporary moralists as no better than brothels. Knutsson's warning against them is probably based on the dangers of sexual intercourse as well as on the general risks posed by crowds.

infected the air in various parts of the world and, when breathed in by people, suffocated them and suddenly snuffed them out. I can bring two pieces of evidence in support of my proposition, both securely grounded in natural science. The first is that when air which is full of vapours and earthy fumes is enclosed and shut up for a long time in the prison of the earth it becomes so corrupted that it constitutes a potent poison to men. This is especially marked in caverns or deep inside the earth, where there is no fresh air supply, as is often seen in the case of wells which have been unused for a long time and have remained sealed up for many years. For when such wells are opened in order to be cleaned out it often happens that the first man to enter is suffocated, and sometimes in turn those who follow him. And the common people are so ignorant that they blame this on a basilisk lurking inside.[24]

It is a matter of scientific fact that earthquakes are caused by the exhalation of fumes enclosed in the bowels of the earth. When the fumes batter against the sides of the earth, and cannot get out, the earth is shaken and moves. I say that it is the vapour and corrupted air which has been vented – or so to speak purged – in the earthquake which occurred on St Paul's day, 1347, along with the corrupted air vented in other earthquakes and eruptions, which has infected the air above the earth and killed people in various parts of the world; and I can bring various reasons in support of this conclusion:

1. In Germany the mortality first began in Carinthia after an earthquake there in which the vapour and air enclosed deep in the mountains violently burst forth and hurled down mighty mountains into the valleys, demolished the entire town of Villach, and buried numerous villages. And then the same mortality in turn invaded Austria, Hungary, Bavaria, Moravia, Bohemia, the Rhineland, Swabia and other provinces of Germany. Its progress followed no logical pattern; instead the filthy disease took a wandering and irregular route from place to place, as if blown along by the wind – something which can only be explained as the effect of corrupt air, expelled from the earth by the earthquake.

2. Houses near the sea, as at Venice and Marseilles, were affected quickly, as were low-lying towns on the edge of marshes or beside the sea, and the only explanation of that would seem to be the greater corruption of the air in hollows near the sea.[25]

24 Basilisks were mythical beasts believed to be able to kill by sight; see further 61 below.

25 When corrupted air condensed (see note 21 above) it became wet and heavy and

3. In all the places where the mortality has persisted for a long time, and still persists, there have been more fogs and stinks than in other years at the times when the sun is low in the sky, that is at its rising and setting, when it falls below the meridian, or whenever it is lower than at the summer solstice, that is in autumn, winter and spring. And this is because the air there is fuller of earthy vapours and fogs than in other years.

4. It can be deduced from the corruption of fruit such as pears.

5. It can be deduced from the flooding of rivers, although this has been brought about by the heavy rain.

6. In every place where the mortality has persisted, virtually every victim has been afflicted as follows. For several days they spend most of each day asleep, weighed down by drowsiness, their heads made thick by a kind of fume, such as they might derive from eating or drinking fumous things.[26] Most die within three days, although a few last for four. What happens is that when the poisonous fumes have gathered in the empty parts of the human body, especially in the chest, they rise into the head and trouble the animal spirits, which is one way of causing sleep.

7. In every place visited by the mortality the poor and common people die first, in great numbers, and the better off die later. But it is well known that the planets look down on rich and poor alike. The explanation would seem to be that the poor, who do not consume rich food or strong drink, do not generate heat or fumes inside themselves as the rich do, who are full of hot food and fumous drink. Therefore the rich do not so easily absorb fumes from outside, for what is inside them leaves no room for such fumes and blocks their entry. That is also the reason why men who eat and drink moderately are more likely to be

---

would thus naturally collect in hollows. Conversely, the direct rays of the sun evaporated the moisture, making the vapours thinner and lighter so that they rose into the middle air where they would do less damage. It therefore followed that corrupt air would be particularly dangerous at night, and at dawn and dusk when the sun's rays were slanting and weak. On the same argument, spring, autumn and winter were also dangerous, although some authors felt that a *dry* winter would be healthy because it would counter the wetness of the poisonous vapours. Hence the anxieties about recent wet winters expressed by li Muisis and the Paris medical faculty.

26 Rich food and drink were thought to generate fumes, which (in modern terms) had an intoxicating effect. The author is not saying that such fumes are poisonous; on the contrary, he later claims that they are beneficial and that filling the body with such fumes makes it more difficult for poisonous air to enter. Most contemporaries disagreed and argued that rich food and drink opened the pores and made the entry of bad air *more* likely.

struck down quickly by this mortality than are the gluttonous, although they cannot hold it at bay indefinitely.

8. As Avicenna and Albertus Magnus rehearse, any earthquake has the power of turning men to stone, and notably into salt, because of the very powerful mineral virtue which exists in earthy vapours.[27] It therefore seems possible that in other circumstances men might die, infected by the vapours spread across the earth.

Because of this, and for other reasons too, it seems to me that air, infected and poisoned by the corrupt vapours and poisonous exhalations vented in earthquakes, is and has been the cause of the mortality discussed here. But doubts have been expressed about this opinion:

1. In some parts of the world the mortality began without an earthquake, which would suggest that earthquakes cannot be the cause.

2. Such vapour would have soon spread, and once it had dispersed and thinned out could hardly have harmed people over a wide area.

3. The air ought to be infected in this way after every earthquake, and so every earthquake ought to be followed by mortality among men, but this is not borne out by chronicles.

4. If the air has been infected all the men in one house or one town ought to die, but this does not happen.

5. There seems to be no reason why animals, who breathe, have not been struck down by the epidemic when men have been killed by it.

6. Such mortality ought to have been less strong in summer than in winter and other times of the year, because such thick, earthy vapours should have been thinned by the heat of summer and drawn up into the middle air, where they could do less harm to man. When the sun is low in the sky, by contrast, the vapours, inspissated and thickened by cold, ought to have descended into the lower atmosphere, nearer the earth, and so harmed more people. But several places have experienced the opposite, and there has been grief and lamentation during the dog days, and peace and tranquillity during the period when the sun's rays were oblique.[28]

27 The reference to salt is presumably to Lot's wife [Genesis 19], who looked back at the destruction by earthquakes of Sodom and Gomorrah and was turned into a pillar of salt.

28 The dog days occur at the height of summer, when Sirius, the dog star, rises in the day time (and is consequently, of course, invisible).

To the first doubt I say that we need to take into account not only the earthquake which did so much damage in Carinthia and in other parts of Germany, but also those which occurred afterwards beyond the Alps and in Italy and in the city of Ravenna. And I would add that over a long period before that great earthquake occurred, the spirits confined in the earth had built up enormous pressure within the earth, since it was not easy for them to topple a mass of such weight, and the intensity of the pressure forced out a significant amount of spirit or vapour through cracks in the earth before the earthquake and infected the air in various places.

To the second it may be said that there was a lot of that earthy smoke, which affected the length and breadth of the earth, not just one place at one time, and accordingly it could not thin out and disappear so quickly, and thus we may deduce that although it is steadily dispersing, it is doing so over a long period, and it is not possible to know to the minute when it will disperse entirely – and we can see that this is the case, for a very great mortality still persists in some parts of Germany and in several places has begun for the first time.

To the third doubt I say that it is not necessary for mortality to follow every earthquake, for a reason which is sufficiently obvious.

To the fourth I say that men differ in their constitution, for some are sturdier and stronger and less sensitive, so that they do not easily sink under any external attack; while others, on the contrary, are of a delicate and soft constitution and readily succumb. And this is why some people die of these things and others never do. Different life styles make their contribution too, as we see when something which is nutritious food for one man is poison to another.

To the fifth it may be said that man has a nobler and weaker nature than all other animals, and therefore what does no harm to brute beasts does have the power to harm men.

To the sixth I say that that poisonous matter has behaved, and is still behaving, according to the rules governing the movement of strong poisons, being driven now to one place, now to another; appearing now in summer, now in winter, now here, now there, and fluctuating at other times of the year.[29] And where it is argued that the summer heat ought to draw it upwards, I say that although the effect of the day may

29 The author is comparing the earth to a human body which, when attacked by poison, tries to expel it: a process described in 62. His opening description of earthquakes is similarly anthropomorphic.

be to thin it somewhat, when night comes it is on the contrary thickened, and when morning comes people ingest such matter into their empty bellies. To which I might add that the matter could be drawn into large numbers of men in spring or winter or at some other time of year and then lie hidden in their bodies until it has penetrated and finally pierced the house of the heart. And thus before men knew that the damage had been done, they were already carrying death within them, which finally launched its attack on that treasure house of life, the heart. As soon as this happened those infected fell dead.

61. The transmission of plague

These extracts are from a treatise on the epidemic written in 1349 by a doctor of Montpellier. The work is loosely based on the report of the Paris medical faculty [56], but the attempt to explain how the plague was transmitted is the author's own.

L-A-Joseph Michon (ed), *Documents inédits sur la grande peste de 1348*, thèse pour le doctorat en médecine, Paris, 1860, pp. 46-52.

This epidemic, according to some people, has the power to kill large numbers by air alone, simply by the breath or the conversation of the sick. They say that the air breathed out by the sick and inhaled by the healthy people round about wounds and kills them, and that this occurs particularly when the sick are on the point of death. But that would kill gradually, after an interval rather than straight away; and the greater strength of this epidemic is such that it kills almost instantly, as soon as the airy spirit leaving the eyes of the sick man has struck the eye of a healthy bystander looking at him, for then the poisonous nature passes from one eye to the other.[30] And this occurs particularly when the sick are at the point of death.

No one who has seen the theories of Euclid concerning burning glasses, and concave and reflecting glasses, will be surprised by this, but will appreciate that the origins of this epidemic and its ability to pass from the sick to the healthy and to kill them, are natural and not miraculous; for something is only 'miraculous' when it does not have a natural reason or cause. The airy and subtle nature which issues from

30 The preferred medieval explanation of sight was that it involved spirit passing from the eye of the observer to the thing observed. After being created in the heart (see note 8 above), spirit passed along the arteries to the brain, where it was transformed into animal spirits which carried the power of seeing along the optic nerve (believed to be hollow) to the eye: N. G. Siraisi, *Medieval and Early Renaissance Medicine*, Chicago, 1990, p. 108.

the heat and brightness of the sun is immediately kindled and flares up when reflected by two mirrors. This is achieved by condensing thin air just using the brightness generated by the sun's rays and the mirrors. That brightness can be used to burn and destroy nearby buildings, houses, castles and trees, and an example of this can be found in Euclid's book. In the same way the corruption of the air has an impact on human bodies, and it has a more immediate impact on them than on other things because of the soft primary matter of which they are compounded.

[The writer then discusses the planetary conjunction in Aquarius, and concludes that one consequence for the northern hemisphere was that the dominance of Saturn, a cold planet, meant that plants did not ripen but had to be eaten when under-ripe.]

And such food inevitably brings sickness, because it ferments in the stomach to create a dangerous viscid and windy moisture, and draws the blood into the liver, which inevitably causes sickness and poisoning. This corrupt matter often forms a windy ulcer, and this is why many such ulcers form on the right side of the body rather than the left. And then man is epidemic [sic].

When the windy moisture has filled one place, it ascends via the jugular vein to the brain, and when it reaches the lungs it fills the pulmonary canals, stopping the movement of the lungs so that they cannot ventilate the heart to cool it. And then the heart grows hot, causing a pestilential fever, and that fever stirs up the humours, which erupt into internal and external ulcers, some of which are caused by the humours and others by wind. Then the brain, in sympathy with the heart because of its motion and sponginess, draws the windy and poisonous moisture from the lungs to itself and then ejects it through the ears. The sufferer experiences a terrific din, like a door being smashed down, which is caused by the primary windiness failing to escape, and then the victims die soon afterwards. But sometimes the brain expels the windy and poisonous matter via the optic nerves at the eyes. This is agony, and the sick man stares fixedly ahead, as if he cannot move his eyes. Amazingly, as it stands in the eyes, the primary windiness assumes the characteristics of a poisonous vapour, and seeks a new home in some other body, which it can enter and be at rest. And if a healthy person sees this visible vapour, he is stamped with the pestilential illness. The man is poisoned faster than air can leave the sick man, for the thin poison moves faster than the heavy air.

Take the example of the basilisk. Whenever one of these creatures chances upon a healthy person who is looking at it, a visible poisonous vapour passes from the eyes of the basilisk into the eye of the observer, and immediately, without warning, poisons him, or works upon him in some other way so that he is sure to die. And it is a characteristic of the basilisk that it always looks upon the brightest member, that is, the eye. Accordingly, someone who wants to capture a basilisk lights a lantern and sets it above his head, and holds something in front of his eyes, and then the basilisk will choose to look at the light and not at the eyes of his captor, and so can be grabbed and killed. This is also why the weasel, arming itself with rue leaves to protect its eyes, can boldly attack the serpent and kill it. Similarly, the book which Aristotle wrote for Alexander includes the story of a serving girl who was fed on poison by a queen who then sent her to Alexander to kill him by her look and embrace alone. When Aristotle saw the girl he knew by her eyes that she was poisonous and warned Alexander to stay away from her, which he did. They then made a stranger sleep with her, and he died immediately.

From this we may conclude that we should above all take precautions against the gaze and breath of people in the throes of illness. This explains why those in the company of the sick, or employed about them, die so quickly.... Therefore when a doctor, priest or friend wants to visit an invalid he should persuade him to close his eyes and then blindfold him with a linen cloth. When this has been done the visitor can treat him, listen to him and handle him in confidence, if he also holds a sponge soaked in vinegar to his nose in hot weather or, in cold weather, keeps his nose in a handful of rue and cummin. And let him also avoid the breath of the invalid.

62. The treatise of John of Burgundy, 1365

Medical treatises on the Black Death survive in huge numbers, many aimed explicitly at a non professional readership. That of John of Burgundy was one of the earliest, and was much copied.

In the translation which follows the ingredients of the remedies, but not the quantities, have been given.

Karl Sudhoff, 'Pestschriften aus den ersten 150 Jahren nach der Epidemie des 'schwarzen Todes' 1348: III', *Archiv für Geschichte der medizin* V, 1912, pp. 62-9.

Everything below the moon, the elements and the things compounded of the elements, is ruled by the things above, and the highest bodies are believed to give being, nature, substance, growth and death to everything below their spheres. It was, therefore, by the influence of the heavenly bodies that the air was recently corrupted and made pestilential. I do not mean by this that the air is corrupted in its substance – because it is an uncompounded substance and that would be impossible – but it is corrupted by reason of evil vapours mixed with it. The result was a widespread epidemic, traces of which still remain in several places. Many people have been killed, especially those stuffed full of evil humours, for the cause of the mortality is not only the corruption of the air, but the abundance of corrupt humours within those who die of the disease. For as Galen says in the book of fevers, the body suffers no corruption unless the material of the body has a tendency towards it, and is in some way subject to the corruptive cause; for just as fire only takes hold on combustible material, so pestilential air does no harm to a body unless it finds a blemish where corruption can take hold. As a result, cleansed bodies, where the purgation of evil humours has not been neglected, remain healthy. Likewise those whose complexion is contrary to the immutable complexion of air remain healthy.[31] For otherwise everybody would fall ill and die whenever the air is corrupted.

It follows that corrupt air generates different diseases in different people, depending on their different humours, because it always develops according to the predisposition of the matter it has entered. And therefore there are many masters of the art of medicine who are admirable scholars, well-versed in theories and hypotheses, but who are too little experienced in the practicalities and are entirely ignorant of astrology: a science vital to the physician, as Hippocrates testifies in his *Epidemia*, where he says that no one ought to be put under the care of any physician who is ignorant of astrology. For the arts of medicine and astrology balance each other, and in many respects one science supports the other in that one cannot be understood without the other. I am as a result convinced by practical experience that medicine – however well it has been compounded and chosen according to medical rules – does not work as the practitioner intends and is of no benefit to the patient if it is given when the planets are contrary. Thus if medicine is given as a laxative it should be with reference to the

---

31 The complexion is the balance of contraries within a body. Since air was hot and wet, people of a cold dry complexion were least susceptible to disease caused by poisoned air. The human complexion was thought to get colder and drier as the body aged, and so corrupted air was likely to be more damaging to the young.

planets if the patient is to empty his bowels successfully, and also if he is not to have an adverse reaction to the medicine. Accordingly those who have drunk too little of the nectar of astrology cannot offer a remedy for epidemic diseases. Because they are ignorant of the cause and quality of the disease they cannot cure it; for as the prince of doctors says: 'How can you cure, if you are ignorant of the cause?' And Avicenna in *Concerning the cure of fevers* emphasises: 'It is impossible that someone ignorant of the cause should cure the disease'. Averroes also makes this point, saying: 'It is not to be understood, except by grasping the immediate and ultimate cause'. Since, therefore, the heavens are the first cause, that is the cause it is necessary to understand, since ignorance of the highest cause entails ignorance of the subsequent cause, and also because the primary cause has a greater impact than the secondary cause.

It is accordingly obvious that physic is of little effect without astrology, and as a result of a lack of advice many succumb to disease. And therefore I, John of Burgundy, otherwise known as Bearded John, citizen of Liège and practitioner of the art of medicine, although the least of physicians, produced a treatise at the beginning of this epidemic on the causes and nature of corrupt air, of which many people acquired copies. I also published a treatise on the difference between epidemic and other illness. Anyone who has copies will find many things in these treatises about lifestyle and cures – but not everything about cures. Because the epidemic is now newly returned, and will return again in future because it has not yet run its course, and because I pity the carnage among mankind and support the common good and desire the health of all, and have been moved by a wish to help, I intend, with God's help, to set out more clearly in this schedule the prevention and cure of these illnesses, so that hardly anyone should have to resort to a physician but even simple folk can be their own physician, preserver, ruler and guide.

CONCERNING PREVENTION

First, you should avoid over-indulgence in food and drink, and also avoid baths and everything which might rarefy the body and open the pores, for the pores are the doorways through which poisonous air can enter, piercing the heart and corrupting the life force. Above all sexual intercourse should be avoided. You should eat little or no fruit, unless it is sour, and should consume easily-digested food and spiced wine diluted with water. Avoid mead and everything else made with honey, and season food with strong vinegar. In cold or rainy weather you should light fires in your chamber and in foggy or windy weather you should inhale aromatics every morning before leaving home: ambergris, musk, rosemary and similar things if you are rich; zedoary, cloves, nutmeg, mace and similar things if you are poor. Also once or twice a week you should take a dose of good theriac the size of a bean. And carry in the hand a ball of ambergris or other suitable aromatic. Later, on going to bed, shut the windows and burn juniper branches, so that the smoke and scent fills the room. Or put four live coals in an earthenware vessel and sprinkle a little of the following powder on them and inhale the smoke through mouth and nostrils before going to sleep: take white frankincense, labdanum, storax, calaminth, and wood of aloes and grind them to a very fine powder. And do this as often as a foetid or bad odour can be detected in the air, and especially when the weather is foggy or the air tainted, and it can protect against the epidemic.

If, however, the epidemic occurs during hot weather it becomes necessary to adopt another regimen, and to eat cold things rather than hot and also to eat more sparingly than in cold weather. You should drink more than you eat, and take white wine with water. You should also use large amounts of vinegar and verjuice in preparing food, but be sparing with hot substances such as pepper, galingale or grains of paradise. Before leaving home in the morning smell roses, violets, lilies, white and red sandalwood, musk or camphor if the weather is misty or the air quality bad. Take theriac sparingly in hot weather, and not at all unless you are a phlegmatic or of a cold complexion. Sanguines and cholerics should not take theriac at all in hot weather, but should take pomegranates, oranges, lemons, or quinces, or an electuary made of the three types of sandalwood, or a cold electuary or similar.[32] You should use cucumbers, fennel, borage, bugloss and spinach, and avoid garlic, onions, leeks and everything else which generates excessive heat, such as pepper or grains of paradise, although ginger, cinnamon, saffron, cummin and other temperate substances can be used. And if you should become extremely thirsty because of the hot weather, then drink cold water mixed with vinegar or barleywater regularly, for this is particularly beneficial to people of a cold and dry complexion and to thin people, and thirst should never be tolerated at such times.

---

32 An electuary is a paste made by mixing powdered ingredients with honey or some other syrupy substance. A cold electuary is one with a cold complexion, not one applied at a low temperature.

If you should feel a motion of the blood like a fluttering or prickling, let blood from the nearest vein on the same side of the body, and the floor of the room in which you are lying should be sprinkled two or three times a day with cold water and vinegar, or with rose water if you can afford it. The pills of Rasis, if taken once a week, are an outstanding preventative and work for all complexions and in all seasons, but Avicenna and others recommend that they should be taken on a full stomach. They loosen the bowels a little, but the corrupt humours are expelled gradually. They should be made as follows: take socotra aloes, saffron, myrrh and blend them in a syrup of fumitory. Anyone who adopts this regimen can be preserved, with God's help, from pestilence caused by corruption of the air.

CONCERNING THE CURE OF THE SWELLING

Now if anyone should contract epidemic disease for lack of a good regimen it is necessary to look at remedies and at how he should proceed, for these epidemic diseases take hold in twenty four hours and it is therefore vital to apply a remedy immediately. But first it should be understood that there are three principal members in the human body: the heart, the liver and the brain, and that each of these has its emunctory, where it expels its waste matter. Thus the armpits are the emunctories of the heart, the groin for the liver, and under the ears or beneath the tongue for the brain. Now it is necessary to know that it is the nature of poison to descend from the stomach, as is shown by the bite of a serpent or other venomous creature. And thus poisonous air, when it has been mixed with blood, immediately seeks the heart, the seat of nature, to attack it. The heart, sensing the injury, labours to defend itself, driving the poisoned blood to its emunctory. If then the venomous matter finds its way blocked, so that it cannot ascend back to the heart by some other path, it seeks another principal member, the liver, so that it can destroy that. The liver, fighting back, drives the resinous matter to its emunctory. In the same way it lays claim to the brain. By means of these events, which are signs to the physician, it is possible to tell where the poisonous matter is lurking and by what vein it ought to be drained.

For if the infected blood is driven to the armpits it can be deduced that the heart is oppressed and suffering, and so blood should be let immediately from the cardiac vein, but on the same side of the body, not the opposite side, for that would do double damage: firstly, the good and pure blood on the uncorrupted side would be drained away; secondly, the corrupt and poisoned blood would be thereby drawn to the healthy side of the body, with the result that the blood on both sides would become corrupted. What is worse, in the process the venomous blood would pass through the region of the heart and infect it, and thereby cause the rapid onset of illness. If, however, the patient feels prickings in the region of the liver, blood should be let immediately from the basilic vein of the right arm (that is the vein belonging to the liver, which is immediately below the vein belonging to the heart) or in the cephalic vein of the right hand, which is between the third and little fingers.

If the liver expels matter to the groin, and it becomes visible next to the privy member towards the inside of the leg, then a vein should be opened in the foot on the same side of the body, between the big toe and the toe next to it, for if blood was let in the arm it would again draw the matter to the heart, which would be a major error. If the poison manifests itself more towards the flank, and further from the genitals, then open a vein in the foot on the same side of the body between the little toe and the toe next to it, or the vein next to the ankle or heel of that foot, or scarify the leg next to the tumour with pitch.[33] If the poison appears at the emunctories of the brain, let blood from the cephalic vein above the median vein in the arm on the same side of the body, or from the vein in the hand between the thumb and index finger, or scarify the flesh with pitch between the shoulder blades.

When the blood has been extracted in this way, and the principal members purged, strengthen them with a cold electuary to offset any febrile cardiac inflammation. Make the electuary thus: take a preparation of roses including the three kinds of sandalwood, cold tragacanth, powder to encourage moistness, add candied rose petals and make an electuary in pill form, which should be taken several times by day and night. If you are poor, make a distilled water from dittany, pimpernel, tormentil and scabious by blending the herbs and mixing them with an equal quantity of water, and a spoonful of the mixture should be taken in summer. If the patient is choleric or sanguine, stir a pennyweight of camphor into the water until it is dissolved. If he is weak, six spoonsful should be taken in twenty four hours as soon as he feels himself

33 The reference is to the practice of cauterisation: the raising of blisters by the application of hot iron, acid or (as here) boiling pitch. The formation of liquid in the blisters was seen as a way of draining dangerous humours from the body, and medieval doctors equipped themselves with cautery charts, which showed them where blisters should be raised on the human body to treat particular diseases.

gripped by illness. In illnesses of this kind, this is the very best and surest medicine.

Diet in these illnesses should be as in the case of fevers, since the illness is always accompanied by fever. Therefore no meat should be eaten, except occasionally a small chicken poached in water and verjuice. Patients should eat small scaly fish, grilled on a gridiron with vinegar or verjuice, and soup of almonds, and drink barley water or small ale. If the patient demands wine, he should be given vinegar mixed with plenty of water. Occasionally, however, he can be given, to cheer him up, white wine diluted with plenty of water.

Place this plaster, called Emanuel, on the tumour. Take the root of the greater valerian, ammoniac, the root of dwarf elder, the root of *somerib* [unidentified], seeds of rue and oil of camomile. They should be bound together with a little wax and a touch of pine resin. And let the plaster be made like an ointment, but not too runny, and let it be renewed two or three times a day. For this ointment draws the venomous matter to itself, coagulates it and mortifies it, so that the matter is kept from approaching the principal members or harming them. If the tumour remained there for a lifetime, it would do no harm once it had been mortified. But if someone wants the swelling removed entirely let him place on it ripening and dissolving agents, with which all surgeons are amply provided.

Also anyone who wishes can use this powder, which is a powerful preventative, and is the very best medicine and cure, stronger in this respect than theriac. It is called the imperial powder, because gentile emperors used it against epidemic illness, poison and venom, and against the bite of serpents and other poisonous animals, and in Arabic it is called Bethzaer, which is to say 'a freeing from death'. Make this powder from these herbs: take St John's wort, dittany, tormentil, pimpernel, scabious, philadelphia, ammoniac, medicinal earth from Lemnos. Concerning this powder, I can say this, that I have proved it a hundred times and that however it is used – whether it is simply rubbed on or drunk with wine – it immediately clears the poison and expels it through the bite. Anybody can protect himself from all poisons and cure himself of snakebite as effectively as emptying the veins of blood. But few apothecaries are aware of these herbs, and nor do our authors make more than a brief mention of them, because they were not expert in such matters. And all the gentile physicians agree that however this powder is used, it makes it impossible to die of poison.

STATEMENT OF THE TIMES FOR BLOOD LETTING

Certain lords have sought from me a schedule of what ought to be known to perform bleeding, and whether it should be done immediately or on the first or second day, and they are the people to whom I have addressed these things concerning the onset of illness.

I say that these pestilential illnesses have a short and sudden beginning and a rapid development, and therefore in these illnesses those who wish to work a cure ought not to delay, and bleeding, which is the beginning of the cure, should not be put off until the first or second day. On the contrary, if someone can be found to do it, blood should be taken from the vein going from the seat of the diseased matter (that is, in the place where morbidity has appeared) in the very hour in which the patient was seized by illness. And if the bleeding cannot be done within the hour, at least let it be done within six hours, and if that is not possible then do not let the patient eat or drink until the bleeding has been done. But do not by any means delay the bleeding for longer than twelve hours, for if it is done within twelve hours, while the poisonous matter is still moving about the body, it will certainly save the patient. But if it is delayed until the illness is established, and then done, it will certainly do no harm but there is no certainty that it will rescue the patient from danger, for by then the bad blood will be so clotted and thickened that it will be scarcely able to flow from the vein. If, after the phlebotomy, the poisonous matter spreads again, the bleeding should be repeated in the same vein or in another going from the seat of the diseased matter. Afterwards three or five spoonsful of the herbal water, made as above, should be administered.

And if not as much as that is available, let one spoonful be given morning and evening, and one spoonful should always be given after consumption of the electuary described above, whether by day (when it can be given at any hour) or by night. Or let the patient be given this confection, which strengthens the heart, expels harmful flatulence from it and quenches fever. Take conserves of violets, roses, bugloss, borage and oranges, powdered roses and sandalwood, cold tragacanth, an electuary of the three sandalwoods, powder to encourage moistness, a cold electuary, camphor and candied roses, mix them together without applying heat and place them in a box, and if the patient is of a hot complexion, or if the fever is intense, add six or seven grains of camphor. If the patient is rich and can afford it, pearls, gold leaf, pure silver, jacinths, emeralds, and the bone from the heart of a stag should be added.[34] In the course of more than twenty four years of experience in places where the epidemic held sway it has been certainly and frequently demonstrated that such an electuary, together with the prescribed regimen, can save the patient from death. And many people have been cured by one bleeding alone, performed at the right time, without any other medicine. But where people delay bleeding beyond the development of the disease, it is doubtful whether it will lead to a cure or not. For while nature keeps the matter in motion, and the heart by its expulsive virtue drives the noisome and infected blood to its emunctory, phlebotomy should be performed because it helps nature, in that the extraction and evacuation of blood strengthens the expulsive virtue of the heart and diminishes the quantity of unhealthy matter, whereby nature is made more powerful against what remains and medicine becomes more efficacious.

I have never known anyone treated with this type of bleeding who has not escaped death, provided that he has looked after himself well and has received substances to strengthen his heart. As a result I make bold to say – not in criticism of past authorities, but out of long experience in the matter – that modern masters are more experienced in treating pestilential epidemic diseases than all the doctors and medical experts from Hippocrates downward. For none of them saw an epidemic reigning in their time, apart from Hippocrates in the city of *Craton* and that was short-lived. Nevertheless, he drew on what he had seen in his book on epidemics. However, Galen, Dioscorides, Rhazes 'Damascenus', Geber, Mesue, Copho, Constantine, Serapion, Avicenna, Algazel and all their successors never saw a general or long-lasting epidemic, or tested their cures by long experience; although they draw on the sayings of Hippocrates to discuss many things concerning epidemics. As a result, the masters of the present day are more practised in these diseases than their predecessors, for it is said, and with truth, that experience makes skill. Moved by piety and by pity for the destruction of men, I have accordingly compiled this compendium and have specified and set out the veins to bleed in these epidemic diseases, so that anyone may be his own physician. And because these illness run their course very quickly, and the poisonous matter rages through the body, let the bleeding be done without delay according to my advice, for in many cases delay brings danger.

34 Medieval authorities believed that such a bone 'is passing profitable against many evils of the body': M. C. Seymour (ed), *On the Properties of Things: John Trevisa's translation of Bartholomaeus Anglicus De Proprietatibus Rerum*, 3 vols, Oxford, 1975-88, II p. 1178.

I have composed and compiled this work not for money but for prayers, and so let anyone who has recovered from the disease pray strongly for me to our Lord God, to whom be the praise and glory throughout the whole world for ever and ever, amen. Here ends the valuable treatise of Master John of Burgundy against epidemic disease.

63. A fifteenth-century treatise on the pestilence

From a fifteenth-century compendium of medical and astrological texts, where it follows an English translation of John of Burgundy's treatise. The Latin is corrupt in places and some of my readings are speculative.

British Library, Sloane MS 965, fos. 143-5.

It should be known to all Christians that pestilence, and every other manifestation of God's vengeance, arises because of sin. It was for that reason that God first took vengeance in Heaven, when Lucifer fell; secondly in paradise, when Adam was driven out; thirdly throughout the whole world when all living things, except for those saved in Noah's ark, were destroyed in a cataclysm; fourthly when Sodom and Gomorrah were submerged by a river of fire; fifthly when Lot's wife was turned into a pillar of salt; sixthly when God took vengeance on the Egyptian pharoah and his people on numerous occasions, as can be found in the book of Exodus, and finally drowned him and his people in the Red Sea when he was pursuing Moses and Aaron and the children of Israel; seventhly when a powerful pestilence reigned in the land of David because it had not obeyed the commands of God, to which King Solomon referred: 'He that sweareth much shall be filled with iniquity: and a scourge shall not depart from his house' [Ecclesiasticus 23.12]. And it therefore follows from these examples that pestilence arises from a multitude of sins, but most especially from swearing worthless, deceitful and meaningless oaths.

If I am asked what is the cause of pestilence, what is its physical cause and by what means can someone save himself from it, I answer to the first question that sin is the cause, as set forth above. To the second question I say that it arises from the sea, as the evangelist says: 'There shall be signs in the sun and in the moon and in the stars; and upon the earth distress of nations, by reason of the confusion of the roaring of the sea and of the waves'.[35] For the devil, by the power committed to

35 Luke 21.25. This occurs in a list of the signs which will precede Christ's second coming and the end of the world.

him, when the seas rise up high, is voiding his poison, sending it forth
to be added to the poison in the air, and that air spreads gradually from
place to place and enters men through the ears, eyes, nose, mouth,
pores and the other orifices. Then if the man has a strong constitution,
nature can expel the poison through ulcers, and if the ulcers putrify,
are strangled and fully run their course the patient will be saved, as
can be clearly seen. But if the poison should be stronger than his
nature, so that his constitution cannot prevail against it, then the
poison instantly lays siege to the heart, and the patient dies within a
short time, without the relief which comes from the formation of
ulcers.

To the third question I say that during the pestilence everyone over
seven should be made to vomit daily from an empty stomach, and twice
a week, or more often if necessary, he should lie well wrapped up in a
warm bed and drink warm ale with ginger so that he sweats copiously,
and he should never touch the sheets after that until they have been
cleansed of the sweat, for if the person sweating had been in contact
with the pestilence a healthy man could catch the plague from the
sheets unless they have been well washed. And as soon as he feels an
itch or prickling in his flesh he must use a goblet or cupping horn to
let blood and draw down the blood from the heart, and this should be
done two or three times at intervals of one or two days at most.[36] And
if he should feel himself oppressed deep within the body, then he
should let blood in the nearest veins, either in the arms or in the main
veins of the feet. Likewise something which is extremely poisonous in
itself may be of service in excluding the plague. And if a healthy adult
does as I have described, they can save themselves whenever a great
pestilence occurs.

64. Ordinances against the spread of plague, Pistoia, 1348

These are the fullest extant civic ordinances, and are particularly interesting
in that they show the city rethinking and amending its strategy as the plague
developed. The sections translated below are primarily concerned with
preventing the spread of infection. A fourth set of ordinances, not printed
here, addresses the problem of providing for the defence of the city given the
much reduced population. The translation omits the preambles and the

---

36 Cupping involved placing heated cups, or special cupping horns, mouth downwards
   on the skin. As the air inside cooled and contracted the suction it created was
   thought to draw bad humours to the surface of the skin, where they could more
   easily be removed by bleeding or some other method.

concluding formalities of each set of ordinances, and also slightly abbreviates the text by reducing some of the formalities and repetitions. In particular note that references to Pistoia and other cities always include the *contado* (the adjoining countryside over which the town ruled) and district as well as the city itself; and that the penalties are to be levied on each offender for every breach of the ordinances.

A. Chiappelli (ed), 'Gli Ordinamenti Sanitari del Comune di Pistoia contro la Pestilenza del 1348', *Archivio Storico Italiano*, series 4, XX, 1887, pp. 8-22.

[2 May, 1348]

1. So that the sickness which is now threatening the region around Pistoia shall be prevented from taking hold of the citizens of Pistoia, no citizen or resident of Pistoia, wherever they are from or of what condition, status or standing they may be, shall dare or presume to go to Pisa or Lucca; and no one shall come to Pistoia from those places; penalty 500 pence. And no one from Pistoia shall receive or give hospitality to people who have come from those places; same penalty. And the guards who keep the gates of the city of Pistoia shall not permit anyone travelling to the city from Pisa or Lucca to enter; penalty 10 pence from each of the guards responsible for the gate through which such an entry has been made. But citizens of Pistoia now living within the city may go to Pisa and Lucca, and return again, if they first obtain permission from the common council – who will vote on the merits of the case presented to them. The licence is to be drawn up by the notary of the *anziani* and gonfalonier of the city.[37] And this ordinance is to be upheld and observed from the day of its ratification until 1 October, or longer if the council sees fit.

2. No one, whether from Pistoia or elsewhere, shall dare or presume to bring or fetch to Pistoia, whether in person or by an agent, any old linen or woollen cloths, for male or female clothing or for bedspreads; penalty 200 pence, and the cloth to be burnt in the public piazza of Pistoia by the official who discovered it.[38] However it shall be lawful

37 The official rulers of Italian cities were the commune (a word which does not have its modern egalitarian connotations). They appointed a *podestà*, often a nobleman from outside the region, as their salaried chief executive. By the fourteenth century this arrangement was mirrored in many cities by the more broadly based *popolo*, represented by a governing council of *anziani* (elders). The *capitano del popolo* corresponded, in background and role, to the *podestà* of the commune.

38 Later outbreaks of plague in Italian cities were often associated with the movement of cloth, and this requirement suggests that the connection may already have been noted. Contemporaries – who were not aware of the role played by fleas in the transmission of the disease – explained the connection as due to the trapping of corrupt air within the folds of fabric.

for citizens of Pistoia travelling within Pistoia and its territories to take linen and woollen cloths with them for their own use or wear, provided that they are in a pack or fardle weighing 30 lb or less. And this ordinance to be upheld and observed from the day of its ratification until 1 January. And if such cloth has already been brought into Pistoia, the bringer must take it away within three days of the ordinance's ratification; same penalty.

3. The bodies of the dead shall not be removed from the place of death until they have been enclosed in a wooden box, and the lid of planks nailed down[39] so that no stench can escape, and covered with no more than one pall, coverlet or cloth; penalty 50 pence to be paid by the heirs of the deceased or, if there are no heirs, by the nearest kinsmen in the male line. The goods of the deceased are to stand as surety for the payment of the penalty. Also the bodies are to be carried to burial in the same box; same penalty. So that the civic officals can keep a check on this, the rectors of the chapels in Pistoia must notify the *podestà* and *capitano* when a corpse is brought into their chapel, giving the dead man's name and the contrada in which he was living when he died; same penalty. As soon as he has been notified, the *podestà* or *capitano* must send an official to the place, to find out whether this chapter of the ordinances is being observed, along with the other regulations governing funerals, and to punish those found guilty. And if the *podestà* or *capitano* is remiss in carrying out these orders he must be punished by those who appointed him; same penalty. But these regulations should not apply to the poor and destitute of the city, who are dealt with under another civic ordinance.

4. To avoid the foul stench which comes from dead bodies each grave shall be dug two and a half armslength deep, as this is reckoned in Pistoia;[40] penalty 10 pence from anyone digging or ordering the digging of a grave which infringes the statute.

5. No one, of whatever condition, status or standing, shall dare or presume to bring a corpse into the city, whether coffined or not; penalty 25 pence. And the guards at the gates shall not allow such bodies to be brought into the city; same penalty, to be paid by every guard responsible for the gate through which the body was brought.

---

39 The bodies of ordinary people were generally buried in shrouds, although they might be carried to church in a coffin. This ordinance probably implies that they were to be buried in a coffin, as people certainly had to be in Tournai [6].

40 A *bracchio* in Pistoia measured between two and two and a half feet.

6. Any person attending a funeral shall not accompany the corpse or its kinsmen further than the door of the church where the burial is to take place, or go back to the house where the deceased lived, or to any other house on that occasion; penalty 10 pence. Nor is he to go the week's mind of the deceased; same penalty.[41]

7. When someone dies, no one shall dare or presume to give or send any gift to the house of the deceased, or to any other place on that occasion, either before or after the funeral, or to visit the house, or eat there on that occasion; penalty 25 pence. This shall not apply to the sons and daughters of the deceased, his blood brothers and sisters and their children, or to his grandchildren. The *podestà* and *capitano*, when notified by the rector as in chapter 3, must send an official to enquire whether anything has been done to the contrary and to punish those responsible.

8. To avoid waste and unnecessary expense, no one shall dare or presume to wear new clothes during the mourning period or for the next eight days; penalty 25 pence. This shall not apply to the wife of the deceased, who may if she wishes wear a new garment of any fabric without penalty.

9. No crier, summoner or drummer of Pistoia shall dare or presume to invite or summon any citizen of Pistoia, whether publicly or privately, to come to a funeral or visit the corpse; nor shall anyone send the same summoner, trumpeter, crier or drummer; penalty 10 pence from each crier, trumpeter, summoner or drummer, and from the people by whom they have been employed.

10. So that the sound of bells does not trouble or frighten the sick, the keepers of the campanile of the cathedral church of Pistoia shall not allow any of the bells to be rung during funerals, and no one else shall dare or presume to ring any of the bells on such occasions; penalty 10 pence, to be paid by the keepers who allowed the bells to be rung and by the heirs of the dead man, or his kinsmen should he have no heirs. When a parishioner is buried in his parish church, or a member of a fraternity within the fraternity church, the church bells may be rung, but only on one occasion and not excessively; same penalty.

11. No one shall presume or dare to summon a gathering of people to escort a widow from the house of her dead husband, but only from the

41 This last sentence refers to a ban on attendance at the commemorative mass one week after a death.

church to his burial place. But it shall be lawful for the widow's kinsmen to send up to four women to escort the widow from her husband's house at other times. No one shall dare to attend such a gathering; penalty 25 pence, paid by those invited and by those who issued the invitation.

12. No one shall dare or presume to raise a lament or crying for anyone who has died outside Pistoia, or summon a gathering of people other than the kinsfolk and spouse of the deceased, or have bells rung, or use criers or any other means to invite people throughout the city to such a gathering; penalty 25 pence from each person involved.

However it is to be understood that none of this applies to the burial of knights, doctors of law, judges, and doctors of physic, whose bodies can be honoured by their heirs at their burial in any way they please.

13. So that the living are not made ill by rotten and corrupt food, no butcher or retailer of meat shall dare or presume to hang up meat, or keep and sell meat hung up in their storehouse or over their counter; penalty 10*d*.[42] And that the rulers of the craft of butchery must investigate these matters on every day when slaughtering occurs, and immediately denounce any offenders to the lords, *podestà* or *capitano*, or to one of their officials; same penalty from the rulers of the craft if they fail to carry out these things in person or by deputy. The *podestà* and *capitano* must each send someone to look into these matters, and punish those found guilty, along with the rulers of the craft if they have failed to denounce them. The word of any official who finds an infringement of the regulations shall be taken as sufficient evidence.

14. Butchers and retailers of meat shall not stable horses or allow any mud or dung in the shop or other place where they sell meat, or in or near their storehouse, or on the roadway outside; nor shall they slaughter animals in a stable, or keep flayed carcasses in a stable or in any other place where there is dung; penalty 10 pence. An official of the *podestà* or *capitano* is to enquire closely into such matters, and his word is to be taken on any infringement of these ordinances.

15. No butcher or retailer of meat shall dare or presume to keep on the counter where he sells meat, meat from more than one ox, calf, or cow

---

42 The word I have translated as 'to hang up' is *gonfiare* which, in modern Italian, means to swell or blow up. This might suggest that butchers were being forbidden to sell carcasses already distended by the gases generated by corruption, but the phrasing seems to suggest that it is the display of carcasses which is being banned. Perhaps both implications are present: that to minimise the risk of corruption *whole* carcasses are not to be displayed, but only joints of meat.

at once, although he can keep the meat of an ox or cow alongside that of a calf; penalty 10 pence. The rulers of the craft must investigate the matter on every day on which animals are slaughtered, and denounce any offenders to the *podesta* or *capitano* of the city; same penalty.

16. In May, June, July and August butchers and retailers of meat shall slaughter meat on the days on which meat can be eaten, including Sundays and feast days, and sell it on the same day to those wishing to buy; the animals to be vetted by the civic officials appointed for the purpose.[43]

17. No butcher or retailer shall dare or presume to kill any ox, cow or calf without first obtaining permission from officials of the *podestà* or *capitano*. As soon as the official's approval has been requested he shall go and see the animal, to decide whether it is healthy or not. When permission has been given the butcher himself must slaughter the animal properly in the official's presence; penalty 10 pence.

18. No butcher or any other retailer of meat shall kill any two- or three-year old boar or sow between 1 March and 1 December; penalty 25 pence.

19. Butchers or retailers shall flay every two- or three-year old boar or sow killed between 1 December and 1 March before putting it on sale. If they wish to salt it down, that is permissible, but it must be flayed first; penalty 25 pence.

20. [Provisions for the election of officials to set the retail price of meat.]

21. For the better preservation of health, there should be a ban on all kinds of poultry, calves, foodstuffs and on all kinds of fat being taken out of Pistoia by anybody; penalty 100 pence and the confiscation of the things being carried contrary to the ban. And whoever can capture such carriers and the things carried, and take them to the gaol of the commune of Pistoia shall have half of the fine and of the value of the goods, after the fine has been paid and the goods sold to the highest bidder.

22. To avoid harm to men by stink and corruption, there shall in future be no tanning of skins within the city walls of Pistoia; penalty 25 pence.

23. [Provisions for enforcement including the proviso that anyone can

43 In other words, the importance of ensuring a supply of fresh meat meant that slaughtering could take place on days when it was usually banned.

denounce an offender before the *podestà* or *capitano*, and receive a quarter of the fine if the accusation is upheld; the word of one man worthy of belief is to be sufficient evidence of guilt, or the statements of four men testifying to the common belief.]

[Revisions of 23 May]

Chapter 1 to be entirely revoked.

Chapter 19 to continue: After the pigs have been shaved or singed the butcher or retailer must flay them before taking them to his home or storeroom; once flayed it is permissible for him to take the carcasses into his storeroom or house, but otherwise not; penalty as specified in chapter 19.

Chapter 21 to be entirely revoked and replaced with: There should be a ban on all kinds of poultry, goats and sheep, and no one shall take them or cause them to be taken out of the contada of Pistoia; penalty 5 pence, to be put to the common use by the *podestà* or *capitano*. And anyone who is able to capture someone doing the contrary, and deliver them to the gaol of the commune of Pistoia shall have half the penalty.

Chapter 22 to be amended by the addition of: That skinners and tanners shall be allowed to tan skins as at present in their tanneries from the day on which these ordinances are ratified until 15 June. Moreover tanneries shall be permitted within the walls of the city, but only in the following places: in the houses along the road which goes from the house of the canons of Pistoia at the chapel of Santa Maria del Nuova to the gate of San Pietro, and in that contrado, and on the land outside the gate. And in those places they may peg out skins and do everything else necessary to tanning, as they wish. And this may also be done below the Castell Traiecti up to the Carmelite friary and in the houses, gardens and grounds round about. And if anyone does the contrary, let him be punished or fined as in the said chapter.

It is also provided and ordained that:

24. So that no corruption or stench should harm people's bodies, within the city the rendering down of dripping or suet should be done in houses at least 25 arms length from their neighbours and nowhere else; penalty 25 pence.

25. That the tanning of gut, to make strings, shall only be done outside the city; penalty 25 pence.[44]

---

44 Animal entrails were tanned and twisted ('spun') to form various types of cord, including the strings for musical instruments and tennis rackets. The generic term

[26-28 Three chapters regulating the meat trade in the city and region.]

29. The *podestà* and *capitano* shall make enquiry into all the matters contained here, and also act on accusations and denunciations made by anyone else before them, and punish and fine offenders as set out above.

[Revisions of 4 June]

30. At the burial of anyone no bell is to be rung at all, but people are to be summoned and their prayers invited only by word of mouth; penalty 25 pence from the heirs or next of kin of the deceased.

31. When the corpse has been carried to the church, everyone who accompanied it there ought to withdraw, and when the next of kin leave no one ought to accompany them except their spouses and the neighbours, and also the dead man's next of kin on his mother's side. These people may go to the house of the dead man, or wherever the body is, but may not enter the building. 'Neighbours' are to be understood as people who lived within 50 arms length of the dead man during his lifetime; penalty 25 pence.

32. The *anziani* and gonfalonier shall choose at least sixteen men from each quarter of the city, and repeat the process as often as seems necessary to maintain the number. These men are to take corpses from houses or dwellings and carry them to church and to burial, and no one else shall dare to enter a house or other place in which a person has died or carry the body to burial; penalty 25 pence. And anybody who asks someone else to remove or carry a corpse shall incur the same penalty. Those who carry the corpse shall have 16 pence between them for their labour, the money to be paid from public funds; and the chamberlains of the commune of Pistoia shall make the payment within two days of the burial; penalty 25 pence. A written receipt from one of the brethren of the place where the burial occurred, or from a priest or one of the keepers of the fabric of the church where the burial took place, or from the rector of the hospital if the burial was at a hospital, is to be taken as sufficient proof that the portering was carried out. And it shall be sufficient for the receipt to say: I, N, have written this. The men chosen and appointed to act as porters must go

---

for the product was catgut, although cats were not, in fact, the source of most of the gut used. As this regulation implies, the process was thought more noxious than the tanning of skins, which could still be carried out within the city walls during the plague.

when anybody asks them, and if they refuse they are to be punished with a fine of 10 pence. An oath on the sacrament by the person who made the request is to be taken as sufficient proof of their refusal.

However, the *disciplinati*[45] of a particular society in the city, who wear the garments of *disciplinati*, shall be allowed to remove and carry the bodies of the dead if this is done without charge, for the good of their souls; for certain good men, in search of salvation, have made themselves porters of the bodies of the poor and destitute, and they shall be allowed to enter houses and other places and take the bodies to burial whenever they wish.

33. Since wax for honouring the corpses of the dead cannot be found on sale, candles are not to be given, but instead it shall be permissible for anyone to give between 6 and 12 pence, at most, as he sees fit to each priest and friar who attends a funeral, in lieu of the candles and money which they were accustomed to give. But canons of the great church of Pistoia, prebendaries, priors, wardens and provosts of churches and of the orders of friars of Pistoia may be given twice that amount; penalty 25 pence.

34. The keepers of the fabric of each church in the city shall keep a supply of wax torches to be carried at the burial and to be held, alight, while the corpse is buried. And no other torches or wax lights should be held or carried at a burial; penalty 25 pence. And after the burial the torches shall be taken back and restored to the keepers, and they shall be reimbursed at the going rate for the wax used, with an additional 5 pence for the good of the dead person's soul.

35. For the support of the church where burial takes place, and of the rector of the church where the dead man was a parishioner, when the burial is in a friary church the friars should be given between 16 and 20 pence in lieu of candles; and the same should be given to the rector of the church where the dead man was a parishioner. And if he is buried in his parish church, the rector should be given the same amount, and so should the keepers of the fabric. However, it shall be left to the discretion of the friars, rectors and keepers of the fabric to take less from the poor and destitute, depending on the status of the deceased.

36. [The *podestà* and *capitano* and their officials should enquire into these matters weekly and punish those doing the contrary; penalty 50 pence. Anyone can bring an accusation before them.]

45 *Disciplinati* were members of a penitential fraternity; in this case, those who had taken on the role of burying the dead.

These ordinances are to be observed until 1 September, or until 1 November at the discretion of the *anziani* and gonfalonier. Saving that anything in them which is contrary to the liberty of the church shall be null and void, and of no effect.

65. Plague regulations of Bernabò Visconti, lord of Milan, 1374

Chronicon Regiense, ed. L. A. Muratori, *Rerum Italicarum Scriptores* XVIII, Milan, 1731, col.82.

Wishing, as far as we can, to preserve our subjects from contagious illness, we have made certain decrees which we send to you enclosed in this, and which we wish to be observed in Reggio and to be enrolled in the volume of our statutes. Milan, 17 January 1374.

To the noble man, the *podestà* of Reggio. We wish that each person who displays a swelling or tumour shall immediately leave the city, castle or town where he is and take to the open country, living either in huts or in the woods, until he either dies or recovers.

Item, those in attendance upon someone who died shall wait ten days before returning to human society.

Item, parish priests shall examine the sick to see what the illness is, and shall immediately notify the designated searchers under pain of being burnt alive.

Item, all the goods, both movable and immovable, shall be put to the use of the lord's treasury.

Item, the goods of anyone who carries the epidemic from another place shall likewise be put to the use of the lord's treasury, and no restitution shall be made.

Item, under pain of forfeiture and death no one shall enter service from attending upon the sick, except as above.

Let all our subjects be informed of these matters.

66. London butchery regulations, 1371

This attempt to ban the dumping of entrails and blood within the city of London is justified in terms of the diseases which arise from corrupt air, and was presumably a deliberate attempt to play upon public anxieties about the plague. It was not, however, a serious attempt to prevent the spread of disease – and two major city shambles were almost immediately exempted from its operation. Two years earlier, in the plague year of 1369, an attempt to stop the butchers of St Nicholas Shambles dumping offal in the river had made no specific reference to the risk of disease, but only to the 'corruption, and grievous stenches, and abominable sights' which assailed residents along the butchers' route from the shambles to the river.

H. T. Riley, *Memorials of London and London Life in the XIIIth XIVth and XVth Centuries*, London, 1868, pp. 356-8 [note: I have modernised Riley's translation to bring it into line with the style of the other translations in this volume].

Edward by the grace of God etc to the mayor and sheriffs of London, greeting. The air in the city has lately been greatly corrupted and infected by the slaughtering of animals in the city, because of the putrefied blood running in the streets and the dumping of entrails in the river Thames, and as a result appalling abominations and stenches have been produced, and sicknesses and other maladies have befallen residents and visitors to the city. Wishing to take precautions against such dangers, and to provide for the decency of the city and the safety of our subjects, we ordained in our parliament at Westminster, with the assent of our council, that all oxen, sheep, swine and other large animals slaughtered for the provision of our city should be taken to Stratford le Bow on one side, and Knightsbridge on the other and slaughtered there, and their entrails cleaned; and if any butcher rashly presumed to do the contrary, the meat and animals should be forfeited and he should be imprisoned for a year. And we ordered that you should make public proclamation of the said ordinance in the places you thought appropriate, and should see that it was observed and punish all butchers doing the contrary.

Afterwards, we were informed by our judges, chancery clerks and other officers, as well as by other reputable men living in Fleet Street, Holborn and Smithfield in the suburbs of the city, that certain city butchers, ignoring the ordinance and proclamation, had subsequently slaughtered large animals within the city and dumped the blood and entrails in various places near Holborn Bridge and elsewhere in the suburbs, and as a result of that abomination and the stenches which infected the air, sickness and other maladies had befallen our officers and other residents and visitors, and would subsequently befall them too, unless some remedy could be devised. We accordingly ordered you frequently to have the ordinance publicly proclaimed in the city and suburbs, and to see that it was observed, and punish all butchers offending against it, or else to tell us why you neglected our frequent commands. We have heard that you have not bothered to do these things, or even to tell us why not, in manifest contempt of us and our commands, and to the considerable damage and annoyance of our officers and others. We greatly marvel at this, and now order you again to have the ordinance publicly proclaimed in the city and suburbs, in such places as you think best, and that you punish all butchers doing the contrary, or that you appear before us in person, wherever we happen to be within England, within three weeks of Michaelmas next.

Westminster, 26 September 1371.

67. Parliamentary statute of 1388

The 1388 parliament met in Cambridge, and this statute may well have been prompted by the notorious state of the King's Ditch which surrounded the city and was not scoured by a proper flow of water.

A. Luders *et al* (ed), *Statutes of the Realm 1101-1713*, 11 vols., London, 1810-28, pp. 59-60.

Because so much dung and other ordure – the offal and entrails of slaughtered animals – along with other filth is thrown and dumped into ditches, rivers and other waters, and also in many other places within or near various cities, boroughs and towns and their suburbs, with the result that the air there is greatly corrupted and infected, and many illnesses and other intolerable diseases daily befall both the inhabitants and residents of the said cities, boroughs and towns, and others visiting or passing through them, to the great harm, damage and danger of the said inhabitants, residents, visitors and travellers, it is accorded and agreed that it is to be proclaimed within the city of London and as necessary within other cities, boroughs and towns within the realm, within franchises as well as outside them, that everybody who throws or dumps such harmful matter, dung, offal, entrails and other ordure into ditches, rivers, waters or other places should be responsible for having it completely cleaned up, removed and carried away, between now and the Michaelmas following the end of this parliament, upon pain of £20 payable to the king; and that the mayors and bailiffs of every such city, borough and town, and the bailiffs of franchises, should enforce it under the same penalty. And if anyone objects that this has not been carried out in the manner described, let him complain to the chancellor after Michaelmas and he shall have a writ compelling the person complained of to come into Chancery to show why the said penalty should not be levied upon him, and if he cannot duly excuse himself the penalty shall be levied upon him. And it shall also be proclaimed in the city of London and in the other cities, boroughs and towns that no one, regardless of status, shall cause any such harmful matter, offal, dung, entrails and ordure to be dumped or thrown into the aforesaid ditches, rivers, waters and other places, and if anyone does so he shall be summoned by writ before the chancellor, at the suit of whoever has made complaint, and if he is found guilty he shall be punished at the chancellor's discretion.

V: Human agency

68. Well-poisoning

A brief contemporary account by a Franciscan friar from Franconia, Herman Gigas. His chronicle ends in 1349.

J. G. Meuschen (ed), *Hermanni Gygantis, ordinis fratrum minorum, Flores Temporum seu Chronicon Universale ab Orbe condito ad annum Christi MCCCXLIX*, Leiden, 1750, pp. 138-9.

In 1347 there was such a great pestilence and mortality throughout almost the whole world that in the opinion of well-informed men scarcely a tenth of mankind survived. The victims did not linger long, but died on the second or third day. The plague raged so fiercely that many cities and towns were entirely emptied of people. In the cities of Bologna, Venice, Montpellier, Avignon, Marseilles and Toulouse alike, a thousand people died in one day, and it still rages in France, Normandy, England and Ireland. Some say that it was brought about by the corruption of the air; others that the Jews planned to wipe out all the Christians with poison and had poisoned wells and springs everywhere. And many Jews confessed as much under torture: that they had bred spiders and toads in pots and pans, and had obtained poison from overseas; and that not every Jew knew about this wickedness, only the more powerful ones, so that it would not be betrayed. As evidence of this heinous crime, men say that bags full of poison were found in many wells and springs, and as a result, in cities, towns and villages throughout Germany, and in fields and woods too, almost all the wells and springs have been blocked up or built over, so that no one can drink from them or use the water for cooking, and men have to use rain or river water instead. God, the lord of vengeance, has not suffered the malice of the Jews to go unpunished. Throughout Germany, in all but a few places, they were burnt. For fear of that punishment many accepted baptism and their lives were spared. This action was taken against the Jews in 1349, and it still continues unabated, for in a number of regions many people, noble and humble alike, have laid plans against them and their defenders which they will never abandon until the whole Jewish race has been destroyed.

69. The persecution of the Jews

The author of this account, Heinrich Truchess (or *dapifer*) von Diessenhoven, was a canon of Constance who had been a chaplain of Pope John XXII (d.1334).

J. F. Boehmer (ed), *Fontes Rerum Germanicarum*, 4 vols, Stuttgart, 1843-68, IV pp. 68-71.

The persecution of the Jews began in November 1348, and the first outbreak in Germany was at Sölden, where all the Jews were burnt on the strength of a rumour that they had poisoned wells and rivers, as was afterwards confirmed by their own confessions and also by the confessions of Christians whom they had corrupted and who had been induced by the Jews to carry out the deed. And some of the Jews who were newly baptised said the same. Some of these remained in the faith but some others relapsed, and when these were placed upon the wheel[1] they confessed that they had themselves sprinkled poison or poisoned rivers. And thus no doubt remained of their deceitfulness which had now been revealed.

Within the revolution of one year, that is from All Saints [1 November] 1348 until Michaelmas [29 September] 1349 all the Jews between Cologne and Austria were burnt and killed for this crime, young men and maidens and the old along with the rest. And blessed be God who confounded the ungodly who were plotting the extinction of his church, not realising that it is founded on a sure rock and who, in trying to overturn it, crushed themselves to death and were damned for ever.

But now let us follow the killings individually. First Jews were killed or burnt in Sölden in November, then in Zofingen they were seized and some put on the wheel, then in Stuttgart they were all burnt. The same thing happened during November in Landsberg, a town in the diocese of Augsburg and in Bueron, Memmingen and Burgau in the same diocese. During December they were burnt and killed on the feast of St Nicholas [6 December] in Lindau, on 8 December in Reutlingen, on 13 December in Haigerloch, and on 20 December in Horw they were burnt in a pit. And when the wood and straw had been consumed, some Jews, both young and old, still remained half alive. The stronger of them snatched up cudgels and stones and dashed out the brains of those trying to creep out of the fire, and thus compelled

---

1 Breaking on the wheel was a form of torture.

those who wanted to escape the fire to descend to hell. And the curse seemed to be fulfilled: 'his blood be upon us and upon our children'.[2] On 27 December the Jews in Esslingen were burnt in their houses and in the synagogue. In *Nagelten* they were burnt. In the abovesaid town of Zofingen the city councillors, who were hunting for poison, found some in the house of a Jew called Trostli, and by experiment were satisfied that it was poison. As a result, two Jewish men and one woman were put on the wheel, but others were saved at the command of Duke Albrecht of Austria, who ordered that they should be protected. But this made little difference, for in the course of the next year those he had under his protection were killed, and as many again in the diocese of Constance. But first those burnt in 1349 will be described in order.

Once started, the burning of the Jews went on increasing. When people discovered that the stories of poisoning were undoubtedly true they rose as one against the Jews. First, on 2 January 1349 the citizens of Ravensburg burnt the Jews in the castle, to which they had fled in search of protection from King Charles, whose servants were imprisoned by the citizens after the burning. On 4 January the people of Constance shut up the Jews in two of their own houses, and then burnt 330 of them in the fields at sunset on 3 March. Some processed to the flames dancing, others singing and the rest weeping. They were burnt shut up in a house which had been specially built for the purpose. On 12 January in Buchen and on 17 January in Basel they were all burnt apart from their babies, who were taken from them by the citizens and baptised. They were burnt on 21 January in Messkirch and Waldkirch, on 25 January in Speyer, and on 30 January in Ulm, on 11 February in Überlingen, on 14 February in the city of Strassburg (where it took six days to burn them because of the numbers involved), on 16 February in Mengen, on 19th of the month in Sulgen, on 21st in Schaffhausen and Zurich, on 23rd in St Gallen and on 3 March in Constance, as described above, except for some who were kept back to be burnt on the third day after the Nativity of the Virgin [11 September].

They were killed and burnt in the town of Baden on 18 March, and those in the castle below, who had been brought there from Rheinfelden for protection, were killed and then burnt. And on 30 May

2 Matthew 27.24: the people's response to Pilate's statement, 'I am innocent of the blood of this just man [Christ]. Look you to it'.

they were similarly wiped out in Radolfzell. In Mainz and Cologne they were burnt on 23 August. On 18 September 330 Jews were burnt in the castle at Kyburg, where they had gathered from Winterthur and Diessenhoven and the other towns of their protector the Duke of Austria. But the imperial citizens did not want to go on supporting them any longer, and so they wrote to Duke Albrecht of Austria, who was protecting his Jewish subjects in the counties of Pfirt, Alsace and Kyburg, and told him that either he had them burnt by his own judges or they would burn them themselves. So the Duke ordered them to be burnt by his own judges, and they were finally burnt on 18 September.

And thus, within one year, as I said, all the Jews between Cologne and Austria were burnt – and in Austria they await the same fate, for they are accursed of God. And I could believe that the end of the Hebrews had come, if the time prophesied by Elias and Enoch were now complete; but since it is not complete, it is necessary that some be reserved so that what has been written may be fulfilled: that the hearts of the sons shall be turned to their fathers, and of the fathers to the sons.[3] But in what parts of the world they may be reserved I do not know, although I think it more likely that the seed of Abraham will be reserved in lands across the sea than in these people. So let me make an end of the Jews here.[4]

70. Measures taken against the Jews in Lausanne

This and the following two texts are taken from material in the Strassburg archives. The city (in common with other towns, see also 72 and 74) wrote round to neighbouring cities enquiring whether they had evidence that

---

3 A reference to Malachias 4.5-6: 'Behold I will send you Elias the prophet, before the coming of the great and dreadful day of the lord. And he shall turn the heart of the fathers to the children and the hearts of the children to their fathers: lest I come and strike the earth with anathema'.

This text was taken to mean that after the coming of Antichrist the prophets Enoch and Elias would reconvert the apostates as a preliminary to the second coming of Christ and the Last Judgement. At the same time they would convert the Jews to Christianity. Heinrich's point is that because the second coming is not yet imminent, contemporary Jews could not be entirely wiped out or converted, because some had to survive to be converted by Enoch and Elias in the Last Days.

4 The sentence is ambiguous and, given the anti-semitism of the author, probably deliberately so. Its surface meaning is that he has come to the end of the two chapters devoted to the Jews and is now about to turn to other matters. But it could also be taken to mean that he hopes to see the extermination of the Jews in Europe, as there are likely to be enough elsewhere to meet the prophetic conditions laid down for Christ's second coming (see note 3 above).

Jews were poisoning wells, and what steps they were taking against the perpetrators. The city received eleven replies in all. The formal courtesies at the beginning and end of the letters have been omitted here.

Urkunden und Akten der Stadt Strassburg: Urkundenbuch der Stadt Strassburg, V, Strassburg 1896, pp. 164–5.

Rodolphe d'Oron, knight, lord of *Artales*, bailiff of Lausanne, and Michel de Vevey, esquire, *sautier* of Lausanne[5] on behalf of the citizens of Lausanne, to Conrad von Winterthur, the bürghermeister of Strassburg, and the city councillors. Lausanne, the Saturday after St Martin in winter [15 Nov, 1348].

We have received your gracious letters with pleasure, and have accordingly sent you in writing under our seals the confessions made by a Jew called Bona Dies. He was condemned to be set on the wheel, where he survived for four days and nights. While he could still speak he held unvaryingly to his first story. And we have informed you that in the lordship of the Count of Savoy many Jews, and Christians as well, have confessed to the same appalling crime. Accordingly they were condemned to punishment by burning and impalement.[6] The confessions they made have been communicated to our friends the officials and councillors of Bern and Fribourg at their request.

71. Examination of the Jews captured in Savoy

The confessions extracted by torture from a group of Jews living in the county of Savoy were evidently widely circulated as evidence of an international conspiracy. Unidentified place names have been printed in italics.

Strassburg Urkundenbuch, pp. 167–74.

The Castellan of Chillon, deputy of the bailiff of Chablis there, to the officials, councillors and citizens of Strassburg.

I understand that you want to know about the confessions of the Jews and the proofs brought against them. I am writing to tell you that the people of Bern have a copy of the inquisition and confession of the Jews dwelling in their neighbourhood who were involved in putting poison into the wells there and in several other places, and that that copy

---

5 Lausanne was largely under the control of its bishop. The bailiff headed the civic hierarchy; the *sautier* was a judicial official. In the published list of officers the name of the *sautier* is given as Michod de Vennes: M. Reymond, *Les Dignitaires de L'Église Notre-Dame de Lausanne jusqu'en 1536*, Lausanne, 1912, p. 130.

6 The word used is *scitote*, which is perhaps related to the Italian *stichata*, a palisade.

contains a detailed acount of the truth of the matter. Many Jews have been tried after being put to the question or, in some cases, making confession without it, and have been condemned to be burnt. Some Christians, to whom Jews gave poison for use against Christians, have also been put on the wheel and tortured. For the burning of Jews and the torturing of Christians has gone on in numerous places within the county of Savoy. May God keep you.

The confession made on the 15 September 1348, in the castle of Chillon, by the Jews of Villeneuve imprisoned there on the charge of poisoning the wells, springs and other places; and putting poison into food in order to destroy and wipe out the entire Christian religion.

I. Balavigny, a Jewish surgeon who lived at Thonon, was arrested at Chillon after being found in the neighbourhood. He was briefly put to the question and, when it was over, he confessed, after a long interval,[7] that, about ten weeks earlier, the Rabbi Jacob (who had come from Toledo and had been living at Chambéry since Easter) sent him, by a Jewish boy, some poison (about the size of an egg) in the form of a powder, enclosed in a leather bag, accompanied by a letter, commanding him on pain of excommunication and by the obedience he owed to the Jewish law, to put the poison into the larger public wells of the town – the ones most commonly used – in order to poison the people using them; and not to tell anybody at all. The letter also said that rabbis had given orders for the same thing to be done in various other places.

He confessed that one evening he secretly put the poisonous powder under a stone in a spring on the shore at Thonon. He further confesses that the boy showed him many identical letters addressed to numerous other Jews, specifically some addressed to Mossoiet, Banditon and Samolet of Villeneuve; to Musseo, Abraham and Aquetus of Montreux, Jews residing at La Tour de Vevey; to Beneton and his son at St Maurice; and to Vivian, Jacob, Aquetus and Sonetus, Jews at Évian les Bains. Several letters of a like nature were sent to Hebrea and Musset, Jews at Monthey. The boy told him that he had taken many others to various places, a long way away, but he (Balavigny) does not know to whom they were addressed. He further confessed that after he had put

---

7 To be put to the question is the standard circumlocution for torture. Because confessions made while torture was actually being applied were – for obvious reasons – suspect, the clerk (with only one exception) stresses that the confession was made after the torture session had finished. The period of torture is variously defined as brief or moderate.

the poison in the spring at Thonon, he expressly forbade his wife and children to use the spring, but without telling them why. In the presence of many credible witnesses he confessed by the Jewish law and by the five books of Moses that everything he had said was true. On the next day, Balavigny, voluntarily and without torture, maintained the truth of his confession, repeating it word for word in the presence of many credible witnesses and further confessing, of his own accord, that one day, on his way back from La Tour de Vevey, he had put into a spring below Montreux, namely the spring *de la Conereyde*, a quantity of poison about the size of a nut, wrapped in a rag, which he had been given by Aquetus of Montreux, who lives in La Tour. He told Manssionnus the Jew, who lives at Villeneuve, and Delosatz, son of Musselotus, what he had done and warned them not to drink from the spring. He describes the poison as red and black in colour.

On 19 September Balavigny confessed, without being put to the question, that three weeks after Pentecost[8] Mussus the Jew of Villeneuve told him that he had put poison in the public drinking fountain of his own town, namely in the custom-house there, and that afterwards he did not drink its water, but only drank from the lake. He also confessed that Mussus told him that he had likewise placed poison in the public drinking fountain at Chillon, namely in the custom-house under some stones. The spring was then investigated and some poison found. Some of it was given to a Jew, who died, thereby proving that it was poison. He said further that rabbis had instructed him and other Jews not to drink water for nine days after poison had been put in it, and he said that as soon as he had put poison in the spring he immediately warned other Jews.

He confesses further that a good two months earlier he had been at Évian and, while talking the matter over with a Jew called Jacob, had asked him, among other things, whether he had had a letter and poison like the others; to which Jacob replied that he had. Afterwards he asked him whether he had obeyed the instructions, to which Jacob replied that he had not placed the poison himself but had given it to Savetus the Jew who had put it into the spring *de Morer* at Évian. He urged on Balavigny the wisdom of dealing with the instructions in the same way.

He confesses that Aquetus of Montreux told him that he had put poison into the spring above La Tour which he uses regularly when he is staying there. He confesses that Samolet told him that he had put the

8 Pentecost, or Whitsun, fell on 8 June in 1348.

poison which he had received into a spring, but refused to tell him which.

Balavigny, speaking as a surgeon, says further that if anyone suffering the effects of the poison comes into contact with someone else, especially while sweating, the other person will be infected; and that the infection can be transmitted by breath as well. He believes this to be the case because he has heard many experienced physicians say so, and is certain that the other Jews cannot acquit themselves of the charge, for they knew perfectly well what they were doing and are guilty.

Balavigny was taken across the lake from Chillon to Clarens, to identify the spring in which he had confessed putting the poison. Upon arrival he was taken to the spot and as soon as he saw the spring he said, 'This is the spring where I put the poison'. The spring was examined in his presence and the linen rag or cloth in which the poison had been wrapped was found in the channel going from the spring by Henri Gérard, a notary public, in the presence of many people, and shown to the Jew. He confirmed that it was the linen cloth or rag in which the poison had been enclosed when he put it in the spring; adding that the poison was of two colours, black and red. The linen cloth or rag was taken away and is in safe keeping.

Balavigny confesses everything recorded here, adding that he believes that the poison is derived from the basilisk, for he has heard it said that the poison would not be efficacious otherwise and is convinced that that is the case.

II. Banditon, a Jew of Villeneuve, was likewise briefly put to the question on 15 September and, when it was over, he confessed, after a long interval, that he had put a quantity of poison, about the size of a large nut, which had been given to him by Musseus, a Jew of La Tour de Vevey, into the spring of Carutet, to poison people.

The next day, Banditon, voluntarily and without being put to the question, confirmed that what he had confessed was true, confessing also that Rabbi Jacob, who had come from Toledo at Easter and was living at Chambéry, sent him, at *Pilliex*, by a Jewish boy, some poison about the size of a large nut, together with a letter which told him to put the poison into springs on pain of excommunication. He had put the poison, which was in a leather bag, into the spring of *Cerclitus de Roch*. He further confesses that he saw many other letters addressed to Jews, which the boy was carrying, and that he saw him deliver one letter to Samolet the Jew of Villeneuve outside the upper gate. He says also that Massoletus the Jew told him that he had put poison in the spring near the bridge at Vevey, namely on the side towards Évian.

III. The said Mamson, a Jew of Villeneuve, when he was put to the question on 15 September, confessed nothing about these matters, maintaining his total ignorance. But on the next day he voluntarily, of his own volition and without being put to the question at all, confessed in the presence of many people that one day in the fortnight after Pentecost he travelled from Monthey in the company of a Jew called Provenzal, and as they went along Provenzal said to him, 'You're going to put the poison which I'll give you into that spring, or it'll be the worse for you'. And this was the spring of *Chabloz Cruyez* between Vevey and Muraz. So Mamson took a quantity of poison, about the size of a nut, and put it in the well. He believes that all the Jews round about Évian held a meeting before Pentecost to discuss the poisoning. He says that Balavigny told him one day that he had poisoned the spring *de la Conereyde* below Montreux. He says moreover that none of the Jews can acquit themselves of the charges, because they were all in it together and are guilty. When Mamson was brought before the commissioners on 3 October he changed none of his testimony, except that he had not put the poison into the spring.

Before their execution, all these Jews confessed by the Jewish law that all these things were true, insisting that no Jew above the age of seven could acquit himself of the charges, because they all knew everything that was going on.

IV. On 8 October Belieta, the wife of Aquetus the Jew was briefly put to the question, and when it was over she confessed that around midsummer last the said Provenzal, who had been arrested and then released at Vevey, although she does not know on what grounds, gave her some poison (about the size of a large nut, and tied up in a linen rag or cloth) in front of the house where he was living. She was to put the poison into springs to poison the people using them, and she handed it on to Mamson and his wife for them to do it.

On 18 October Belieta was put to the question, and when it was over she confessed that Provenzal had given her some poison, about as much as a large nut, to put in springs so that people using the water would fall sick and die. And she took the poison and did as she was told. Asked whether any Jew knew about the poisoning she says that Geney the Jewess and Jocet of La Tour knew about it very well.

V. Aquetus son of Belieta the Jewess was put to the question to a moderate extent, and when it was over accused Aquetus the son of Banditon, who lived in Villeneuve; saying that he overheard through a window of his house Aquetus saying to his father Banditon that a Jew called Provenzal, whom he didn't know, had, twelve weeks previously, given him some poison in a paper cornet and told him to put the poison in some well-used spring; and he heard his father answer that he should put the poison in the first spring he could find, and afterwards he heard Aquetus tell his father that he had sprinkled the poison into the spring of *Cerclitus de Roch.*

When the accused Aquetus was brought before the two commissioners, he denied the accusations to Aquetus' face. Aquetus the accuser replied that that was what he had heard and he wasn't making it up. And immediately he confessed that everything set out here was true, and that he had sprinkled poison in the spring, so that the people using it would die; and that he had revealed the matter to his father. Asked whether his father and the other Jews in Villeneuve know about the poisoning, he says that he is sure they do, because the leading members of the Jewish community always discuss matters among themselves outside the upper gate of Villeneuve, and the humbler Jews do the same. And he confessed these things without being put to the question, adding that the poison was green and black. And he confessed that this was true by the Jewish law and the five books of Moses; adding that, by his soul, the Jews richly deserved to die, and that indeed he had no wish to escape death, for he too richly deserved to die.

On Friday 10 October 1348 in the castle at Châtel an investigation was held on the authority of the court of the illustrious prince, our lord Amadée, Count of Savoy, into the accusations noised abroad by public fame and clamour against the Jews of both sexes imprisoned there. They were shown to be guilty of trying to kill Christians by poisoning springs, wells and other things used by them, and were accordingly punished. Their confession was made in the presence of many credible witnesses.

I. Agimetus, a Jew, who had been staying at Geneva and was imprisoned in the castle there, was put briefly to the question and then afterwards, after a long interval, he was put to the question again, this time to a moderate extent, whereupon he confessed in the presence of many credible witnesses the things unfolded below. Firstly that in last Lent the trading house of Claus de Rances sent him to Venice to buy silk and other things. When this came to the ears of Rubi Peyret, the

rabbi at Chambéry, Rabbi Peyret sent for Agimetus, and when he had
come into his presence said to him: 'It has come to our knowledge that
you will be going to Venice to buy merchandise. Here's a sachet of
poison, folded up in a bag of thin leather. Put a little in the wells,
cisterns and springs at Venice, and at the other places on your route,
to poison the people using the water.'

Agimetus took the sachet full of poison and took it with him to Venice,
and when he arrived he scattered some of the poison into a well or
cistern of fresh water near the house of the said Germans to poison the
people using it, affirming that that was the best source of fresh water
in the town. He affirms also that Rubi Peyret promised him, Agimetus,
that he could name his own reward for the deed. Moreover he
confesses voluntarily that he left as soon as he had done it, to avoid
being arrested by the burgesses and others, and that he went to
Calabria and Apulia and threw poison into numerous wells there, and
that he put poison into the spring in the piazza of Barletta, into the
public spring at Toulouse and into springs along the coast. Asked
whether anyone died in the places where he put poison, he says that he
does not know, because he always took himself off in a great hurry.
Asked whether any Jews in those places were guilty, he says he does
not know. And he confessed the truth of all these things on the five
books of Moses and a Jewish roll, and that he had lied about none of
the things that had happened to him.

II. Jocetus the Jew, an inhabitant of Châtel, put briefly to the question,
after a long interval confessed, in the presence of many credible
witnesses, that a good fourteen weeks ago Rubi Peyret, the rabbi at
Chambéry, met him near his house and handed him a quantity of
poison about as big as a fist in a piece of net, and he could see through
the little holes that it held powder and that the powder was black. And
he transferred the powder to a large paper cornet and put some into a
spring in the middle of the road from Vevey to Châtel, which was used
by everybody passing that way, and left the rest under a clod of grass
and earth near a tower. And Rubi Peyret gave Jocetus five gold
shillings for doing it. He confesses moreover that Rubi Peyret gave
him two bags, each the size of an egg, with two letters which he was
to deliver to two Jews living in La Tour de Vevey, Aquetus and
Abraham, to poison people with; telling them to put the poison into
springs. The two Jews received the bags from him in their houses at
La Tour and said that they were prepared to carry out the instructions
in their letters.

III. Iconetus, a Jew who once lived at Bas but now at Châtel and was arrested there, was put to the question to a moderate degree, and when it was over confessed after a long interval that two years ago Abuget, one of the richest and most powerful Jews in Bas, gave him some poison (which was white, and about the size of two fists) outside his house, saying to him, 'Go to Brussels and Hainault and put this poison in the best springs in that area, to poison the people using them'; and he gave him two florins for doing it, and said that he should put the poison secretly and stealthily into the springs and tell nobody. When Iconetus had taken the poison he left, and travelled to the places specified. And when he had reached Brussels he left two lots of poison in springs in the town of Tinimont and at the top of the town, placing it stealthily under a large stone at about noon, and then he retreated hastily and, leaving the town, headed for Hainault and there stealthily left another bag in a beautiful spring near the market town of Mons in Hainault, leaving it as before under a large stone to poison the people using the water, and again leaving immediately to go begging for bread elswhere. Asked whether he knows what the poison was made of, he says he does not, and confesses that all these things are true, on the five books of Moses.

IV. Aquetus Rubi, a Jew born in *Warembon* but now living in Châtel, was put briefly to the question and afterwards confessed that a year ago he was at Le Pont-de-Beauvoison and had lost all his money at dice and was planning to leave for the region around Geneva when Salamin the Jew, an inhabitant of Le Pont-de-Beauvoison, came to him and said, 'You've lost all your money and you've got nothing. Go to those parts, but take this poison with you and put it into springs and wells in the big and middling towns, and I'll give you six shillings in Savoy money'. Aquetus took the poison, about as much as two fingers, in a piece of leather, together with the six shillings, and one day put the bag full of poison under a big stone in a spring at *Perioso* near the drinking fountain at the *Maison du Chat*, to poison people using water from the spring. Asked if he had put poison anywhere else he said not. He also said he did it for a laugh, but now he was sorry for what he had done. Asked whether any of the Jews in La Tour, Évian, Villeneuve and Châtel knew anything about the posionings he said that he did not know, and that everything he had confessed was true, on the Jewish law.

VI. Aquetus son of Jocetus the Jew, living at Châtel, was put to the question to a moderate extent on 11 October and when it was over confessed truthfully, after a long interval, that a good year ago he was staying at Chambéry and studying in the house of Peyret, the rabbi in Chambéry, and one day the rabbi called him and took him to his chamber and said, 'Look, here's poison in a paper cornet, take it, and put it in the well of *Korvellus* near the house of Rabbi Peyret' and he ordered him under pain of excommunication to do this and so poison the people who drank the water, and not to tell anybody. Aquetus took the poison, which was a powder, and straightaway put it deep in the said well. He says also that afterwards he did not drink the water, but left Chambéry with his father and went to live at Châtel. And he confessed on the Jewish law that these things were true.

The Jews confessed all these things in the presence of two notaries public and many other eminent people and others specially summoned for the purpose.

Very dear friends, after receiving and reading your letters, I had a transcript made of these confessions, but there are many other accusations and proofs against those Jews and against other people elsewhere in Savoy, both Jews and Christians, who have now been punished for this appalling crime, which I do not have by me at the moment and so cannot include. You should know that all the Jews living in Villeneuve have been burnt by due legal process, and at Augst three Christians were flayed for their involvement in the poisoning – I was myself present on that occasion. Many Christians have been similarly arrested for this crime in many other places, notably in Évian, Geneva, La Croisette and Hauteville, who at the very last, on the point of death, confirm that they distributed poison given them by the Jews. Some of these Christians have been quartered, others flayed and hanged. Certain commissioners have been appointed by the Count to punish the Jews, and I believe that none remains alive.

72. Letter from Cologne to Strassburg

The justices, officials and councillors of Cologne to Conrad von Winterthur, the bürghermeister and the officials and councillors of Strassburg. 12 January [1349].

Strassburg Urkundenbuch, pp. 178-9.

Very dear friends, all sorts of rumours are now flying about against Judaism and the Jews prompted by this unexpected and unparalleled mortality of Christians, which, alas, has raged in various parts of the world and is still woefully active in several places. Throughout our city, as in yours, many-winged Fame clamours that this mortality was initially caused, and is still being spread, by the poisoning of springs and wells, and that the Jews must have dropped poisonous substances into them. When it came to our knowledge that serious charges had been made against the Jews in several small towns and villages on the basis of this mortality, we sent numerous letters to you and to other cities and towns to uncover the truth behind these rumours, and set a thorough investigation in train. But we have been unable to get the whole story, either from you or anywhere else – just as you have recently written to us to say that you have still not arrived at the truth of the matter.

If a massacre of the Jews were to be allowed in the major cities (something which we are determined to prevent in our city, if we can, as long as the Jews are found to be innocent of these or similar actions) it could lead to the sort of outrages and disturbances which would whip up a popular revolt among the common people – and such revolts have in the past brought cities to misery and desolation. In any case we are still of the opinion that this mortality and its attendant circumstances are caused by divine vengeance and nothing else. Accordingly we intend to forbid any harassment of the Jews in our city because of these flying rumours, but to defend them faithfully and keep them safe, as our predecessors did – and we are convinced that you ought to do the same.

We know what prudence you show in all your dealings, and it is by way of friendship that we urge you to proceed sensibly and cautiously in this Jewish business, as right and reason demand, and to take steps to guard against any popular rising from which a massacre of Jews and other disturbances might arise; and that the rage which the common people feel against the Jews should be checked before it spreads down the Rhine. You should take the decision to protect the Jews in your city, and keep them safe – as your predecessors did – until the truth is known. For should an uprising occur in your city against the Jews, experience tells us that it will surely spread to every other city and town. It therefore behoves you and us and all the major cities to proceed with prudence and caution in this matter, for the man who does not keep a wary eye on what the future may bring often falls into unexpected dangers.

Farewell. If you have obtained any definite information, either from kings and princes or from or the Jews themselves, let us know it in writing by this messenger.

73. Mandate of Clement VI concerning the Jews

On 5 July 1348 Clement VI reissued the bull *Sicut Judeis*, which extended the church's protection to the Jews. On 26 September 1348 he followed it up with this order notifying all prelates and clergy of the reissue and instructing them to take action against anyone persecuting Jews. On 1 October the order was reissued with the additional comment that the false accusations against the Jews were motivated by a greedy desire to get possession of their wealth. The greeting clause has been omitted from the translation.

S. Simonsohn (ed), *The Apostolic See and the Jews* vol I *Documents: 492-1404*, Toronto, Pontifical Institute of Medieval Studies; Studies and Texts 94, 1988, no. 373.

Although we rightly abhor the deceit of the Jews who, persisting in their imperviousness, refuse to admit the secret wisdom in the words of the prophets and their own writings or to accept the Christian faith and salvation, we are nevertheless mindful that Our Saviour chose to be born of Jewish stock when he put on mortal flesh for the salvation of the human race, and that it is our duty to succour humanity when the help of our protection and the clemency of our Christian piety have been invoked. Accordingly, following in the footsteps of our predecessors of happy memory, Popes Calixtus, Eugenius, Alexander, Clement, Celestine, Innocent, Gregory, Nicholas, Honorius and Nicholas III, we have taken the Jews under the shield of our protection, ordering among the rest that no Christian presume in any wise to wound or kill Jews, or take their money or expel them from his service before their term of employment has expired, unless by the legal judgement of the lord or the officials of the country in which they live; and that anyone who, knowing of these commands, still dares to do the contrary, shall lose his title or office, or suffer the ultimate penalty of excommunication, unless he takes steps to correct his presumption by making due satisfaction, as is set out more fully in the letters.

Recently, however, it has been brought to our attention by public fame – or, more accurately, infamy – that numerous Christians are blaming the plague with which God, provoked by their sins, has afflicted the Christian people, on poisonings carried out by the Jews at the instigation of the devil, and that out of their own hot-headedness they have impiously slain many Jews, making no exception for age or sex; and that Jews have been falsely accused of such outrageous behaviour so that they can be legitimately put on trial before appropriate judges – which has done nothing to cool the rage of the Christians but has rather inflamed them even more. While such behaviour goes unopposed it looks as though their error is approved.

Were the Jews, by any chance, to be guilty or cognizant of such enormities a sufficient punishment could scarcely be conceived; yet we should be prepared to accept the force of the argument that it cannot be true that the Jews, by such a heinous crime, are the cause or occasion of the plague, because throughout many parts of the world the same plague, by the hidden judgement of God, has afflicted and afflicts the Jews themselves and many other races who have never lived alongside them.

We order you by apostolic writing that each of you upon whom this charge has been laid, should straitly command those subject to you, both clerical and lay, when they are assembled in worship at mass, not to dare (on their own authority or out of hot-headedness) to capture, strike, wound or kill any Jews or expel them from their service on these grounds; and you should demand obedience under pain of excommunication, which henceforward you should use against those who disobey. But if they have ground of complaint against the Jews, whether concerning these matters or anything else, these letters in no way remove the power to proceed against them as was their right, but they should prosecute them in proper judicial form for these matters or any other offences before competent judges.

74 Accusations of well-poisoning against the poor; Narbonne 17 April 1348

Jaime Villanueva, *Viage Literario a las Iglesias de España* XI *Viage a Gerona*, Madrid, 1850, appendix of documents, pp. 270-1.

Andre Benezeit, burgess of Narbonne and deputy of Aymer, Vicomte of Narbonne, to the *jurés* of Gerona.

We have received your letters in which, as prudent men wishing to avoid future danger, you asked us to inform you by letter about the mortality of people which God has allowed to start in *Romania*[9] and which has reached the region around Avignon, Narbonne and Carcassonne; whether or not it has been caused by potions or poisons placed in various places by many people; if people have been arrested for this and have confessed; if they were subsequently punished and if so, how; and at whose instigation these things are said to have been done. Concerning these matters we now inform you that in Narbonne,

---

9 *Romania* can mean a variety of places in the middle ages; here it probably refers to Anatolia.

Carcassonne, Grasse and the places round about there has been throughout Lent, and still is, such a great mortality that the common opinion is that it has killed a quarter of the inhabitants. And by the scent of the said potion or poison many beggars and mendicants of various countries were found and arrested for the crime in Narbonne and elsewhere, carrying (as they said and it appeared) powdered substances which they were putting into rivers, houses, churches and foodstuffs to kill people.

Some of them have confessed as much of their own free will, others under torture. They are sticking to their confessions, admitting that they were given the potions in various places by people whose identities and names they say they do not know. But since they were given money to scatter the deadly potions, the most likely explanation is that these things were done on behalf of the enemies of France, although it is still not possible to be absolutely sure. Anyway, those who confessed in Narbonne were torn by red hot pincers, disembowelled,[10] their hands cut off, and then burnt. Justice was done on four in Narbonne, five in Carcassonne, two in Grasse, and many others have been arrested for the same offence.

Although some people still maintain that the mortality has natural causes and arises from the conjunction of the two planets which are now reigning; we believe that it is certainly the combined effects of the planets and the potions which are causing the mortality. The illness brought about by these things is known to be contagious, for when one person dies in a house, their servants, friends and family are afflicted in the same way by the same disease and within three or four days all lie dead together.

May the Almighty deliver you and us from these things. We have written this to you with an exceedingly heavy heart. We are at your service, in true friendship, in these matters and in larger ones and will send you more information as soon as we can.

75 An accusation of well-poisoning

This account comes from the autobiography of the fourteenth-century German mystic Henry Suso (Heinrich Seuse). Henry is the 'Servant' and the 'he' of the narrative, which is written in the third person. The translation is that of the late Professor James M. Clark.

10 *Excartayrati.* In modern French *écarteler* is to quarter, but it seems unlikely that quartering would feature in the middle of a list of tortures, and I have accordingly translated it as disembowelled.

Henry Suso, *The Life of the Servant*, transl. J. M. Clark, London, 1952, chapter
XXV.

Once, when he was about to set out on a journey, a companion was
given to him, a lay brother, who was mentally unbalanced. He was
reluctant to take him with him, for he recollected what trials he had
suffered from his companions in the past. Yet finally he agreed, and
took him with him.

Now it happened that they entered a village before breakfast. That day
there was a fair, and all kinds of people had come to it. It had been
raining, and his companion was wet through; he entered a house and
went up to the fire, saying that he could go no further. He told the
Servant to do his business without him and said he would wait for him
there.

Scarcely had the friar left the house, when his companion got up and
sat at the table, joining some rough fellows and traders who had come
to the fair. They saw that the wine had gone to his head; so when he
got up and stood in the doorway, gaping at them, they seized him and
said that he had stolen a cheese from them. While these wicked men
were brutally ill-treating him, four or five soldiers came up and
attacked him, and said that the evil monk was a poisoner of wells. For
it was at this time that there were great rumours of poisoning abroad.
So they seized him, and made such a commotion that many men ran up
to the place.

When the lay brother saw how things stood, and that he was a
prisoner, he wanted to escape, so he turned round and cried out to
them: 'Stop a while, stand still; let me say what I have to say, and I will
tell you how it happened, for it is, alas, a sad story!' They stopped, and
all listened. He began and said, 'Look and you will all see for
yourselves that I am a fool and an ignorant man, and no one pays any
attention to me. But my companion is a wise and experienced man. His
Order has entrusted to him a bag of poison to sink in the wells, here
and there in the country as far as Alsace, whither he is now bound.
Everywhere he goes he will defile everything with deadly poison. See
to it that you get him soon, or he will commit crimes that no one can
ever undo. He has just taken out a little bag, and he has thrown it into
the village well, so that all those who come to the fair, and drink out
of the well, will be poisoned. That is why I stayed here, and would not
go out, because I do not like it. And as a proof that I am telling the
truth, you should know that he has a large sack, which is full of these

bags of poison and with the gold pieces, that he and his Order have got from the Jews to pay him for committing these crimes.'

When the wild ruffians who had gathered round heard these words, they raged and cried with a loud voice: 'Come along, away with the murderer before he escapes!' One grasped his pike, another his axe, and each took any weapon he could find, and they ran with wild ferocious gestures. They broke open houses and monasteries, searching every place where they thought they might find him, thrusting their naked swords through bedding and straw, so that the whole fair came running along. People from other towns also came up, honourable men who knew the Servant. When they heard his name mentioned, they came forward and persuaded the mob that they were doing him an injustice, that he was a very pious man, who was incapable of committing such a crime. Not finding him, they finally desisted in their search, and took his companion to the judge as a prisoner. The latter ordered him to be locked up in a cell.

This went on until daybreak. The Servant knew nothing of these disturbances. When he thought it time to break his fast, and he hoped his companion had got dry before the fire, he entered the inn to have a meal. But when he entered the tavern, they began to tell him the whole story of what had happened. He ran forthwith in great alarm to the house where his companion and the judge were, and begged for his companion to be liberated. But the judge said this could not be done: he intended to commit him to prison for his crime. This was sad and doleful news for the Servant,who ran hither and thither to get help. But he could not find anyone who would help him. After carrying on his efforts with great shame and grief, he finally procured the man's release by payment of a heavy fine.

He now thought his troubles were at an end, but they were only just beginning. For when, with pain and loss, he had escaped from the authorities, he fell into danger of his life. For, as he was leaving the judge, about the time of vespers, the rumour had spread among the common people and young boys that he was a poisoner. They denounced him as a murderer, so that he did not dare to leave the town. They pointed at him, and said: 'Look, fellows, that is the poisoner! He has kept out of our way all day; he must be put to death! His money won't help him with us, as it did with the judge!' When he tried to escape down the village, they cried out all the louder after him. Some said, 'We will drown him in the Rhine,' for this river flowed past the village. Others cried, 'No, the unclean murderer will pollute all the water; we should burn him alive.'

A huge peasant with a sooty jacket grabbed a pike, pushed between the others and cried, 'Listen to me, gentlemen all! We cannot inflict any more shameful death on the wicked heretic than this: I will thrust this long pike through him, as one does to a venomous toad that one impales. Just let me stick this pike through the naked body of this poisoner. I will lift him up from behind and fix him fast in this fence, and take care that he does not fall. Let his unclean corpse dry in the wind, so that all the people that pass to and fro will have a sight of the murderer, and will curse him after his shameful death, and that he may be all the more accursed both in this world and the next. For the vile scoundrel has well deserved it.'

The wretched Servant heard all this with bitter fear, groaning deeply, and the large tears ran down his face. All those who stood round in a circle, and saw him in his anguish, wept bitterly, and some beat their breasts with compassion, and struck their hands together over their heads. But no one dared to speak, fearing the dreadful rabble would attack them also. At nightfall, he went to and fro, begging with tears that for God's sake someone would have mercy and give him lodging. But he was cruelly driven away. Some kind women would gladly have given him shelter, but they did not dare to do so.

The wretched sufferer was thus in peril of his life, and all human help had deserted him, as everyone was just waiting to see them attack him and kill him. He fell down in anguish and fear of death in front of a fence, raised his wretched swollen eyes to the heavenly Father, saying: 'Alas, Father of all mercies, when wilt thou come to my aid today in my great distress? Alas, merciful heart, why hast Thou forgotten thy mercy to me? Alas, Father, alas, faithful, mild Father, help me, wretched man, in this great misery! I cannot take counsel with my own heart, since it is dead already, whether it would be more tolerable to drown, or to be burnt alive, or to die at the stake, yet I must suffer one of these deaths. I commend to Thee today my wretched spirit. Have mercy on me in the face of the miserable death that threatens me: they are near me who would destroy me.' This sorrowful lament came to the ears of a priest, who ran vigorously to him, dragged him out of their hands, took him to his house and kept him overnight, so that no harm came to him. Early the next morning he helped him to escape from all his troubles.

PART THREE: CONSEQUENCES

'In truth, this great pestilence was a turning point in the national life. It formed the real close of the Mediaeval period and the beginning of our Modern age.'[1] The words are Cardinal Gasquet's, and the quotation enshrines the perception of the late-nineteenth-century historians who rediscovered the plague as a subject of historical research that the mortality of 1348-49 set the world on a new course. Gasquet himself was primarily interested in the impact of the disease on religious behaviour, but he also saw the mortality among the working classes as bringing 'nothing less than a complete social revolution': 'to use a modern expression, labour began then to understand its value and assert its power'.[2] Not all contemporaries shared Gasquet's views in detail, but there was widespread agreement that the plague had wrought a cataclysmic change, not only in society but within the individual. All the old certainties of the 'high' middle ages had been swept away: the feudal system collapsed; respect for social hierarchy and order was undermined; and the intellectual authorities of the past ceased to be believed. The new world which emerged was presented as one of violent and paradoxical extremes: 'So violent and motley was life, that it bore the mixed smell of blood and roses. The men of that time always oscillate between the fear of hell and the most naive joy, between cruelty and tenderness, between harsh asceticism and insane attachments to the delights of this world'. Huizinga's famous evocation of the late middle ages stands in the same tradition as Jusserand's description of the religious scepticism which followed the plague: 'It is a violent movement of the whole nature which feels itself impelled to burn what it adores; but the man is uncertain in his doubt, and his burst of laughter stuns him; he has passed as it were, through an orgy, and when the white light of morning comes he will have an attack of despair, profound anguish with tears and perhaps a vow of pilgrimage and a conspicuous conversion'.[3]

1 F. A. Gasquet, *Great Pestilence*, London, 1893, p. xvi.

2 *Ibid.* p. 195.

3 J. Huizinga, *The Waning of the Middle Ages*, Harmondsworth, 1968 (original publication 1924), p. 25; J. J. Jusserand, *English Wayfaring Life in the Middle Ages*, 1891, pp. 382-3, cited (with approval) by P. Ziegler, *The Black Death*, Harmondsworth, 1969, p. 288.

Not surprisingly, such extravagance produced a backlash. In the course of the twentieth century historians generally became much less willing to ascribe sweeping cultural or psychological changes to the plague. By 1977 Philippe Ariès, in his influential study of changing attitudes to death, could address the subject with hardly a reference to the plague, other than a brief statement of its irrelevance.[4] This is an extreme example, but other historians were clearly suspicious of the plague as an explanation of change – in part, perhaps, because it had come to seem too easy an explanation, but also because *any* such radical change was now felt to be unlikely. The emphasis instead was firmly on cultural continuities, with the plague allowed (at most) a supporting role as the intensifier of existing patterns of thought.

Alongside this re-assessment of the plague's impact went a revision of the accepted levels of plague mortality. Compiling accurate mortality figures from medieval sources is – as every historian who has tried it agrees – virtually impossible. Lists of deaths exist. In England the richest source are the manorial court rolls which record the deaths of customary tenants [81] and other records exist which purport to give the numbers of deaths in a particular region, although their accuracy is difficult to evaluate [82].[5] But such raw figures mean nothing unless the size of the group within which the deaths occurred is also known, and that (broadly speaking) becomes less likely the larger the group. Thus the percentage of English noblemen who died can be calculated with extreme accuracy, as can the deaths within a particular religious house [18, 80]. Given full records it is also possible to arrive at a fairly accurate percentage figure for deaths among the beneficed clergy in a particular diocese or the customary (heriot-paying) tenants of a single manor. But it is not possible to obtain reliable percentage figures for *all* the residents of a manor, let alone of a village or city or county.[6]

4 P. Ariès, *The Hour of Our Death*, Harmondsworth, 1983, pp. 124-7.

5 Translations of manorial documents covering the plague period include: L. F. Salzman (ed), *Ministers' Accounts of the Manor of Petworth, 1347-1353*, Sussex Record Society, LV, 1955; J. L. Fisher, 'The Black Death in Essex', *Essex Review* LII, 1943, pp. 13-20.

6 There are apparently no surviving records of deaths or burials for any English town. A very few note wills proved during the plague, but wills were made by such a small proportion of the population (and probably not all of those made could be proved during the emergency) that this is an extremely problematic source in trying to arrive at the total number of deaths in an area. Colchester recorded 110 wills in 1348-9 (compared with 25 the following year): Fisher, 'Black Death in Essex' p. 20. The figure is worth comparing with the wills estimated to have been made in Amounderness during the plague: see 82. For a French parish register covering the plague period see 'Le registre paroissial de Givry', *Bibliothèque de l'école*

Any attempt to arrive at regional or national percentages thus relies
on the historian's judgement of whether the figures for specific groups
may be taken as representative of the population at large, and is
accordingly at best speculative and at worst entirely subjective. But for
that very reason the national percentages bandied about during the
last century provide a useful measure of the importance which their
compilers attached to the plague.

Gasquet had been convinced that the first outbreak of plague had
carried off half the English population. This soon came under attack.
As early as 1916, Dr Elizabeth Levett pointed out the dangers of
Gasquet's anecdotal approach. It is not enough to pile up individual
references to tenant deaths or the non-payment of dues as proof of the
enormity of the mortality; some sort of objective yardstick has to be
found. Her own preferred yardstick was the degree of administrative
dislocation, and she argued that the apparent lack of such disruption
within the estates of the bishopric of Winchester must have meant that
the mortality levels were lower than hitherto thought; probably less
than one third, although she insisted that it was otiose to look for
precise figures.[7] Most later writers continued this downward revision,
although few were prepared to go as low as J. C. Russell, who argued
for a death rate of 20%, or J. F. C. Shrewsbury, who opted for an
incredible 5% (on the basis that bubonic plague finds it difficult to
secure a foothold within the human population).[8] By the late 1960s the
'safe' estimate was generally taken to be a national death rate of around
one third: a figure which avoided on the one hand the 'credulity' of
nineteenth-century historians and on the other Russell's
disconcertingly arbitrary figures.[9]

A death rate of one third in less than two years is still, of course,
shockingly high. Even so, relatively few of the writers who adopted
that figure felt that the plague had an immediate impact on the

---

des Chartes C, 1939, pp. 295-308. Between 1 August and 19 November 1348 there
were 615 recorded deaths; more than in the previous 20 years.

7 A. E. Levett and A. Ballard, 'The Black Death on the estates of the see of
Winchester', in P. Vinogradoff (ed), *Oxford Studies in Social and Legal History* V,
Oxford, 1916, pp. 72-80. Ballard, by contrast, argued for two thirds mortality in
some of the Winchester manors: pp. 199, 213.

8 J. C. Russell, *British Medieval Population*, Albuquerque, 1948, pp. 230, 367. The
figure of 20% is first suggested as the death rate for 10-35 year-olds, but in the
conclusion it has become the overall mortality level. J. F. D. Shrewsbury, *A History
of the Bubonic Plague in the British Isles*, Cambridge, 1970, pp. 36, 123.

9 This figure was given wider currency by its adoption by Ziegler, *Black Death*, pp.
235-9.

medieval economy. It came to be the accepted wisdom that surprisingly little changed in the short term: wages remained at their low, pre-plague levels, prices did not fall and vacant land holdings soon found takers. It was only in the mid 1370s that change became perceptible: wages rose, holdings stood empty and landlords lost interest in the direct cultivation of their estates – harbingers of an economic malaise which was to last into the fifteenth century, In other words, it was the population's failure to recover (however that was to be explained), rather than its initial downturn, which was thought to have done the real economic damage. One of the few dissenters was J. M. W. Bean, who not only argued that the first visitation of plague had direct consequences which deserve to be considered a serious crisis, but also, in an influential article, claimed that the English population had begun to recover by the 1370s, on the grounds that all but the first two outbreaks of plague were too slight, and too localised, to have a major effect on the population.[10]

The belief that the loss of one third of the population could be absorbed without immediate economic distress rested on the assumption that the population of pre-plague England had become too large for the available resources. The result was under-employment, low wage levels and fierce pressure on land: a state of affairs which, broadly speaking, benefited land owners at the expense of tenants and wage earners. Low wages also meant a stagnant demand for services and manufactured goods, except at the luxury end of the market. On this interpretation, the people killed in 1348-49 were – to put it much too crudely – surplus to economic requirements. Far from triggering a crisis, their removal actually benefited the economy in the short term, notably by allowing a more satisfactory balance between demand and the available land.[11]

The most influential proponent of the over-population theory was Professor Michael Postan, although not all his arguments met with

---

10 J. M. W. Bean, 'The Black Death: the crisis and its social and economic consequences' in Williman, *The Black Death*, pp. 23-38; *idem*, 'Plague, population and economic decline in England in the later middle ages', *Economic History Review*, 2nd series XV, 1963. For a criticism of the latter see J. Hatcher, *Plague, Population and the English Economy, 1348-1530*, London and Basingstoke, 1977, pp. 15-19. The continuing demographic effect of later outbreaks does now seem to be established, although there is a growing insistence that this cannot be the whole story and that fertility must be added to the demographic equation. An important contribution on the fertility side of the argument is L. R. Poos, *A rural society after the Black Death: Essex 1350-1525*, Cambridge, 1991, part III.

11 J. L. Bolton, *The Medieval English Economy, 1150-1500*, London, 1980, pp. 57-63.

acceptance. For Postan, the plague pulled population levels down dramatically, and then delayed their recovery well into the fifteenth century, but it did not originate the downturn. That had started much earlier, probably by the turn of the century, as a consequence of a series of 'natural' checks brought into play by the pressures of over-population, including a tendency to delay marriage, reduced crop yields due to soil exhaustion, and a sensitivity to natural disasters such as famine.[12] Subsequent writers have generally been willing to accept that by the early fourteenth century the population had reached its ceiling, with a resulting increase in the number of people living on the subsistence level, but there has been much less agreement that this resulted in a sustained downturn in the population. The consensus of opinion has been, rather, that although the famine years of 1315-17 brought crisis mortality levels (perhaps of the order of 10-15%) this constituted a temporary setback from which the population had been able to recover by the middle of the century.[13] The plague thus struck a population which was near to its medieval peak, an argument which makes the 'delayed action' effect of the plague even more understandable.

Postan's own view was an early manifestation of what has probably been the most sophisticated downgrading of the plague's importance: the perception that the 'crisis' of the fourteenth century was rooted within the existing social and economic structure and was thus independent of the plague – which becomes, on this reading, merely an intensifying or complicating factor in the situation. In other words, and to use the modern jargon, economic and social change in the fourteenth century was endogamous (it came from flaws or tensions *within* the system) rather than exogamous (caused by outside factors). Not all the historians who share this perception have agreed on the nature of that fatal flaw, or on the point at which it began to make its presence felt. Where Postan and his followers saw agrarian production as the key factor, others have looked to the bullion supply and its effect on the patterns of trade and manufacturing, or to the artifical social

12 Postan's views are conveniently summarised in *The Medieval Economy & Society*, Harmondsworth, 1975, pp. 40-44. Plague itself cannot be included in the category of natural disasters to which the population was sensitive. It has sometimes been assumed that plague must have been particularly dangerous to the weak, but there is no evidence that this was the case. The poor died in greater numbers than the rich because they were more likely to come into contact with rats and their fleas, not because they were malnourished.

13 e.g. Z. Razi, *Life, Marriage & Death in a Medieval Parish: economy, society and demography in Halesowen 1270-1400* , Cambridge, 1980, p. 94.

structures characteristic of feudalism.[14] Where they all agree is in their insistence that the plague's contribution to the crisis was only superficial – in the sense that the plague's effects (although possibly dramatic in themselves) were superimposed on deeper trends.

By the 1970s the plague had thus been cut down to size. It was generally accepted that the first outbreak killed an uncomfortably large number of people, but not as many as credulous writers had once believed; and in any case England could stand the loss, and may even (in the short term) have benefited from the pruning. There was a widespread sense that the plague had simply intensified or complicated existing trends, and that the identification of the causes underlying those trends was a more important task for the historian than trying to quantify the plague's contribution. This ruthless downgrading of the plague's importance necessarily denied the validity of contemporaries' own views of the situation. In 1968 Jacques Heers, claiming that belief in a fourteenth-century catastrophe had been discredited for almost twenty years among 'better informed writers', chided earlier historians for their 'excessive faith in certain contemporary witnesses, men of the church often unaccustomed to handling figures, quite naturally inclined to magnify the losses and the problems, to present a distorted, fictionalized image ... to lend credence to a kind of black legend of their time.'[15] Even writers arguing that the plague did constitute a crisis took it as axiomatic that contemporary comment must be mistrusted.[16]

Many medieval estimates of mortality are indeed suspect, but they are testimony to a sense of dislocation and shock which it is unduly (and offensively) arrogant to ignore, whatever the actual mortality levels may have been. In recent years English assessments of the mortality in 1348-49 have also been rising steadily back towards a death rate of almost one in two, providing a context in which any contemporary exaggeration seems entirely understandable. By 1975 informed opinion had come to feel that the figure of one third mortality lay towards the bottom of any likely range. Five years later, 40% or more was offered as the best estimate, and even this now seems too cautious. It has recently been claimed that many areas lost about half their

14 The various 'flaws' are usefully surveyed by B. F. Harvey, 'The 'crisis' of the early fourteenth century' in Campbell, *Before the Black Death*, pp. 1-24.

15 Quoted in Ariès, *Hour of Our Death*, p. 125.

16 Bean, 'The Black Death' p. 32.

inhabitants.[17] An average mortality of 47% or 48% no longer seems unreasonable.

This upward revision has not been prompted by major discoveries, so much as by a new willingness to take existing figures at face value. Even when the trend was to minimise the national death rate, local studies were regularly yielding mortality figures of 40% and more. One of the earliest such studies, an analysis by Hamilton Thompson of the clerical vacancies recorded in the episcopal registers of York and Lincoln, suggested a death rate of about 40% among beneficed clergy during the first outbreak.[18] Attempts to adjust the figure downwards proved unavailing, and many writers therefore took refuge in the assertion that the death rate among the clergy must have been higher than among the population at large, either because of their higher age profile (although there is no firm evidence that the first plague was age-specific) or because of their increased exposure to infection.[19]

Figures for the death rate among manorial tenants were generally even higher, but proved easier to dismiss as flawed or atypical. Percentages based on the non-payment of rent were easiest of all to discount, on the grounds that administrative dislocation must have facilitated the avoidance of payment by the living. Figures based on heriots − the death duty owed by customary tenants − avoided this problem, but were open to the charge that figures might be inflated by the payment of more than one heriot for a single property, if successive holders died, or by the payment of a heriot when land was transferred between the living. Such criticisms became progressively harder to sustain as historians tightened up their methodology, particularly when more sophisticated techniques were found, on the whole, to produce *higher* mortality rates. As such studies accumulated it also became difficult to argue that the samples all happened to have come from areas of unusually high mortality and that any national average

17 Hatcher, *Plague, Population*, pp. 24–5; Bolton, *Medieval English Economy* p. 61; R. H. Britnell, *The Commercialisation of English Society, 1000-1500*, Cambridge, 1993, p. 155.

18 A. Hamilton Thompson, 'Registers of John Gynewell, Bishop of Lincoln, for the years 1347-50', *Archaeological Journal* LXVIII, 1911; *idem*, 'The pestilences of the 14th century in the diocese of York', *ibid* LXXXI, 1914.

19 Russell, *Medieval Population* p. 230 is the main advocate of the age-specific theory, but this receives no support from contemporary accounts of the first plague. Contemporaries *were* aware that the next two outbreaks were uneven in their impact, and their belief in the universality of the first outbreak can probably be trusted.

would need to be much lower to allow for the less-badly affected regions.

The revised death rate signals a major shift in attitudes towards the plague and its likely impact, but it does not mean that the Black Death is about to be reinstated in its old role as agent of cataclysmic change. The debates of the last fifty years have drawn attention to too many other elements in the situation for any monocausal interpretation of contemporary developments to seem acceptable. There is now a perceptible impatience with attempts to fit the fourteenth century into the strait-jacket of a single 'fatal flaw'. Change is more likely to be seen as the result of a complex interplay of forces, of which the plague is still only one; albeit a more powerful one than has lately been allowed.

The original exponents of a one in two death rate took it for granted that enormous mortality would mean enormous change; just as their critics assumed that modest change must be evidence of modest mortality. That simple correlation no longer exists. In the cultural arena it is now more widely recognised that people under pressure are likely to articulate their anxieties in ways which are already familiar to them, and that cultural continuities spanning the plague cannot therefore be taken as evidence for the insignificance of those anxieties, or of the upheaval which triggered them. Terror is not any less real because it fails to find novel ways of expressing itself – indeed, the reverse is more likely to be true.

Historians over the last forty years have also become adept at explaining why plague mortality had a smaller impact than might have been expected on the contemporary economy. Their solution – surplus population before 1348 – remains valid, but it is very unlikely indeed to be the whole story. The explanation is assuming, in effect, that change did not occur: that gaps in the ranks of tenants and workers were quickly filled and that life continued much as before. But this is barely credible given a death rate of one in three, and becomes progressively less so as the accepted mortality level rises towards one half. A much more persuasive argument is that some change did indeed occur as a direct result of the first outbreak, but that it was, for a time, contained. It was only after two major recurrences of plague in the 1360s that change became unmanageable, so that pressures which can be glimpsed in the period 1349-52 become apparent on a far larger scale in the 1370s.

In the case of central government, change was not so much contained as ignored. The insistence on business as usual is impressive, but there is also something chilling about the refusal to admit the scale of the disaster.[20] The tax assessments, set in 1334, were not altered for about a century, although the proceeds of the statute of labourers were used to offset some of the bill.[21] The exchequer consistently tried to collect money at the same rate as before the plague, and accounting officials found themselves hard pressed to convince exchequer staff that revenues really had fallen [93], or that the death of their subordinates was an adequate excuse for a failure to present their accounts [91]. Not surprisingly, something of a double standard was involved here. Royal officials might only grudgingly admit that royal revenues had dropped below their pre-plague levels, but they were keenly alert to the possibility that the king might be losing out when the priory of Lewes made him a gift of advowsons on the basis of their pre-plague value [100].

As the inquisitions into the Lewes advowsons reveal, the value of land did not invariably fall after the plague. The 20 acres of arable land which comprised the major part of the glebe at Fishlake (Yorks) held their value between 1348 and 1351. What this probably meant in practice was that the rector had a tenant who was prepared to go on paying the same rate. Not all lords were so lucky. One of the arguments for the plague's limited effect is that 'holdings were soon all filled'.[22] This is generally explained as a response to the land hunger of the preceding generations, which had created a queue of people eager to take on more land once it became available.

Certainly such people must have existed. Given the value attached to land in the middle ages it would be surprising if there were not people ambitious to acquire or extend their own holdings – at least once they were confident that the plague had ended. Their *immediate* reaction is more likely to have been that of the tenants of Houghton (co. Durham) who refused to take on any new commitments 'because of the fear of pestilence', or those of Easington 'who flatly refused to make a fine unless they should still be alive after the pestilence' [95]. Many other holdings passed directly to the heirs of the former tenants. In Walsham le Willows few of the known kinsmen of the dead refused the tenancy or failed to appear [81].

20 W. M. Ormrod, 'The English government and the Black Death of 1348-49', in *idem* (ed), *England in the Fourteenth Century*, Woodbridge, 1986, pp. 175-88.

21 R. H. Hilton, *Bond Men Made Free: medieval peasant movements and the English rising of 1381*, 1977, p. 148. For the use of the proceeds from the statute of labourers, see **102**.

22 Bolton, *Medieval English Economy*, p. 62.

Smooth transfers did occur. But it is clear that in many places supply was exceeding demand. It could hardly fail to do so, when on some manors two in three of the customary tenants had died,[23] or when the combination of death and departure had left 'scarcely two' tenants behind [96]. Under such conditions lords who wanted to find tenants had to be prepared to lower their asking price. Many must have decided that any income was better than nothing. In July 1349 a group of new tenants at Easington (co. Durham) were allowed to take a holding on their terms rather than leave it lying fallow in the lord's hands, 'for, as has become apparent, there is no other alternative' [95]. Nor was it only new tenants who were able to bargain down their rents. The tenants of Rudheath (Ches.) secured the remission of one third of their rent by threatening to leave the manor 'unless they were granted such a remission, to last until the world improves and the tenements come to be worth more'. As the lord's officials sadly noted, had the tenants carried out their threat it would have left the lord's tenements empty [94].

In the case of customary holdings, tenants were more interested in using their new bargaining power to reduce their labour services. The importance they attached to this can be seen in an Oxfordshire example, where the handful of surviving tenants forced a renegotiation under threat of abandoning the manor, and ended up paying a substantial cash premium for a very modest reduction in their labour services [96]. The official who recorded the agreement clearly felt that the peasants had come badly out of the settlement, with the cash increment worth more than the services it had replaced. It can also be argued that the replacement of labour service with rent was to prove a poor bargain for tenants in general, since cash rents were not protected by custom and were (as many of the remissions make plain) subject to regular renegotiation. But in the context in which they were first made, such transactions are eloquent testimony to the pressure under which lords found themselves.

The plague had sent wages – particularly agricultural wages – soaring. Customary labour services thus became, almost overnight, a more than usually valuable asset for lords with land to cultivate; and an asset which was carefully protected in the ordinance of labourers [98]. In remitting labour services lords were making a very explicit admission

---

23 For example, at Witney and Cuxham: Levett & Ballard, 'Black Death on estates of Winchester', p. 199; P. D. A. Harvey, *A Medieval Oxfordshire Village: Cuxham, 1240-1400*, Oxford, 1965, pp. 135-6.

of weakness. The chronicler Henry Knighton was absolutely clear about this: when lords negotiated a reduction in labour services it was because it was their only hope of securing *any* work from their customary tenants [21]. Knighton's account is relatively late (it was produced in the early 1390s) but is borne out by more nearly contemporary references. When the steward of Aldham (Suffolk) negotiated a reduction in labour services in 1351 he was careful to emphasise that this was done as a mark of lordly favour to tenants who now lacked the power to perform the customary services, but it is also made quite clear that he was doing it 'because the lord's interests made it necessary' [97]. A Durham remission of labour services to the tenants of Killerby in return for a cash rent is more honest: 'let it be done in secret, because of the bad example it sets to the other villages' [118].

A readiness to compromise did not always have the desired effect, as the Bishop of Coventry and Lichfield found.[24] Where it failed, more devious means might be employed. The Bishop of Durham's solution was to make empty land the financial responsibility of the vill in which it lay, or of an individual official. The bishop got his rent, and the community was put under very effective pressure to cooperate in finding new tenants; which they duly tried to do – reporting, for instance, on local people with enough resources to take on land [118].

By the mid 1350s the combination of sticks and carrots had generally had its effect. This is not to say that all holdings had found takers, but most had done so and lords no longer felt it necessary to offer inducements to secure tenants. In some cases the late 1350s even found lords trying to move rents back upwards to their pre-plague levels. Where this was not possible, lords were turning to other methods to make good the shortfall – notably by stepping up the level of fines and amercements levied in their courts.[25] Tenants had demonstrably lost their chance of negotiating more favourable terms, and this denial of the possibility of further change generated resentment. There are suggestions from several areas that relations between lords and their tenants became more confrontational as a result. Attempts by the serfs of Wawne to secure a reduction in their labour

24 E. Fryde, 'The tenants of the bishops of Coventry and Lichfield, and of Worcester after the plague of 1348-9' in R. F. Hunnisett and J. B. Post (eds), *Medieval Legal Records*, HMSO, 1978, p. 233.

25 Hilton, *Bond Men*, pp. 156-7; R. H. Britnell, 'Feudal reaction after the Black Death in the palatinate of Durham', *Past & Present* CXXVIII, 1990, pp. 28-47; C. Dyer, 'The social and economic background to the rural revolt of 1381' in R. H. Hilton and T. H. Aston (eds), *The English Rising of 1381*, Cambridge, 1987, pp. 21-36.

services took the form of a 'rebellion' which was put down by force.[26] The monks' aggression was rooted in fear that any sign of weakness would 'bestow even greater audacity on the troublemakers who wanted to withhold their service' [119]. Lords, as well as their tenants, had not forgotten the consequences of seigneurial weakness in the years immediately after the plague.

Wage movements were contained with even greater promptness. It has long been recognised that, when calculated on a decade-by-decade basis, wages rose less dramatically after the plague than might be expected – and rose, moreover, in step with grain prices so that they were barely rising at all in real terms. It was not until the 1370s that wages parted company with prices, and began a rise in real terms which was to continue into the fifteenth century.[27] But contemporaries were unanimous that in the short term wages rocketed, as workers realised their bargaining power. The degree of venom with which writers like William Dene and Henry Knighton [19, 21] describe the workers' demands may mean that their claims are exaggerated – Dene, for instance, thought that wages tripled – but their fervour suggests that the problem was a real one; as does the speed of the government's reaction [98].

The ordinance of labourers, the government's first response to wage rises, was issued in June 1349. Knighton believed that workers had become so full of themselves that they simply ignored it, and this may well be true. There are relatively few recorded cases brought under the ordinance, and the statute of labourers which followed in 1351 admits to widespread evasion [112]. The need for labour was evidently so acute that men who could afford to pay over the odds had simply continued to do so, leaving lesser employers unable to compete. But the problem was compounded by the fact that the enforcement of the ordinance had been entrusted to the very group who were most likely to take that attitude: the landowners of the shires. The statute, by contrast, gave responsibility to the commissioners of the peace, a body which included royal justices. Presumably it still proved difficult to bring great men to book, although Knighton believed that Edward III targeted them directly and levied swingeing fines. But there seems no

26 M. J. O. Kennedy, 'Resourceful villeins: the Cellarer family of Wawne in Holderness', *Yorkshire Archaeological Journal* XLIV, 1976, pp. 107-17, supplies more details of the episode than appear in the chronicle account printed below.

27 C. Dyer, *Standards of Living in the later Middle Ages: social change in England c1200-1520*, Cambridge, 1989, pp. 211-19.

reason to believe that the legislation failed in its effect – after all, many employers would have been grateful for an excuse to peg wages. The surviving lists of prosecutions certainly suggest that the legislation was being enforced with vigour. The justices seem to have been willing to hunt down seigneurial officials who poached other men's servants, as well as the altogether easier quarry of freelances guilty of over-charging their employers.

It was not only secular employees who seized the chance to secure higher wages for themselves. The plague had carried off large numbers of priests – so many that the Bishop of Bath and Wells felt it wise to remind his flock that confession could, in an emergency, be made to a lay man, or even to a woman [87]. Episcopal registers reveal that bishops were soon taking longer to find suitable candidates to fill parish vacancies,[28] and might have to look to the ranks of regular clergy [89]. The fees demanded by stipendiary priests rose dramatically. In 1349 Edward III ordered the bishops to ensure that such men were paid no more than their accustomed salary and did not leave their employer in search of higher wages [99]. In 1350 the Archbishop of Canterbury reiterated the command, prefacing it with a blistering attack on clerical greed [108]. In 1362 it was reissued, with an explicit admission of failure to date and a handy list of suitable wages.

The bishops were not complaining only of clerical avarice, but of clerical laziness as well. The specific charge levelled against the clergy was that they preferred to earn easy money singing masses for the dead than to take on the onerous responsibilities of a parish, particularly when parochial revenues were falling due to the reduction in the numbers of parishioners; a reduction which was sufficiently severe in some cases to lead to the amalgamation of parishes [105]. Langland was to make the same point in *Piers Plowman* [110] and the reality of the problem is confirmed by a case from the diocese of York where a mass priest positively refused to take on the job of parish chaplain in his local church [109]. But even the job of chantry priest was not invariably attractive. In 1365 Roger of Chesterfield, himself a rector and so presumably well-informed about clerical attitudes, thought it prudent to limit the demands made on the priest of his own chantry foundation in order to make it more attractive to future applicants for the job. The liturgical round was curtailed, and the incumbent was permitted occasional trips to the local ale-house [107].

28 R. A. Davies, 'The effect of the Black Death on the parish priests of the medieval diocese of Coventry and Lichfield', *Historical Research* LXII, 1989, pp. 88-90.

Secular employees were also accused of living in idleness. In their case
the accusation brought against them immediately after the plague was
that some of them had turned to beggary, realising that they could
make a respectable living from funeral doles. Given the desperate shortage of agricultural labourers it is not surprising that attitudes to able
bodied beggars hardened dramatically, and successive revisions of the
labour legislation progresively tightened up definitions of acceptable
mendicancy, until by 1388 pilgrims and students were expected to
provide themselves with references if they did not want to be put in the
stocks for refusing to work [117]. By this date it was not only beggars
who were attracting the indignation of employers. Wages had by now
begun to rise markedly (one of the purposes of the 1388 additions to
the statute was to endorse a number of wage increases) and it was
becoming evident that many workers were responding by working
shorter hours. Hence the sideswipe at frivolous leisure pursuits; hostility
which was to develop in the fifteenth century into a paternalistic
distaste for workers 'wasting' their money in drinking and gambling.[29]

As this implies, the attacks on the greed and laziness of workers had
a powerful moral component. They were in danger of damning their
own souls, whether through avarice, envy or pride. But the fact that
the lower orders were getting above themselves – first by refusing to
obey their betters and then by acquiring the means to enjoy an inappro-
priately comfortable lifestyle – was also seen as symptomatic of a wider
malaise. It represented an inversion of the natural order: the world
turned upside down [19]. Most writers came to feel that mankind had
been made worse by the plague, and the vehemence with which they
urge the point may well be rooted in disappointment. The plague had
been widely seen as God's merciful intervention to draw mankind
away from sin: an act of destruction and renewal analogous to the
Flood. Gilles li Muisis had pointed with satisfaction to dice-makers
turning their skills and their raw material to the manufacture of prayer
beads, or to burgesses making honest women of their mistresses [6].
But, as Jean de Venette sadly concluded, if the world had been renewed
it had not been made any better by its renewal [7]. Accounts of the
post-plague world are laments for a missed opportunity: men were
more greedy and quarrelsome [7]; women became sexually degenerate
[25d]; clergy haunted taverns and gambling dens [108]; little men
bustled about to make themselves the equals of their betters [120].

---

29 Dyer, *Standards of Living*, pp. 223-5; M. Bailey, 'Rural society' in R. Horrox (ed),
    Fifteenth-century Attitudes, Cambridge, forthcoming.

It is impossible to know whether the plague really did bring a widespread decline in moral standards; although it is worth noting that moralists had produced an almost identical list of failings by way of explaining the plague's arrival – the only significant addition after 1349 being the arrogance of the lower orders. Nor is it possible to generalise about the plague's immediate impact on contemporary *mores*. Many chroniclers believed that it brought a widespread breakdown in law and order, and it is possible to find individual examples of looting and violence.[30] But there are also plenty of accounts of intense personal piety and a desire to make reparation for past wrongs [92]. Human beings react in different ways to disaster. Their reactions are also open to different interpretation by observers. Boccaccio's famous account of unbridled hedonism, for instance, strikes a very different note from the account in the Neuberg chronicle of men seeking a sort of half-happiness by holding parties to cheer themselves up; but the motives, and perhaps the behaviour, are unlikely to have been so very different [2, 9].

For contemporary chroniclers, the behaviour of the lower classes after the plague was a clear sign of the world plunging further into sin. Modern readers, who generally do not share the medieval commitment to social hierarchy as an expression of divine order, are unlikely to agree. In any analysis of the plague's impact the increased bargaining power of workers, and the adjustment of the balance of power between lords and their tenants, are now more likely to be seen as benefits. Although these changes were contained with some success in the short term, the recurrence of plague in the 1360s and 1370s made them irresistible. Nationally, it is possible to see the fifteenth century as a period of economic decline or stagnation; but there can be very little doubt that most individuals saw their standard of living rise. It was also a period in which many people enjoyed a greater degree of self-determination. The fifteenth century has been seen as the golden age of the labourer; serfdom was becoming an irrelevance; and opportunities in manufacturing and what would now be called service industries widened. Social mobility is always difficult to quantify, but contemporary attempts to codify the trappings appropriate to each social group [121] strongly suggest that society was thought to be becoming more open; as does a rear-guard action by a handful of

---

30 Fryde, 'Tenants', p. 229; A. Jessopp, 'The Black Death in East Anglia' in *idem, The Coming of the Friars and other historic essays*, London, 1889, pp. 233-9 (I have been unable to trace the source of Jessopp's examples).

theorists who insisted, in the teeth of practical experience, that status and behaviour were innate, and the upwardly mobile were therefore bound to make fools of themselves.[31]

Enumerating the benefits of the plague must always seem faintly distasteful – if not positively fatuous, as in the case of Russell's suggestion that the plague raised the general level of health in England.[32] We cannot ask contemporaries whether they thought the price worth paying, and if we could they would probably be unable to answer – there are some balance sheets which cannot be struck. But there are hints that they were aware that their new prosperity was, in effect, being paid for by crisis mortality; or, to put it in more personal terms, that the increased expectations of the survivors derived ultimately from the deaths of family and friends.[33] In the post-plague world the survivors felt both vulnerable and guilty. The vulnerability is the easiest to document. The later middle ages had a very powerful sense of the fragility of success. It is the dark side of the familiar view of the period as an age of ambition, in which anything was possible. The two aspects come together in the image of Fortune's Wheel, omnipresent in fifteenth-century writing and art. One message of the wheel is that man can rise if he chooses, but the other is the inevitablity of failure: what rises will fall, and there is nothing the individual can do about it.

The element of guilt is more speculative, but would help to explain the late-medieval obsession with human mortality. This was not, of course, new. The Church had always emphasised the transience and corruptibility of the body as against the immortality and incorruptibility of the soul, and had urged Christians to meditate on death in order to get their priorities right. But there is an unmistakable change of emphasis after the plague. One dimension of this relates to the sense of vulnerability mentioned above. The unpredictability of death is hammered home endlessly: 'ther is nothing more suer or more certeyn to any creature in this wrecchid world leving then deth, which every creature leving inevitably most suffre, and nothing more onsuer and uncerteyn than the dredfull oure therof'.[34] Alongside this goes an obsessive emphasis on the corruption of the body, not now juxtaposed against the immortality of the soul, but against images of the pride of

---

31 R. Horrox, 'Service' in *Fifteenth-century Attitudes*, forthcoming.

32 Russell, *Medieval Population*, p. 233.

33 This develops a point first made by Hatcher, *Plague, Population*, p. 73.

34 Will of John Coket, 1483: Public Record Office, Prob 11/7 fo. 170v.

life, as in the story of the Three Living and the Three Dead or in *transi* tombs, with the cadaver lying beneath a representation of the deceased in all their glory.[35] This may be where guilt comes in. There is certainly a sense here that the good things of life come with a price tag attached – and inherent in such images is often the idea that the dead person is conscious of their terribly altered state.

Both these aspects of the late-medieval view of death can be rationalised in terms of a response to the plague. Most plague victims lingered for several days, with time to prepare themselves for a good death; and a few chroniclers actually point to this as a sign of divine grace [7]. But contemporaries put much more stress on the fact that apparently healthy people might be struck down without warning. The association of plague with an unprepared death was one of its particular terrors. The other aspect of plague mortality which almost every chronicler mentions is the lack of respect with which the bodies of the dead were treated: carted off by louts looking to earn some quick money, allowed the most cursory of exequies, and then tumbled into a grave pit. In fact the excavation of mass plague burials in London shows that bodies were deposited with some care; but the heavy emphasis which gilds and fraternities subsequently put on providing a decent funeral for their members suggests that (even if the gilds themselves were not a response to anxieties raised by the plague) contemporary sensibilities must have been bruised by conveyor-line burials.[36]

It is the scarcely imaginable scale of plague mortality which contemporaries stressed. But that mortality was made up of individual deaths, individual bereavements. This aspect is the hardest of all for the historian to bring into focus – especially the medieval historian, with

35 The story of the three living and the three dead relates how three young aristocrats out hunting meet themselves in a state of death – not (as in the nineteenth-century romanticised version) as interestingly pale and emaciated bodies, but as decomposing corpses. The story is first recorded in the previous century, but gained wider currency after the plague. There are examples in Polzer, 'Fourteenth-century iconography'. For more general discussion of attitudes to death, see P. Tristram, *Figures of Life and Death in Medieval English Literature*, London, 1976, chapter V; E. Duffy, *The Stripping of the Altars: traditional religion in England 1400-1580*, New Haven, 1992, chapter 9.

36 D. Hawkins, 'The Black Death and the new London cemeteries of 1348', *Antiquity* LXIV, 1990, pp. 637-42, a reference I owe to Keith Murdoch. Boccaccio [2] supports the careful layering of bodies in mass graves. For the gilds' attitudes to burial see C. M. Barron, 'The parish fraternities of medieval London' in C. M. Barron and C. Harper-Bill (eds), *The Church in Pre-Reformation Society*, Woodbridge, 1985, pp. 24-5.

relatively few personal records to work on.[37] It is rare to be able to see a single death among so many. John Constable of Halsham in Holderness made a death bed disposal of his land: 'being of good memory but afflicted with great weakness for the four days preceding, at the time of the mortality then raging in those parts, languishing *in extremis* about that hour of day called Midovernone, made his charter concerning the said manor'.[38]

The bereaved rarely find a voice – and when they do it is usually a public, not a private, voice. Edward III, writing to the family of his dead daughter's fiancé, suggests that 'inward desolation' has been balanced by gratitude at having an intercessor in heaven [77]. The rawness of Petrarch's loss is expressed in elegantly polished Latin [76]. Agnolo di Tura does no more than briefly mention how he buried his five children with his own hands. But their bleak dignity is not only a matter of public decorum. The suffering was simply too great to take in: 'It seemed to almost everyone that one became stupefied by seeing the pain.... There was no one who wept for any death, for all awaited death'.[39] Gabriele de' Mussis agreed: 'Our hearts have grown hard now that we have no future.... The survivors can weep if they want' [1]. Boccaccio noted that people in Florence stopped weeping at funerals and started cracking jokes instead – a phenomenon he seems to have regarded unsympathetically, although it is a common enough form of emotional self-defence [2].

The fear of death proved a potent solvent of other social norms. The ruler of Sicily roamed wild and uninhabited places like a fugitive because he was afraid of death [4]. City dwellers went and camped in the fields. The sick and dying were shunned. A medieval deathbed was normally attended by family and friends, as well as by a priest; now, according to Boccaccio, when the poor died in their homes the first anyone knew of it might be when their bodies began to stink. Parents abandoned dying children; children refused to visit dying parents – a negation of human affection which was clearly thought profoundly shocking. When chroniclers wanted a single image to express the horror of the plague this was often the one they chose. Humans were

37 For early-modern reactions see P. Slack, *The Impact of Plague in Tudor and Stuart England*, Oxford, 1990, pp. 17-21.

38 W. Rees, 'The Black Death in England and Wales, as exhibited in manorial documents', *Proceedings of the Royal Society of Medicine* XVI, 1923, section of the history of medicine, p. 33 (note 4).

39 All quotations from Agnolo di Tura are taken from the translation by W. M. Bowsky in *European Problem Studies: The Black Death*, New York, 1971, pp. 13-14.

reduced to the level of beasts: 'the sick are treated like dogs by their families' [5]; 'no more respect was accorded to dead people than would nowadays be shown towards dead goats' [2]. For those who, in di Tura's phrase, 'escaped and regained the world', that world could never have been quite the same again.

VI: The impact of the plague

76. Petrarch on the death of friends

Petrarch's 'Letters on Familiar Matters' were dedicated to his friend Louis Heyligen, the author of the letter printed in 5, whom Petrarch nicknamed Socrates. Three extracts, all addressed to Socrates, are printed here. The first is the opening of the preface to the collection, written in 1350, in which Petrarch laments all that the plague took from him – including, although she is not mentioned explicitly, Laura, the great love of his life. The other two extracts come from letters written in May-June 1349, when Petrarch was at Parma.

(a) Preface: Petrarch, *Epistolae de Rebus Familiaribus et variae*, ed. Joseph Fracassetti, Florence, 1859, I p. 13.

What are we to do now, brother? Now that we have lost almost everything and found no rest. When can we expect it? Where shall we look for it? Time, as they say, has slipped through our fingers. Our former hopes are buried with our friends. The year 1348 left us lonely and bereft, for it took from us wealth which could not be restored by the Indian, Caspian or Carpathian Sea. Last losses are beyond recovery, and death's wound beyond cure. There is just one comfort: that we shall follow those who went before. I do not know how long we shall have to wait, but I know that it cannot be very long – although however short the time it will feel too long.

(b) Letter from Parma: *Ibid*, pp. 442-3 (book VIII.7).

Scarcely a year and a half has passed since I returned to Italy and left you weeping on the banks of the Sorgues, so I am not asking you to cast your mind back a long way, but to count up those few days and consider what we were, and what we are. Where are our dear friends now? Where are the beloved faces? Where are the affectionate words, the relaxed and enjoyable conversations? What lightning bolt devoured them? What earthquake toppled them? What tempest drowned them? What abyss swallowed them? There was a crowd of us, now we are almost alone. We should make new friends – but how, when the human race is almost wiped out; and why, when it looks to me as if the end of the world is at hand? Why pretend? We are alone indeed.... How transient and arrogant an animal is man! How shallow the foundations on which he rears his towers! You see how our great band of friends has dwindled. Look, even as we speak we too are slipping away, vanishing like shadows. One minute someone hears that another has gone, the next he is following in his footsteps.

(c) Another Letter: *Ibid*, pp. 443-5 (Fracassetti prints this as a continuation of VIII.7, but modern editors prefer to make it a separate letter: VIII.8).

There remained to me at least something salvaged from the wreck of last year: a most brilliant man, and (you must take my word for it) one great in action and counsel, Paganino da Milano, who after numerous proofs of his virtue became very dear to me, and seemed worthy of your friendship as well as mine. He was on the way to becoming another Socrates, displaying almost the same loyalty and good fellowship, and that friendship which lies in sharing good and bad fortune and in baring the hidden places of the heart in a trusting exchange of secrets.

How much he loved you, how much he longed to see you – you whom he could see only with the eyes of imagination. How much he worried about your safety during this shipwreck of the world. I was amazed that a man unknown to him could be so much loved. He never saw me graver than usual without becoming anxious himself and asking, 'Is something wrong? How is our friend?' But when he heard that you were in good health he would cast aside his fears with wonderful alacrity.

And this man (I speak it with many tears, and would speak it with more but my eyes are drained by previous misfortunes and I should save some tears for whatever may befall in the future), this man, I say, was suddenly seized by the pestilence which is now ravaging the world. This was at dusk, after dinner with his friends, and the evening hours that remained he spent talking with us, reminiscing about our friendship and shared concerns. He passed the night in extreme pain, which he endured with an undaunted spirit, and then died suddenly the next morning. None of the now-familiar horrors were abated, and within three days all his children and household followed him.

Go, mortals, sweat, pant, toil, range the lands and seas to pile up riches you cannot keep; glory that will not last. The life we lead is a sleep; whatever we do, dreams. Only death breaks the sleep and wakes us from dreaming. I wish I could have woken before this.

77. The death of Princess Joan

Joan, the daughter of Edward III of England, was to have married Pedro, the heir to Castile, but died of plague at Bordeaux on 2 September 1348, on the way to her wedding. On 15 September her father sent letters to Alfonso, King of Castile (from which this extract is taken), the Queen of Castile and Pedro the Infante. The rest of the letter, not printed here, discusses what should be done about Joan's dowry.

Thomas Rymer (ed), *Foedera, Conventiones, Litterae, et cujuscunque generis acta publica*, 20 vols, London, 1704–35, III pp. 39–40.

We are sure that your magnificence knows how, after much compli-cated negotiation about the intended marriage of the renowned Infante Pedro, your eldest son, and our most beloved daughter Joan, which was designed to nurture perpetual peace and create an indissoluble union between our royal houses, we sent our said daughter to Bordeaux, *en route* for your territories in Spain. But see (with what intense bitterness of heart we have to tell you this) destructive Death (who seizes young and old alike, sparing no one, and reducing rich and poor to the same level) has lamentably snatched from both of us our dearest daughter (whom we loved best of all, as her virtues demanded).

No fellow human being could be surprised if we were inwardly desolated by the sting of this bitter grief, for we are human too. But we, who have placed our trust in God and our life between his hands, where he has held it closely through many great dangers – we give thanks to him that one of our own family, free of all stain, whom we have loved with pure love, has been sent ahead to heaven to reign among the choirs of virgins, where she can gladly intercede for our offences before God himself.

78. The Wakebridge family

In three months in 1349 William de Wakebridge of Derbyshire lost his father, his wife, two brothers, two sisters and a sister in law. Their deaths are listed in the cartulary of the chantries which Wakebridge later endowed in the parish church of Crich (Derbys). The first chantry, in honour of SS Katherine and Nicholas, was planned in 1350. Not all the family members commemo-rated there had died in the plague – William's mother Joan, for instance, had died in 1344 – but many of the friends listed had probably done so.

(a) Family deaths in 1349.

British Library, Harleian MS 3669, fos. 98-103.

18 May	Nicholas, son of Peter de Wakebridge [the founder's brother]
27 June	Elizabeth de Aslaccon, the sister of the wife of William de Wakebridge
16 July	Robert, son of Peter de Wakebridge, formerly vicar of Crich [the founder's brother]
5 August	Peter de Wakebridge and Joan his daughter [the founder's father and sister]
10 August	Joan, wife of William de Wakebridge and Margaret his sister
15 August	John de Wakebridge, chaplain

(b) The souls to be commemorated in the Wakebridge chantry.

Ibid, fo. 22v.

[The keeper of the chantry and his successors] are to celebrate masses every day for ever, unless there is a lawful impediment, for the below-written souls, that is to say for the souls of Nicholas de Wakebridge and Joan his wife; Nicholas, the son of that Nicholas; Joan, Amice and Sarah, the sisters of Nicholas the son of Nicholas; Peter de Wakebridge and Joan his wife [the parents of the founder]; Robert, Nicholas and Peter, the sons of Peter; Joan and Elizabeth, my wives; John de Wakebridge, chaplain; Matilda de Wakebridge; William Cosyn and Eleanor his wife; John Cosyn, chaplain; Cecily and Alice, the daughters of William [Cosyn]; John de la Pole and Cecily his wife; Henry de Coddington and Margery his wife; their parents; Roger de Chester-field, cleric; Henry de Chaddesden; Nicholas de Chaddesden; Richard de Tissington; William de Ballidon; Roger Beler and Margaret his wife; Alice Beler; Cecily Wyn; Ralph Frechevill; and their heirs, and for the souls of all my friends and all the benefactors of the chantry.

79. The death of Abbot Michael of St Albans

H. T. Riley (ed), *Gesta Abbatum Monasterii Sancti Albani*, 3 vols, Rolls Series, 1867-9, II pp. 369-70, 381, 382.

And now, when the industry of Abbot Michael should have been most useful to the monastery, the pestilence (which almost halved mankind) intervened, and a very untimely death halted his career. The fabric of his life was cut short when it seemed that the weaver had only just begun the cloth. To the detriment of the monastery he was one of the first of his monks to be struck by that deadly illness. He felt bodily distress on Maundy Thursday, but out of devotion to the feast, and wishing to commemorate the Lord's humility, he solemnly celebrated high mass before dinner. After mass he washed the feet of his poor with due humility and reverence,[1] and after dinner bathed and kissed the feet of all his brothers, and he performed every one of the day's offices alone, without help.

On the next day, his illness increasing, he took to his bed and, when he had made confession from a contrite heart, he received the last sacrament of unction like a true catholic; and thus he lingered in sorrow and lamentation until nones on Easter Day. Then, while the convent was at dinner, he saddened all their hearts by passing away. He was translated from the distortions of this world of shadows to the true light, from unceasing toil to rest, and from lamentation to the ineffable joy of his Lord.

There died at this time, not counting the many who died in daughter houses, 47 monks, outstanding in religion and remarkable in learning, and who moreover, for the most part, had no equals in virtue.

[The chronicler returns to Abbot Michael's death in the biography of his successor:]

Meanwhile, by the dominion of Saturn, or rather at the will of God, pestilence arose, which snatched many mortals from their mortal matters and parted plenty of prelates from their preferments. Among them was the lord abbot of St Albans, Michael, of blessed memory; worthy, we believe, by his spiritual life to be the minister of that Michael who is the minister of God's Majesty. At the same time Nicholas, the prior of the monastery, died, as did the subprior.

[A new abbot is elected, and prepares to leave for Avignon.] The time

---

1 On Maundy Thursday (the day before Good Friday) the medieval church commemorated Christ's washing of the feet of his disciples: John 13. 4-15.

came when all the necessary preparations had been made for the journey and Thomas de la Mare, the abbot-elect, was ready to set out for the Curia. With him went two of the brethren who were to accompany him to the Curia: Brother Henry of Stukeley and Brother William of Dersingham, religious and very learned men. But when they reached Canterbury, William of Dersingham was infected by the fatal plague and, taking his leave of mortal things, was buried there.

80. Deaths among the nuns of Malling

This series of entries from the episcopal register of Hamo Hethe, Bishop of Rochester, gives a vivid sense of the death rate once the plague took hold in an enclosed community. The final extract, from later in the same year, hints at the continuing difficulties experienced by the much-diminished community.

C. Johnson (ed), *Registrum Hamonis Hethe diocesis Roffensis*, Canterbury and York Society XLVIII, 1948, II pp. 869-73, 898.

Memorandum that on Wednesday 6 May 1349 at Trottiscliffe it came to the notice of Hamo, by the grace of God Bishop of Rochester, that the lady Isabel de Perham, Abbess of the house of Malling, had died the previous night; and promptly, in the morning of the same day, the bishop sent the following letter to the precentress, the subprioress (since the house was then lacking a prioress) and the convent.

Brother Hamo, by divine permission Bishop of Rochester, to our beloved daughters in Christ the precentress and subprioress (the house lacking a prioress) and convent of Malling, greeting, grace and blessing. Since lady Isabel de Perham of happy memory, the last abbess of your house, has rendered her spirit to its creator, and the house still remains bereft of the comfort of an abbess, we order (as is our right by custom) that you should be present at the chapter meeting on Thursday 7 May (a date chosen because of the various grave dangers which we can clearly see are likely to arise because of your lack of an abbess) along with all of your sisters who are entitled to attend and who are willing and able, without inconvenience, to be present, and whom you have had summoned, to discuss with us or someone delegated by us the future choice of an abbess. And the meeting is to be prorogued from day to day until the choice has been made. Warn the sisters beforehand that the procedure will be carried out at the stated time whether or not they are present, according to ancient custom; and the same will be true if the choice is deferred until another day. At the stated day, time and place you are to notify us or our commissary in writing, sealed with your common seal, of what you have done or caused to be done in the matter, along with the names of each and every one of the vowed sisters summoned to take part. Given at Trottiscliffe, 6 May 1349.

[Because of his illness, the bishop delegated the Prior of Rochester, John de Sheppey, to oversee the election, which was to be by secret ballot.]

On the following Thursday, 7 May, in the chapter meeting in the chapter house of Malling, the precentress and subprioress and the nuns of the house entered and presented themselves before the prior, who had some of the bishop's clerks helping him. He first preached a sermon and was then shown by the precentress, in her name and that of the convent, a certain certificate sealed under the common seal which read as follows.

To the venerable father and lord in Christ, lord Hamo, by the grace of God Bishop of Rochester, and to his commissary, his humble and devoted daughters, the precentress and subprioress of Malling and the convent there, give the obedience, reverence and honour due to such a father. We have lately received your mandate, reverend father, and by the authority of that mandate we summoned all of our sisters who are entitled, willing and able without inconvenience to attend at the stated time to hold an election and choose an abbess; and we have also tried to do everything required by your mandate. Accordingly the names of the sisters summoned are contained in the schedule appended to this certificate. And thus we have diligently executed your mandate with all reverence, according to its force, form and effect. In witness of which we have attached our common seal to the present document. Given at Malling, Thursday 7 May 1349.

After this certificate had been read and all the sisters named individually in the attached schedule summoned, they all appeared in person before the lord prior except for Joan de Rokesle, Margaret de Hunting-field, Mary de Godwyneston, Benedicta de Grey, Joan de Wye, Christine Nasard, Mary de Norton, Margery de Patshull, Margaret de Northwood and Alice Cotoun, who were then lying gravely ill in the infirmary.

[Then the precentress, as president of the chapter, and all the other nuns present chose the bishop's chancellor, Thomas de Alkham, to read aloud on their behalf the usual order for excommunicates and unauthorised persons to leave.]

And when this had been read by the said lord Thomas, it was decided by the commissary of the Bishop of Rochester and the precentress and all the nuns who were present that they should proceed by ballot. And so the commissary of the bishop, in the traditional way, took his seat as presiding officer in the chapter, with the bishop's clerks sitting around him, and then took the vote of each of them, beginning with the senior nun and proceeding to the others in decreasing order of seniority, in the order in which they had been named in the certificate. Privately (although the clerks could hear, and two of them wrote down the nomination of each nun) the vote of each of them was taken and recorded in writing by the scribes, as is the custom in that house. Then he sent two of the clerks to the rest of the nuns who were absent, as described above, and their votes were taken on the orders of the commissary.

The commissary and the clerks then counted up the votes cast, as is the custom, and found that eleven nuns had voted for Benedicta de Grey, and that the others had each voted for other candidates. The commissary summoned all the sisters and asked them as a group whether they were happy for him to elect as abbess of the house the person who had received the most nominations (without, however, declaring who that was), as was the custom in the election of abbesses in that house. And when they had all answered that they agreed, the said commissary elected the said Benedicta. [The formal statement of election follows.]

Because the abbess-elect was lying sick she could not, as custom dictated, be led or carried to the high altar; but the bishop's chaplain, who was present, began singing the angelic hymn, *Te deum laudamus*, whereupon all the sisters immediately rose to their feet and, taking up the hymn, went in procession to the choir. When the hymn was finished the commissary said an appropriate prayer for the abbess-elect from the altar steps. But on that very night Benedicta, the abbess-elect, died.

[The news of Benedicta's death reached the Bishop of Rochester the next day, 8 May, and the whole process began again, with the new election taking place on 9 May. By this time there were only ten nuns eligible to vote, of whom eight were lying sick: Emma Port, Margaret de Huntingfield, Joan de Wye, Katherine Levenoth, Mary de Norton, Margery de Patshull, Margaret de Northwode and Alice Cotoun. Seven voted for Alice de Tendring, two for Margery de Patshull and one for Joan Colkyn. The election of Alice was confirmed and she went to the bishop at Trottiscliffe to take her vow of obedience.]

On 27 October 1349 the lord Bishop of Rochester directed a formal monition to the Abbess of Malling that from the date of the order she and all her sisters should eat and sleep in one house, and that they should all be present at every one of the daytime and night time offices, remaining until the end of the office, except in cases of bodily infirmity or self-evident necessity. And this is because of the small number of people performing divine worship there, which is the result of the pestilence.

81. Deaths in Walsham le Willows

The court roll lists all the tenants who had died since the previous court – which does not, of course, represent all the deaths on the manor. In each case the entry records the land which they held at their death and the heriot (death duty) paid to the lady of the manor. This was customarily the dead tenant's best beast, and its payment entitled the heir to enter (take possession of) the holding. Where no heriot could be paid, because the tenant had no beasts, the heir would pay an entry fine to have possession. In a number of cases the heir refused to take over the land.

This is based on Mr Ray Locke's transcript of Suffolk Record Office, Bury St Edmunds, HA504/1/5 fo. 14: the record of the court held at Walsham le Willows on 15 June 1349. I am extremely grateful to him for allowing me to use his findings, which are now the subject of an article in *Proceedings of the Suffolk Institute of Archaeology and History*, XXXVII, part 4, 1992.

John le Syre held a messuage and 12 acres; heriot, a cow before calving; heir, Adam his son, who enters.

Adam Hardonn held a cottage and garden; heriot, a mare; heir, William his brother, who does not come.

Nicholas le Fraunceys held a messuage, 3 acres and 1½ roods;[2] heriot, a cow after calving; heir, Alice, daughter of Margaret Fraunceys, and wife of John Hamund, a free man of Bury St Edmunds, who enters.

Emma Fraunceys held a cottage and garden and 1 rood; no heriot because she had no beast; heir, John Fraunceys her brother, who declines to hold the tenement.

Matilda Robbes held a bakehouse and half an acre; no heriot because she had no beast; heir, John her brother, who does not come.

John Deeth held a cottage; no heriot because he had no beast; heir, Katherine his daughter, who pays 3*d* for entry.

2 A rood is a quarter of an acre and there are 40 perches in a rood. The perch was also a linear measurement: see note 17 below.

Walter Deneys held a messuage, 5 acres and half a rood; heriot, a cow after calving; heir, Robert his son, who has died. After his death the lord had as heriot a ewe after lambing and before shearing; heir, John his son, who enters.

William Deneys held half a messuage and 7½ acres; heriot, a stot;[3] heir, Nicholas his brother, who enters.

Avice le Deneys held 5 acres; heriot, a cow after calving; heir, Nicholas her son, who enters.

Juliana Deneys held 1 acre and 1 rood; no heriot because she had no beast; heir, Nicholas le Deneys her kinsman, who comes and declines to hold the tenement.

Walter Noreys held a messuage, 3 acres and 2½ roods; heriot, a cow; heir, Walter his son, who died before the court was held and no one comes to receive the tenement.

Walter Payn held 3 messuages and 30 acres; heriot, a mare; heir, Robert his son, who enters.

William Payn held a messuage and 24 acres; heriot, a mare; heirs William and John, sons of Robert Lene, who enter.

Walter son of Geoffrey Payn held a messuage and 5 acres; no heriot; heirs, William and John his sons, who enter by a fine of 2s.

William Hawys held a messuage and 40 acres; heriot, a stot; heirs, Robert and John his sons, who enter.

John Hawys held a tenement; heriot, a cow; heirs, William and Robert his sons, who enter.

Thomas Dormour held 1 acre and 1 rood; heriot, a cow after calving; heir unknown.

Edith, wife of the aforesaid Thomas held a messuage and 12 acres; heriot, a cow; heir, William Swift her kinsman, who enters.

Walter Osbern held part of a tenement; heriot, a stot; no one comes to receive the tenement.

Bartholomew Jerico held a messuage and 6 acres; heriot, a stot; heir, John his kinsman, who does not come.

John Osbern held a cottage and 2½ acres; no heriot; heir, Elyanor his kinswoman, who does not come.

---

3 A stot is a bullock: a castrated ox.

William Cranemere held a messuage and tenement; heriot, a stot; heir, William his son. Afterwards William died holding the tenement; heriot a stot; heirs, Robert and William his sons. Afterwards Robert died; heriot, a cow.

William Rampolye held a messuage and tenement; heriot, a cow; heirs, William, Robert, Walter and John his sons, who enter.

John, William and Roger, the sons of Simon Rampolye, held a messuage and tenement; heriot, a ewe after lambing and before shearing; heir, Alice their sister, who enters.

William le Tayllour surrendered a messuage held in villeinage to Walter Rampolye, who paid a fine of 2s for entry and afterwards died, holding the said tenement and 4 acres; heriot, a mare; heirs, Robert Rampolye his brother, Alice daughter of Simon Rampolye, and the four sons of William Rampolye; of whom Robert, Alice and two of the sons enter, the other two sons refuse.

William Wyther held a messuage and 5½ acres; heriot, a mare; no heir comes.

John Pynfoul held a messuage and 13 acres; heriot, a stot; heir, Illary his daughter, who enters.

Agnes Longe, wife of William Swon, held part of a messuage and 1½ roods; no heriot; heir, John her son, but William her husband has a life interest.[4]

John le Tayllour held a life interest in a tenement called Checers; no heriot; it escheats to the lady because John's former wife Katherine, who held the land, was a bastard.

Joan, Katherine and Christian, daughters of Henry Crane, held 1 acre, 1 rood and a quarter of a messuage; no heriot; heirs, Elyanor Wyndelgard and Nicholas son of Thomas le Fuller, of whom Nicholas comes and surrenders his right to Elyanor, who enters by a fine of 6d. Before Joan died she surrendered 3 roods of land in villeinage to John son of Manser of Shuckford, who enters by a fine of 9d.

William le Smyth held a messuage and tenement; heriot, a mare; heir, William his son, who enters.

---

4 The widower of a woman who had held land in her own right was entitled to hold that land for his lifetime after her death on condition that he had had children by her. In the next entry John le Tayllour's life interest in *The Chequers* was on these grounds.

Richard le Man held 1 acre and 1 rood; no heriot; heir, Thomas his son, who does not come.

Alice, Agnes and Katherine, daughters of William Typetot held certain tenements; heriots, 2 cows and a filly; heirs, Robert and William, sons of Elyas Typetot, who enter.

John le Man held certain tenements; heriot, a mare; heir, Robert his son, who enters.

Richard Qualm held certain tenements; heriot, a cow after calving; heir, Richard son of Walter Qualm, who enters.

Simon Peyntour held a tenement; heriot, a cow after calving; heirs, Richard and John his sons, who enter.

Simon and Simon, sons of Peter le Peyntour, held a messuage and 12 acres; no heriot; heir, their sister Alice, who does not come.

Walter Qualm held 2 messuages and 4 acres; no heriot; heir, Richard son of Walter Qualm, his nephew, who enters by a fine of 20d.

John atte Broke held half a messuage and 7 acres; no heriot; heir, John his kinsman, who does not come.

Agnes, the wife of John Stonham held 2 acres; heriot, a cow after calving; heirs, Illary and Isabel her daughters, but John has a life interest.

John Rampolye held a tenement; heriot, a cow after calving; heir, Simon his brother, who enters.

Agnes, the wife of Robert Rampolye, held a messuage and 14 acres; heriot, a colt; heir, Simon her son, but Robert has a life interest.

Richard Patyl, son of Edmund Patyl, held half a messuage and an acre; no heriot; heir, John his brother, who enters by a fine of 6d.

John Patyl held a tenement; heriot, a cow; heir, Alice his daughter, who enters.

Edmund, son of John Patyl, held half a messuage, 1 acre and 1 rood; no heriot; heirs, Walter his brother and Alice, daughter of John Patyl, who enter by a fine of 8d.

William Patel held a messuage and 1 acre; heriot, a cow after calving; heir, Nicholas his son, who enters.

William son of Walter Patyl held a messuage and 2 acres, 1½ roods, 10 perches; heriot, a cow after calving; heir, Christian his sister, who does not enter because William was in debt to the lady and the land is to be seized.

John Typetot held 3 acres; heriot, a cow after calving; heir, Robert his son, who enters. He held a messuage and 2½ acres of free land @ 5½d p.a., his heir Robert is aged 9.

Cecilia Puddynge held 3 acres; heriot, a cow after calving; heir, Robert, son of John Typetot, who enters.

Walter Hereward held a messuage and 2 acres, 1½ roods; no heriot; heirs, Thomas his son and John son of Robert Hereward, who enter by a fine of 12d.

Robert le Tayllour held a tenement; heriot, a cow after calving; heirs, Peter his son, Sara, daughter of John le Tayllour, and John son of William le Tayllour, who enter.

Katherine, the wife of the said Robert, held a tenement; heriot, a cow after calving; heirs as above, who enter.

Isabel, daughter of William le Meller, held a messuage and 2½ acres; no heriot; heir, Robert the chaplain, son of Matthew Terewald, enters by a fine of 16d. Afterwards Robert surrenders the property to Matilda Robhod and her heirs, with reversion to his heirs.

William Wauncey held 1 acre, 1½ roods; no heriot; heirs, the four sons of John Wauncey, who do not come.

Alice, the wife of Nicholas Kembald, held a tenement; heriot, a cow before calving; heirs, Robert and Thomas her sons, who enter.

William, the son of Alice Helewys, held 1½ acres; heriot, a stot; heirs, Robert and Thomas his brothers, who enter.

Robert le Ku held half a messuage and 17 acres; heriot, a cow before calving; heir, Olivia his daughter, who enters.

Matthew Terewald held a tenement; heriot, a cow; heir, Robert his son, who enters.

Ralph Echeman held a tenement; heriot, a cow; heir, Adam his son, who enters.

Walter Springald held part of a messuage and 2½ acres; heriot, a wether before shearing; heir, Robert his brother, who enters.

Robert Springald held a messuage and 2½ acres; no heriot; heirs, Isabel and Illary, daughters of John Stonham, and Agnes, daughter of Amabilia Springeld (aged 3 years), who enter by a fine of 18d.

Richard Spileman held a messuage and 5 acres; heriot, a cow after calving; heir, Amice his daughter, who enters.

Peter Gilbert held half a messuage and 2 acres; heriot, a filly; heir, Matthew his brother, who enters.

Peter le Neve held a messuage and 2½ roods; no heriot; heir, William son of William le Smyth, who surrenders the land to the use of the lady. Afterwards the lady granted the land to John Spileman, who pays 6*d* for entry.

Richard Patil, villein, held various land; heriot, a stot; heir, his bastard son Matthew who purchased it jointly with him. Matthew is outlawed for felony and the property escheats to the lady during his life; with reversion after his death to Richard, son of Richard Patyl junior.

Richard Patyl junior and William his brother held a messuage and 3½ acres; heriot, a stot and a wether before shearing; heir, Richard, son of the said Richard, who enters.

Walter le Syre held a tenement; heriot, a cow after calving; heir, Adam le Syre his kinsman, who enters.

William le Syre who held a tenement; heriot, a cow; heir, Adam le Syre his kinsman, who enters.

Avice, the wife of John Bonde, held a messuage and 5 acres; heriot, a filly; heirs, her three sons, who enter.

Richard Kebbil held a messuage and tenement; heriot, a colt; heir, John the chaplain, his son, who enters.

Idonea Sare held 2½ acres; no heriot; heir, Robert her son, who enters and the fine is waived.

Roesia Stronde held 5 acres and a quarter of a messuage; no heriot; heir, Robert son of Robert Sare, who enters and the fine is waived.

Robert le Man held a messuage and 1 acre; heriot, a cow after calving; heir, Robert his son, who enters.

Walter le Meller held 1 acre, 3 roods; heriot, a cow after calving; heir, his son John, who enters.

Robert Lenne held 4 perches; no heriot; no one comes.

Alice Lenne held 1 rood; no heriot; no one comes.

Stephen le Cupper held a tenement; heriot, a cow after calving; heir, Robert son of Edmund Lene, who enters.

Peter le Taillour held a tenement; heriot, a cow after calving; heirs, Alice his daughter and Alexander son of Isabel Taillour, who enter.

Alice, the wife of Matthew Gilbert, held a cottage and 5 acres; heriot, a cow after calving; heir, Robert Terewald, chaplain, but Matthew has a life interest.

Thomas le Fuller held a messuage and tenement; heriot, a cow before calving; heir, Nicholas his son, who enters.

Alice the wife of Thomas le Fuller surrendered 3 roods of land and a rood of woodland with a cottage to Agnes her daughter in villeinage; she enters by payment of a fine of 12*d*.

Alice, wife of Thomas le Fuller, held a tenement; heriot, a cow after calving; heir, Nicholas her son, who enters.

Walter le Fuller held a messuage and tenement; heriot, a stot; heir, Alice, daughter of John Elys, who enters.

Agnes, wife of Henry Albry, held a messuage and 12 acres; no heriot; heir, William Alwyne her kinsman, who enters by payment of a fine of 3*s*.

Nicholas Goche held a messuage and 14 acres; heriot, a filly; heir, William Alwyne his kinsman, who enters.

Peter Margery held a tenement @ 16½*d*; heirs, John and Robert his sons, who perform fealty.

John Warde and John his brother held a messuage and 16 acres; no heriot; heirs, Robert and William, the sons of Peter Warde, who enter by payment of a fine of 3*s* 4*d*.

Peter le Jay held a messuage and 16 acres, with Nunnescroft; heriot, a cow after calving; heirs, William and Robert his sons, who declined to take the tenement.

John le Taillour and William his son held various land; heriot, a cow after calving; the aforesaid John and William were bastards and therefore the land escheats to the lady.

Robert Hereward held half a rood; heriot, a cow after calving; heir, John his son, who enters.

82. The plague in Lancashire

This document is an inquiry into the money claimed by the Archdeacon of Richmond from the Dean of Amounderness, in Lancashire. The dean was responsible for collecting the revenues of vacant churches, the fees paid for the granting of probate, and money arising from the administration of the goods of those who died intestate. The archdeacon accused the dean of concealing money raised from these sources in the last four months of 1349 and the dispute was put to a local jury. The body of the document (in French) is the archdeacon's version, detailing the extra money he thought he should have received. The jury's figures follow in square brackets.

The archdeacon's account is manifestly not an accurate tally of the number of deaths in the deanery, but it is of interest as an example of what an informed observer thought a likely death rate. The jury's downwards revision of the figures may say more about the difficulties of collecting money in troubled times than about the scale of the archdeacon's exaggeration.

I have abbreviated the entries slightly, notably by omitting the repeated statement that testators and the intestate had goods worth more than £5 – poorer people were not expected to make wills.

A. G. Little, 'The Black Death in Lancashire', *English Historical Review*, V, 1890, pp. 524-30.

The period of the account of the said Sir Adam de Kirkham is from the feast of the Nativity of Our Lady [8 September] 1349 to the following 11 January.

The vicarage of Kirkham and the chapelry of Goosenargh were vacant twice during that time, and Sir Adam de Kirkham received all the mortuaries and oblations during that period, £12 more than in the account [the jurors say that he had 20s].

The vicarage of Poulton and the chapelry of Bispham were vacant during the pestilence and Sir Adam received all the mortuaries and offerings during that period to the value of £14 [the jurors say 40s].

The church of Lancaster and the chapelry of Stalmine were vacant in that period and Sir Adam received all the mortuaries and offerings during that time to the value of 20 marks [£13 6s 8d] [the jurors say 100s].

The vicarage of Garstang was vacant twice during that time and Sir Adam received all the mortuaries and offerings during that time to the value of 10 marks [the jurors say 40s].

The priory of Lytham was vacant during that time and Sir Adam received all the mortuaries and offerings during that time to the value of £10 [the jurors say 50 marks, i.e. £33 6s 8d].

Within the parish of Preston, 3,000 men and women died, of whom 300 made wills; Sir Adam received 20 marks [£13 6s 8d] more than appears in his account for proving the wills [the jurors say £10].

That is to say: from the executors of William Mirresson and his wife, half a mark; the executors of Thomas Mareschal and his wife, 6s; the executors of Robert Litester and his wife, 40d; the executors of John

Tilleson and his wife, 4s; the executors of William de Wrokhol and his wife, 40d; and from many others amounting to 20 marks.

Sir Adam received, or ought to have received according to the right and custom of the church, £11 in acquitances for the wills, for which he did not account.

200 parishioners of Preston died intestate and the administration of their goods pertains to the Archdeacon of Richmond; value £10, for which he made no account.

That is to say, from the goods of Robert de Witeneye and his wife 60s; the wife of Long Aubrey 100s; Richard Waddere and his wife 60s; Jakke o'the Hill 40s; and from the goods of many others who died intestate.

Within the parish of Kirkham 3,000 men and women died, of whom 600 made wills, and Sir Adam received 20 marks [£13 6s 8d] more than appears in his account for proving those wills [the jurors say £4].

Sir Adam received, or ought to have received, £10 in acquitances for the wills, for which he did not account [the jurors say 20s].

100 parishioners of Kirkham died intestate and the administration of their goods pertains to the Archdeacon of Richmond; value 100s, for which he made no account.

Within the parish of Poulton 800 men and women died, of whom 200 made wills, and Sir Adam received 100s more than appears in his account for proving those wills [the jurors say 20s].

That is to say, from the executors of Robert de Thacherstions, 2s; the executors of Richard de Ellale, 3s; the executors of the wife of Roger Pans, 20d; the executors of Richard de Marton, 2s 6d; and from many others, amounting to 100s.

Sir Adam received or ought to have received £4 in acquitances for the wills, for which he did not account [the jurors say half a mark, i.e. 6s 8d].

40 parishioners of Poulton died intestate and the administration of their goods pertains to the Archdeacon of Richmond; value 40s.

Within the parish of Lancaster 3,000 men and women died, of whom 400 made wills, and Sir Adam received 20 marks more than appears in his account for proving those wills [the jurors say £4].

Sir Adam received, or ought to have received, £10 in acquitances for the wills, for which he did not account [the jurors say 20s].

80 parishioners of Lancaster died intestate and the administration of their goods pertains to the Archdeacon of Richmond; value 60s.

Within the parish of Garstang 2,000 men and women died, of whom 400 made wills, and Sir Adam received £10 more than appears in his account for proving those wills [the jurors say 40s].

That is to say, from the executors of John de Staunfgood, 40d; the executors of his wife, 3s; the executors of Adam Hannemagh, 4s; the executors of Robert Taillour, 2s; the executors of the wife of Matthew Walker, 2s; the executors of William de Couper, 2s 6d; and from others, amounting to the abovesaid sum.

Sir Adam received, or ought to have received, 60s in acquitances for the wills, for which he did not account [the jurors say 20s].

140 parishioners of Garstang died intestate and the administration of their goods pertains to the Archdeacon of Richmond; value £10.

Within the parish of Cockerham 1,000 men and women died, of whom 300 made wills, and Sir Adam received £4 10s more than appears in his account for proving those wills [the jurors say 20s].

That is to say, from the executors of William de Fournais, 3s; the executors of the wife of Richard de Guncestre, 18d; the executors of Thomas Belan, 2s; the executors of Roger Hanson, 3s; the executors of the wife of Adam Slauk, 18d; and from others amounting to £4 10s.

Adam received, or ought to have received, 30s in acquitances for the wills, for which he did not account [the jurors say half a mark].

60 parishioners of Cockerham died intestate and the administration of their goods pertains to the Archdeacon of Richmond; value £10.

Within the parish of Ribchester 100 men and women died, of whom 70 made wills, and Sir Adam received 40s for proving those wills [the jurors say 33s 4d].

Adam received, or ought to have received, 30s in acquitances for the wills [the jurors say half a mark].

40 parishioners of Ribchester died intestate and the administration of their goods pertains to the Archdeacon of Richmond; value 100s.

Within the parish of Lytham 150 men and women died, of whom 80 made wills, and Sir Adam received 100s for proving those wills [the jurors say half a mark].

Adam received or ought to have received 20s in acquitances for the wills [the jurors say 40d].

80 parishioners of Lytham died intestate and the administration of their goods pertains to the Archdeacon of Richmond; value 100s.

Within the parish of St Michael 80 men and women died, of whom 50 made wills, and Sir Adam received 40s for proving those wills [the jurors say 1 mark].

Adam received or ought to have received 10s in acquitances for the wills [the jurors say half a mark].

40 parishioners of St Michael died intestate and the administration of their goods pertains to the Archdeacon of Richmond; value 40s.

Within the parish of Poulton[5] 60 men and women died, of whom 40 made wills, and Sir Adam received £4 [6 marks] for proving those wills [the jurors say 1 mark].

Adam received or ought to have received [blank] in acquitances for the said wills [the jurors say half a mark].

20 parishioners of Poulton died intestate and the administration of their goods pertains to the Archdeacon of Richmond; value 40s.

83. A new burial ground in London

This account comes from the *Survey* of London compiled by the antiquary John Stow in the second half of the sixteenth century and carries the story of the burial ground beyond the plague itself. I have modernised the spelling but not the syntax.

John Stow, *A Survey of London*, ed. C. L. Kingsford, 2 vols, Oxford, 1908, II pp. 81-2.

And without the bar of West Smithfield lieth a large street or way, called of the house of St John there, St John's Street, and stretcheth towards Islington, on the right hand whereof stood the late dissolved monastery called the Charterhouse, founded by Sir Walter Manny, knight, a stranger born, lord of the town of Manny in the diocese of Cambrai, beyond the seas, who for service done to King Edward III was made knight of the garter. This house he founded upon this occasion. A great pestilence entering this island, began first in Dorsetshire, then proceeded into Devonshire, Somersetshire, Gloucestershire, and Oxfordshire, and at length came to London, and overspread all England, so wasting the people that scarce the tenth

---

5 This second Poulton entry is probably an error for Bispham – the one parish in Amounderness not otherwise included in this list.

person of all sorts was left alive, and churchyards were not sufficient
to receive the dead, but men were forced to choose out certain fields for
burials; whereupon Ralph Stratford, bishop of London, in the year
1348, bought a piece of ground called No Man's Land, which he
enclosed with a wall of brick, and dedicated for burial of the dead,
building thereupon a proper chapel, which is now enlarged and made
a dwelling house; and this burying plot is become a fair garden,
retaining the old name of Pardon churchyard.

About this, in the year 1349, the said Sir Walter Manny, in respect of
the danger that might befall in this time of so great a plague and
infection, purchased thirteen acres and a rood of ground adjoining to
the said No Man's Land, and lying in a place called Spittle Croft,
because it belonged to St Bartholomew's Hospital, since that called the
New church haw, and caused it to be consecrated by the said bishop of
London to the use of burials.

In this plot of ground there was in that year more than 50,000 persons
buried, as I have read in the charters of Edward III; also I have seen
and read an inscription fixed on a stone cross, sometime standing in
the same churchyard, and having these words: 'In the year of Our Lord
1349, during the reign of the great pestilence, this cemetery was
consecrated, in which, and within the boundaries of the present
monastery, there were buried more than 50,000 bodies, not counting
the many buried there since that time; upon whose souls may God have
mercy. Amen'.

In consideration of the number of Christian people here buried, the
said Sir Walter Manny caused first a chapel to be built, where for the
space of twenty-three years offerings were made; and it is to be noted,
that above 100,000 bodies of Christian people had in that churchyard
been buried; for the said knight had purchased that place for the burial
of poor people, travellers, and other that were diseased to remain for
ever; whereupon an order was taken for the avoiding of contention
between the parsons of churches and that house; to wit, that the bodies
should be had into the church where they were parishioners, or
died, and, after the funeral service done, had to the place where they
should be buried.[6] And in the year 1371 he founded there a house of

---

6 Under normal conditions the dead would be buried in their parish churchyard, and
the parish priest would receive the mortuary (payable from the estate of the dead
person), as well as offerings from those attending the funeral mass. The arrangement detailed here: that the body went to the parish church before burial in Pardon
churchyard, was designed to protect the financial rights of the parish priests.

Carthusian monks, which he willed to be called the Salutation, and that one of the monks should be called prior; and he gave them the said place of thirteen acres and a rood of land, with the chapel and houses there built, for their habitation; he also gave them the three acres of land lying without the walls on the north part, betwixt the lands of the abbot of Westminster and the lands of the prior of St John (which three acres were purchased, enclosed, and dedicated by Ralph Stratford, Bishop of London, as is afore showed), and remained till our time by the name of Pardon churchyard, and served for burying of such as desperately ended their lives or were executed for felonies.

84. Burial problems in Worcester

Wolstan de Bransford, Bishop of Worcester, to the Dean of Worcester; Hartlebury, 18 April 1349.

Thomas Nash, *Collections for the History of Worcestershire* I, London, 1781, pp. 226-7.

With heartfelt anxiety we have given careful consideration and frequent thought to the dangerous and (alas) all too numerous burials in the churchyard of our cathedral church of Worcester, which have grievously increased in recent times because of the unprecedented numbers of deaths now occuring. We naturally wish, with God's help, to provide the best remedy, not only for the sake of our brethren devoutly serving God and his most glorious mother in the cathedral, and the citizens and other residents of the city, but also for the sake of all the other people resorting to the city, considering the manifold dangers which in all probability await them from the decomposing bodies. After giving thought to the matter we have ordained, and now do ordain, that a suitable and proper place for the purpose, namely the burial ground of the hospital of St Oswald in Worcester, should supply the deficiency of the cathedral churchyard and should receive bodies for burial during the present time. Accordingly we give you responsibility on our behalf, and straitly charge you, to enjoin and order the sacrist of our cathedral church, and anyone else whom it may concern, that during this mortality the burial of any corpse pertaining to the cathedral burial ground may be, at the sacrist's discretion, in the churchyard of St Oswald, until we can devise some other solution to the problem.

85. A new burial ground at Newark

This order from William Zouche, Archbishop of York, to the perpetual vicar of Newark (Notts) was sent from Cawood on 15 May 1349. It is the earliest licence for the extension of a burial ground in the diocese; many more were to follow in the next three months (see below 86). I have printed only the preamble to the licence, setting out the situation in Newark.

York, Borthwick Institute of Historical Research, Reg. 10, fo. 127v.

The care of the pastoral office pressing on us, urges and leads us to give, with God's help, all possible support to the just desires of our subjects, particularly when they concern the health of souls. A petition put before us on your behalf has shown that the mortality of plague which has been afflicting various parts of the world began to attack the townspeople of Newark some time ago now, and has carried off numerous residents and inhabitants of the town, and is daily gaining in strength there, with the result that the burial ground of the church, because it is small and has no room to expand, is not adequate for the burial of the dead. With all this in mind, you have purchased, at your own expense, a certain plot or piece of land, which is walled and lies in the street called Apiltongate in Newark aforesaid, between the tenements of Peter de Swafeld on one side and Martin le Sadler on the other. With the approval of all those who have an interest in the matter you have petitioned that we should deign to grant a licence and give our authority for the burial of the bodies of the dead there.

86. Consecration of new burial grounds in Yorkshire

Orders from William Zouche, Archbishop of York, to his suffragan the Archbishop of Damascus for the consecration of new burial grounds between June and August 1349. In the letters the greeting and dating clauses have been paraphrased and the order to the suffragan to report action omitted; the memoranda are printed as they stand.

York, Borthwick Institute of Historical Research, Reg. 10, fo. 286-v.

Memorandum that at Ripon on 26 June 1349 a commission was issued to the Archbishop of Damascus to consecrate the churchyard of the chapel of Egton within the parish of Lythe, with the express agreement and at the request of M. John de Bolton, rector of the same.

A like commission to consecrate the churchyard of the chapel of St Thomas by Beverley.

William, Archbishop of York, to Hugh, Archbishop of Damascus; Ripon, 10 July 1349.

By this letter we appoint you in our place to consecrate the chapel of St Oswald at Fulford with its churchyard so that ecclesiastical burial may be performed there, with the consent of the abbot and convent of the monastery of St Mary at York to whose use the parish church of St Mary [recte St Olave] at York (of which the said chapel is a dependency) is canonically appropriated. This is on the understanding, however, that when the pestilence or mortality of men which is now reigning comes to an end, then burial in the said chapel and burial ground shall stop, and on condition that you firmly instruct the residents and inhabitants of the village of Fulford that they should not presume or attempt, by reason of the dedication of the chapel and burial ground, to withdraw anything which may be to the prejudice of the said mother church, and that the burial ground of the chapel should be walled and henceforth kept for ever from any defilement.[7]

Memorandum that on 15 July in the same year a commission was issued to brother Hugh, Archbishop of Damascus, to consecrate the chapel and churchyard of Cleasby, within the parish of Stanwick, with the agreement of Master John de Crakhale, rector of the same parish etc.

William, Archbishop of York, to Hugh, Archbishop of Damascus; Ripon, 17 July 1349.

By this letter we appoint you in our place to consecrate the churchyard of the chapel of Wilton and the chapel itself within the parish of Leatham in our diocese, with the express agreement of Sir Thomas de Thwenges, rector of the parish, so that ecclesiastical burial may be performed there until Christmas (without prejudice to the said church), on account of the pressing pestilence or mortality of men now waxing strong. We want the privilege to stop after Christmas and we have dictated in these letters that it must do so unless the residents and inhabitants of the said village of Wilton obtain an extension. This is provided that the chapel and its burial ground are walled and are henceforth kept (as is fitting for consecrated places) from any defilement, whether by men or animals, for ever.

Memorandum that at Ripon on 23 July 1349 a similar commission was issued for the chapel and churchyard of Seamer within the parish of

---

7 The residents of Fulford evidently found this arrangement far more convenient than using their parish churchyard of St Olave in the suburbs of York, and when the plague was over Zouche had to order them to return to the old arrangement. His command was ignored, and in September 1353 his successor John Thoresby reiterated it, accusing the residents of Fulford of 'taking a foolish delight in novelty': Borthwick Institute, Reg. 11 fo. 11v.

Rudby, with the express agreement of Sir John de Wodhous, now rector of the same church.

Memorandum that on 23 July at Ripon a commission was issued to the suffragan to consecrate the chapel and churchyard of Brotton within the parish of Skelton and a certain plot adjoining the churchyard of the church of Guisborough with the agreement of the prior and convent of Guisborough, to whom the said churches are appropriated. So that ecclesiastical burial may be performed there by reason of the mortality until next Christmas – in the same form as was written over the page for the chapel of Wilton.

Memorandum that at Cawood on 1 August 1349 a commission was issued to brother Hugh, Archbishop of Damascus to consecrate the churchyard of the chapel of Barton within the parish of Gilling in Richmondshire, so that ecclesiastical burial may be performed there as long as the plague is reigning, with the agreement of the abbot and convent of the monastery of St Mary at York and Sir N. Darell, vicar of the same parish, without, however, any prejudice to the church and with the standard clause etc.

Memorandum that on 7 August at Burton by Beverley a commission was issued to the suffragan to consecrate the chapel and churchyard of Easby within the parish of Stokesley with the express agreement and at the request of the rector, Sir William de Feriby.

87. A shortage of priests to hear confession

The Bishop of Bath and Wells to the clergy of his diocese, ordering them to publicise the fact that in an emergency confession may be made to a layman; Winchcombe, 10 January 1349.

D. Wilkins, *Concilia Magnae Britanniae et Hiberniae*, 4 vols, 1739, II, pp. 745-6.

The contagious pestilence, which is now spreading everywhere, has left many parish churches and other benefices in our diocese without an incumbent, so that their inhabitants are bereft of a priest. And because priests cannot be found for love or money to take on the responsibility for those places and visit the sick and administer the sacraments of the church to them – perhaps because they fear that they will catch the disease themselves – we understand that many people are dying without the sacrament of penance, because they do not know what they ought to do in such an emergency and believe that even in an emergency confession of their sins is of no use or worth unless made to a priest having the power of the keys. Therefore, desirous as we must be to provide for the salvation of souls and to call back the wanderers who have strayed from the way, we order and firmly enjoin you, upon your obedience, to make it known speedily and publicly (either in person or through someone else) to everybody, but particularly to those who have already fallen sick, that if when on the point of death they cannot secure the services of a properly ordained priest, they should make confession of their sins, according to the teaching of the apostle, to any lay person, even to a woman if a man is not available. Each rector, vicar or parish priest among you should publicise this within your church, and deans should make themselves responsible for places within their deanery which have no incumbent.

Moreover we urge you, in the bowels of Jesus Christ, that you let it be known at the same time that confession made in this way to a lay person can be wholesome and of great benefit to them for the remission of their sins, according to the teaching and canons of the church. And lest anyone should hesitate or refuse to make confession to a lay person in an emergency, imagining that lay confessors are likely to reveal what was said to them, you should make it known to everybody, and particularly to those who have already heard such confessions or who might hear them in future, that they are obliged by the orders of the church to conceal such confessions and keep them secret, and are forbidden to reveal them by word or sign or in any other manner whatsoever, unless the person making the confession wishes it to be revealed. And if they do otherwise, such offenders should know that they have committed an extremely grave sin and incurred the indignation of Almighty God and of the whole Church by their action.

And because many people are caught out, because they have put off repentance to the last minute, until illness compels it and the fear of damnation becomes overwhelming, we (trusting in the mercy of God and in the merits and prayers of his most glorious mother, our patrons the apostles Peter, Paul and Andrew, and all the saints) grant that during this pestilence all your parishioners who make confession to a priest who holds the keys of the church, and has the power of binding and loosing, while they are still healthy, rather than waiting until they fall ill, should receive forty days of indulgence, as should every priest who urges them to this course and hears the confessions of the healthy.

You should also let it be known that all those who confess their sins to a lay person in an emergency, and then recover, should confess the same sins again to their own parish priest. In the absence of a priest, the sacrament of the Eucharist may be administered by a deacon. If, however, no priest is available to administer the sacrament of extreme unction then, as in other matters, faith must suffice for the sacrament.

You are to take pains to publicise this order, and the points made in it, distinctly and clearly in the vernacular in the usual way in the churches and other places specified above, or ensure that it is done by someone else, letting us know by the feast of St Peter *in cathedra* [22 February] what you have done in the matter.

88. A papal licence for extra ordinations

Clement VI to William Zouche, Archbishop of York; Avignon, 12 November 1349.

James Raine (ed), *Historical Letters and Papers from the Northern Registers*, Rolls Series, 1873, pp. 401-2.

Lest the lack of ministers should mean a reduction in divine service or neglect of the care and rule of souls, we gladly share the help of apostolic goodwill as far as, with God's approval, we are able. Your petition which has been shown to us sets out very clearly that, because of the mortality from plague which overshadows your province at this time, not enough priests can be found for the cure and rule of souls or to administer the sacraments. We want to find an appropriate solution to the problem, because we fervently desire an increase of worship and the health of souls, and have therefore inclined favourably to your request and of our special grace grant you, brother, licence to celebrate four extra ordinations of candidates for both minor and priestly orders at the appointed times within one year of the date of the present letter, either in person or through another catholic bishop in communion with the apostolic see, notwithstanding any decrees to the contrary. Therefore let no one at all break the terms of our grant or rashly dare to go against it, and if anyone should presume to do so, may he incur the displeasure of Almighty God and of his blessed apostles Peter and Paul.

89. The shortage of secular clergy

William Zouche, Archbishop of York, to Brother Thomas de Stodeley, a canon regular of the monastery of St Oswald at Nostell; Burton by Beverley, 8 September 1349.

York, Borthwick Institute of Historical Research, Reg 10 fo. 36v.

At the presentation of the prior and convent of the monastery of St Oswald at Nostell, we have for charity's sake admitted you, in whose merits and virtues we have sincere trust, to the vicarage of Tickhill in our diocese which is vacant by the death of Sir Hugh de Derford, the last vicar there. This is usually ruled by a secular chaplain and we are making an exception on this occasion to make good the lack of secular priests, who have been carried from our midst by the plague of mortality which hangs over us. We institute you canonically as perpetual vicar there with the obligation of personal residence, undertaken on your behalf before us in due form.

90. A failed chantry endowment

This glimpse of the personal dislocation caused by the plague has survived because of its financial implications. Three Bridgnorth men had agreed to pay £10 for a royal licence to make a grant in mortmain, but had died before making payment. The exchequer attempted to extract payment from the town bailiff by charging the sum to his account, and his protest prompted the following inquiry. The royal writ initiating the investigation was sent on 10 June 1355, and the inquiry was held in the following month. I have omitted the names of the jurors.

Public Record Office, Chancery inquisitions miscellaneous, C 145/172/1.

Edward by the grace of God King of England and France and Lord of Ireland, to the sheriff of Shropshire, greeting. On 3 April 1348 Richard Moghale, chaplain, John Dugel, chaplain, and John atte Leghe, the executors of the will of Joan, widow of Nicholas de Picheford, made a fine of £10 for our letters patent granting that the said executors might give and assign rents of 5m in Bridgnorth to the chaplain celebrating mass for the soul of the said Nicholas in perpetuity.[8] The executors died in the last pestilence, and, although our said letters granting them licence still remain, unexecuted, in the hanaper of our chancery, yet the treasurer and barons of our exchequer are charging the said £10 to the account of John Canne, the bailiff of Bridgnorth, on whose behalf we have been asked to provide a remedy in the matter.[9] Our said letters do still remain in the hanaper, as our beloved

---

8 A 'fine' in medieval usage was not (as now) a penalty for wrongdoing, but a payment for permission to be allowed to do something.

9 The hanaper was the financial arm of the royal chancery, responsible for collecting payments made for royal letters. Its accounts were audited by the exchequer, which is why it is exchequer officials who are chasing up the promised payment.

clerk Richard de Thoresby, the keeper of the hanaper, has testified to us, and we accordingly wish to have greater assurance from you that the said executors did die in the said pestilence as has been claimed; and if they did, then when and where. And we order you to make a careful inquiry into the matter by the oath of worthy men of legal standing in your bailiwick, through whom the truth may be better known, and that you send the findings clearly and in full to our chancery before the feast of St Peter *ad vincula* [1 August] under your seal and the seals of the jurors.

An inquisition held before John de Burton, Sheriff of Shropshire, at Bridgnorth on 10 July 1355.

The jurors, carefully examined, say on their oath that Richard de Moghale, chaplain, John Dugel, chaplain, and John atte Leghe, executors of the will of Joan, the widow of Nicholas de Pichford, are dead. Examined as to when and where, they say on their oath that Richard de Moghale, chaplain, died at Bridgnorth on 24 February 1349; John Dugel, chaplain, in the same town on 3 April in the same year; and John atte Leghe in the same town on 7 May in the same year.

91. The deaths of officials

The royal government expected business as usual during the plague, and accordingly fined Aymer fitz Waryn, the Sheriff of Devon, £20 for failing to come to Westminster to render his account in summer 1349. The following is the sheriff's excuse, which was subsequently endorsed by a local jury. The penalty was later waived by the king.

Public Record Office, Exchequer plea rolls, E 13/77 mem 40.

He says that on the day after Trinity Sunday,[10] and both before and after that date, he was lying sick at Marland, and the illness which kept him there was so serious that his life was then despaired of, which meant that he was unable to travel. And he says that Richard de Greencombe, who was his under-sheriff and sub-escheator and responsible for receiving the issues of the county, along with his other ministers and officials (viz Richard de Upcote, clerk, John Furlang, clerk, Richard Wolfe and Robert Taynestor) who had the keeping of the writs, rolls and memoranda which he needed to make up his account, had died suddenly at Marland before that date of the pestilence then raging in the county.

10 This was the day when fitz Waryn was meant to make his account at the exchequer. In 1349 it fell on 8 June.

92. A wrong redressed

The moral impact of plague emerges from the resolution of this long-standing Essex dispute. The entry was made at the foot of the record of proceedings in the court for the manor of Waltham, held at Pleshy on 1 April 1349. Almost all the previous entries are concerned with the deaths of tenants.

Public Record Office, Duchy of Lancaster court rolls, DL 30/64/806 mem 3 dorse.

Roger son of Richard Andrew came into court and requested the court that he might be allowed to have back the horse seized by way of heriot on the death of his father, Richard Andrew, for tenements held in Great Waltham, as appears in the records of the court held on 18 January 1344. He says that the aforesaid tenements do not owe heriot, as appears from the verdict of an inquisition held at Pleshy on 7 February 1317, on which day Richard presented himself to do fealty to the lord for the aforesaid lands and tenements in Waltham. It was then put to him by the constable then in office that the tenements were held by homage and foreign service, and Richard answered and affirmed that Andrew his father and he himself held all the lands and tenements of the lord earl by fealty and suit of court to the lord's court at Waltham, and by the service of a rent of assize[11] of 12s p.a. for all services and secular demands, as set out in the earl's charter. But he was unable to produce the charter in court because, a long time ago, his house had burnt down, and the charter and other muniments had been inside and had been burnt. And he asked for a ruling on the matter by the whole homage.[12] Whereupon the assessors of the court, charged to give an opinion, said on oath that the said charter and other muniments had been burnt, and that the tenements were held of the lord by fealty, suit of court and a rent of assize of 12s as above, and that the aforesaid lands and tenements do not owe heriot by virtue of the aforesaid enrolment and the inquisition newly held by the whole homage.

It seemed to John de Benyngton, then constable of Pleshy, that the taking of the horse as heriot had been wrong; and so, his conscience moved by the deaths and the pestilence which there then was, he paid Roger Andrew 18s as recompense for the horse. This halts the action concerning the taking of heriot from the aforesaid tenements.

11 A rent of assize is a fixed cash rent.

12 The homage was the whole body of men expected to attend the manorial court. The assessors in the next sentence are a narrower and more elite group, usually drawn from the leading inhabitants. Their main role was to assess the level of amercements (penalties for wrongdoing) imposed by the court.

93. An immediate fall in revenue

When the Bishop of Worcester died on 6 August 1349 his temporalities were, as usual, taken into the king's hands during the vacancy of the see and were administered by two royal officials until 28 November. The yield from the land during that period was so much lower than expected that the exchequer launched an inquiry, which vindicated the officials' claims that much of the shortfall was due to plague mortality. In reading the financial details which follow, it should be borne in mind that medieval practice was to make the accounting officials answerable for the money which *ought* to be collected from the source in question, and then leave them to explain any which was missing. It is this process (which was being carried out in 1352) which is recorded in the opening stages of the text. I have silently omitted brief passages relating to another matter on which the exchequer had taken issue with Leo Perton, one of the two officials concerned.

Edmund Fryde, 'The tenants of the Bishop of Coventry and Lichfield and of Worcester after the plague of 1348-9', in R. F. Hunnisett and J. B. Post (eds), *Medieval Legal Records*, HMSO, 1978, pp. 258-60.

Robert Warcop and Leo Perton received the issues of the temporalities of the Bishop of Worcester, which were in the king's hands because of the death of Bishop Wolstan from 28 August 1349 until 28 November following, when they handed over the temporalities to Master William de Fenton and William de Evesham to hold as long as the vacancy should last, on condition that they answered for the issues to John, Bishop of St Davids, to whom the king granted all the issues and other profits which ought to pertain to the king from 28 November.[13] The grant was made under the great seal by a writ dated 28 November, by which the king ordered the keepers to hand over the temporalities to William and William. When their account was audited they were found to owe £238 5s ½d.

Of this they paid £66 13s 4d by tally on 19 October 1350. And they seek allowance of £30 8s 8½d which they paid to William Cusance, treasurer of the king's wardrobe, for the expenses of the king's household, for which they have two receipts in William's name. This leaves owing £141 3s. Of this they challenge £25 5s 7¾d with which they are charged for the farm and other issues of the manor of Stratford upon Avon, which they say they were not able to collect because Wolstan the last bishop, some time before his death, had leased the manor to John Peyto for life, and he held it during the whole

---

13 John Thoresby, the Bishop of St Davids, had been provided to the see of Worcester on 4 September. The temporalities were restored to him on 10 January 1350.

vacancy and still holds it, with the agreement of the cathedral chapter and with the king's permission, and he is due to pay his rent at certain stated terms, none of which happened to fall within the period of account, and they take their oath to that effect. They have been told to ensure that he answers the king for the issues before the quindene of Michaelmas next, and in the meantime they have respite.[14]

And they are charged with £24 6s 5d due from the tithe of sheaves and hay from the church of Hillingdon [Midds] and 6s 8d rent from the same, which they say they were unable to collect because the dean and chapter of London claim to have the fruits of the church during any vacancy at Worcester and have taken it. They have been told to ensure that the dean and chapter answer the king for the money before the quindene of Michaelmas etc.

And they are charged with 33s 4d for a pension of the church of Berkeley payable at Michaelmas for the manor of Hanbury which is part of the temporalities of the bishop, but they say they could not collect it because the prior of Worcester claims the pension and had collected it. They have been told to ensure that the prior answers the king etc.

And they challenge £84 4s ½d with which they say they were overcharged within the account for the rents of assize, customary rents and other lesser rents and services, along with autumn works, boon works, threshing, ploughing and harrowing, carrying and stacking crops, and other rents on various episcopal manors; this was beyond what they were able to collect because of the lack of tenants who used to pay the rent and of customary tenants who used to perform the labour services. They died in the deadly pestilence which raged within the bishop's estates during the period of the account and earlier, and the accounting officials have handed over two rolls listing the names of tenants from whom rent was due and the numbers of virgaters, *noklands*, *arkemen* and cottagers from whom the services were due. And they ask to be discharged of the said £84 4s ½d, calculating that about £85 12s 1¾d could not be collected for the abovesaid reasons, and they maintain that they can prove it. They have been told to obtain a writ from the king to the treasurer and barons of the exchequer discharging them of the amount before the quindene of Michaelmas next. And in the meantime they have respite. And they owe £15 13s 6¾d which is

14 A quindene was the fifteenth day after a feast. Since the day at each end of the fifteen was counted it is the equivalent of a fortnight (fourteen nights). Thus the quindene of Easter (mentioned below) is the second Sunday after Easter, and the quindene of Michaelmas (29 September) is 13 October.

also respited to them until Michaelmas, along with the larger sum.

[Robert Warcop and Leo Perton duly appeared in the exchequer at Michaelmas 1353 to report progress. They presented the following letter from the king, dated 27 October 1352.]

Edward, by the grace of God King of England and France and Lord of Ireland, to the treasurer and barons of the exchequer, greetings. By letters patent of 28 August 1349 we committed the custody of the bishopric of Worcester, then being vacant, to our beloved clerk Robert Warcop and to Leo Perton, on condition that they answered in the exchequer for all the issues, as is more fully set out in the said letters. And although the said Robert and Leo collected and paid over all the services, issues and profits due from the free tenants and villains and from all the lands and tenements of the bishopric, considering the pestilence which was then raging in those parts, yet the auditors of their account, without giving due weight to the reduction in the rents and services of the tenants and the diminution of the value of the land and tenements, charged the said Robert and Leo with the full sum collected from the temporalities during the vacancy in the 31st year of King Edward our grandfather [1302-3]. We, not wishing Robert and Leo to be unfairly charged, order that if it can be proved by inquiry or by some other proper means that Robert and Leo collected all the money possible from the services due from the free and unfree tenants and from the lands and tenements of the bishopric, considering the pestilence, and that they faithfully answered for it at the exchequer, then they should be discharged of the larger sum of money beyond that which they were able to collect.

And the said keepers asked that they might be discharged of the said £84 4s ½d, according to the terms of the writ, asserting that they had been charged with the following sums from the rents of free and customary tenants and from the labour services of the villeins on various episcopal manors, beyond what they were able to collect:

Hartlebury: 102s 8½d beyond the 109s 3¼d received
Northwick: £4 5s 4½d beyond the 23s 10d received
Wick by Worcester: 53s 4½d beyond the £7 12s 5½d received
Kempsey: £4 11s 6½d beyond the 4s 4½d received
Aston: 15s 11½d beyond the 5s ½d received
Hanbury by Wych: £4 10¾d beyond the 2s 7½d received
Alvechurch: £7 9s 5½d beyond the 36s 5¼d received
Fladbury: £6 8s 7d beyond the 35s 6d received
Blockley: £7 5s 6d beyond the 64s 9¼d collected

Ripple: £8 8s 1¼d beyond the 106s 11¼d collected
Bredon: 101s 4d beyond the £4 5s 9¾d collected
Cleeve: £4 15s 4½d beyond the 45s 7¼d collected
Withington: £4 17s 9¾d beyond the 74s 9¾d collected
Bibury: £4 2s 6½d beyond the 25s 5d collected
Bishop's Hampton [Hampton Lucy]: 48s 5¾d beyond the £4 8s 7d
collected
Henbury in Salt Marsh: £12 3s 7d beyond £7 19s 3¼d collected

The keepers calculate that they cannot levy the said £84 4s ½d or
thereabouts for the reasons stated above and they maintain that they
can prove it. And it was found that the said keepers had been charged
with the rents of free and customary tenants and with the labour
services of villeins within the manors at the rate of £123 16s 2d (as
itemised above) on the basis of the account of Humfrey Walden, who
had been keeper of the bishopric during its vacancy in the 30th year of
Edward I [1302]. On the strength of that finding it was agreed to
make inquiry, and that John de Wyndesovere, parson of Cleeve, John
de Sudyngton, Stephen de Dudlegh, parson of Strensham and John
Worthyn, or two or three of them, should be assigned to make inquiry,
and that they should be commanded to return their findings to the
exchequer by the quindene of Easter. And a transcript of the
proceedings and of the two rolls were sent to them under the
exchequer seal for their information, and a day was assigned for the
keepers to hear their findings.

[The findings, gathered at six inquiries, confirmed the accuracy of the
keepers' lists of rents and services due from the surviving tenants and
ruled that they could not have collected more than they did.]

94. Decayed rents

These entries come from the manorial account of the royal manor of Drakelow
in Cheshire for the year Michaelmas to Michaelmas 1349-50. The first extract
is from the income side of the account and is a list of the rents due. As usual
in medieval accounts the property rent is shown as a lump sum, with any
shortfall itemised on the debit side of the account as 'decayed rents' – the
second extract printed here. When a property was left tenantless (whether by
death or abandonment) the lord's only redress was to seize the standing crops
to offset against the rent owed. The first list is of cases where grain had been
set against rents due in the current accounting year (i.e. tenants who had died
or fled after their rent was paid in June 1349); the second list is of tenants who
had died before that date, and who therefore had no assets in the current
accounting year. Neither list includes properties which had been retenanted.

The accounting official (the 'he' of the extracts) was the bailiff John de Wodhull.

Public Record Office, Ministers' accounts, SC 6/801/4.

Rents.

He answers for £51 4s ½d as appears in earlier accounts, received from various tenements belonging to the lord in Rudheath, which lands and tenements are held of the lord for term of years. The rent is due at St Martin [11 November] and the Nativity of St John the Baptist [24 June] in equal shares.

And for the rent of 215 acres, 1 rood and a quarter part of a perch of arable land in Overmarsh, which used to be leased out for 2s an acre, he has received nothing this year because the said land has lain fallow because it has not proved possible to find tenants because of the pestilence last year.[15] Moreover, those tenants who held part of the land last year relinquished it completely at Michaelmas at the beginning of this accounting year.

And for 123 acres, 7¾ perches, nothing because it lies in the common land.

Decayed rents.

He accounts for decayed rents from various below-written tenants of the lord for the term of St Martin because they had nothing except their grain, which was taken into the lord's grange at the lord's expense in lieu of the said rent:

Roger le Cartewrught	6d
John Hardyng	2s
William de Haselyngton	3s
William del Mor	18d
Richard Hardyng	6d
Alice de Twemlowe	6d
John Coudrey	9d
William de Haselyngton	16½d
Henry le Walshman	18d
Henry de Ingelwode	6d
Roger, son of Henry de Whistelhagh	2s 3¾d
Richard Strongbogh	3s 1d
Agnes Lyly	3s 9d

15 That is, the last accounting year, up to Michaelmas (Sept. 29) 1349. The plague was active in the area from late spring 1349.

Philip Hullesson	6d
Richard le Swon	5s 6½d
William, son of John	4s 7½d
Adam le Ward and John de Echeles	7s 10½d
Amise de Sprouston	2s ½d and half a farthing
Philip Pecok	7s 3¾d
Henry le Deye	20d
Robert Pecok	5s 9¾d
Roger, son of Adam	7s 2½d
John Haunesson	5s 10¼d
William, son of William de Lostok	6s
John le Crouther	10s
John le Vernon	5s
Cecilia Gagge	19½d and half a farthing
John Raven	4s 8d
Thomas Haunesson	5s
Robert, son of Stephen	18d
Hugh son of Warin	12¼d and half a farthing
Richard le Smyth	2s 5d
Hugh le Shepherde	13½d

He accounts for decayed rents from various below-written tenants of the lord for the terms of St Martin and the nativity of St John the Baptist, that is for a whole year. These tenants were those who died of the pestilence and from whom the lord had nothing but their grain, which he gathered last year, and the herbage of some of the land with which the receiver was charged earlier in the account:

Randal Hardyng	4s
John le Gardiner	3s 7d
Randal de Merton	28s 4d
Isabel, daughter of Edmund	5½d
John del Cogges	4s 7¾d
Richard de Ravenescroft	8s 6½d
Hugh le Marler	4s 2½d
William, son of Henry	2s 10¾d
Hamo, son of Robert	15s 8½d
Robert, son of John de Croxton	18s
Richard Lovkyn	12d
Robert de Plumlegh	9s 1d
John de Moston	7s 2½d
Robert de Penere	9s

John le Gardiner	14s
John, son of John	3s 8d
Agnes de Multon	10s
William le Porter	12d
William Brette	4s 6d
Henry le Mon and Robert de Crumwell	18d
Hugh de Crumwell	25s 6d
Robert del Bonke	4s
Thomas le Palfreyman	16s 8d
Nicholas le Warde	24s
William de Denhale	3s 6¼d
William le Hunte	4s 7d
Richard de Bradeford, Robert de Bradeford and William de Denhale	4s 10¼d
Robert le Shereman	2s
Roger Sallot	4s
Robert, son of Randal de Bradeford	19½d
Walter Bucke	12d
Robert, son of Randal de Bradeford	5¼d
Hugh le Mon	10s 8d
Lucy de Shipbrok	8s 4d
Hugh Gorst	2s 6d
Richard le Kyng	3s
Robert Gorst	21s
John Vaudrey	6s
William le Maistresson	2s 3d
Richard, son of Nicholas de Wynyngton	3s 10d
Total:	£20 9s 2¼d and half a farthing

Remission of rent.

He accounts for money remitted to the tenants of Rudheath by the justices of Chester and others of the lord's council, that is for a third of their rent which had to be remitted due to the effects of the pestilence. The tenants threatened to leave (which would have left the lord's tenements empty) unless they were granted such a remission, to last until the world improves and the tenements come to be worth more.

95. Unwillingness to take on vacant properties

This selection of cases from the records of the hallmote – the court of the estates of the Bishop of Durham – reflects the immediate dislocation caused by the plague. The bishop continued to have trouble enforcing tenancies, and examples from the following decade are printed below, 118.

I have used a transcript of PRO Durham 3/12 prepared by Dr Richard Britnell; the translations are my own.

[Houghton, 15 July 1349]

Because of the fear of pestilence no one wishes to make a fine for certain land in the lord's hand.

[Easington]

Everyone refuses to make a fine because of the pestilence.

[Easington, 16 July]

5s from Elis Groveson, John Groveson, Richard son of Walter, Nicholas Turner, Hugh son of Margaret, and Walter, son of Elis, for the land which William Gedelyng surrendered at the last hallmote on the surety of all the jurors. And no more because they had no wish to take on the said land, because of poverty and the pestilence, and therefore they flatly refused to make a fine unless they should still be alive after the pestilence or to labour according to the proclamation or on any other terms at all. And it is of more use to the lord that they take it at farm than that the land lie fallow in the lord's hand – for, as has become apparent, there is no other alternative.

[Sedgefield, 17 July]

Half a mark from John Goldyng for a bond tenement which was of William Kyd, one of the lord's serfs, who fled by night with his whole family. And there is no other serf or anyone else who is prepared to make a fine for the said land and therefore the said John has made a fine on his own behalf on the surety of the jurors and Sir John de Cletlam. And afterwards it was said outside the court that the said John Goldyng had connived at the flight of the said William.

[Whessoe, 26 October]

Be it remembered that the steward committed to Akres de Qwessowe a bond tenement which was of John son of Robert, because there were no blood relations. Peter de Hessewell and John Hannsard acted as sureties under pressure from the steward, on the understanding that Akres had accepted the land. And Peter de Hessewell says that Akres utterly refuses to hold the land. And therefore nothing has been received of the fine of 40s.

96. The renegotiation of labour services

This example is taken from the cartulary of Eynsham Abbey. It occurs among the villein services listed in an extent (valuation) of the manor of Wood Eaton (Oxon) drawn up in 1366 but enshrining an agreement made in 1349.

H. E. Salter (ed), *Eynsham Cartulary*, Oxford Historical Society, XLIX & LI, 1907-8, II pp. 19-20.

Walter Dolle, virgater, holds a messuage, 18 acres of arable and 2 acres of meadow. He used to pay, if it was at farm, 5s rent; perform one ploughing (with the lord providing a meal); give one hen; give eggs at Easter; render pannage; harrow for one day (which shall consist of harrowing 3 roods of land); weed for one day with another man; cart hay for a day; and perform three bedereaps[16] with three men in autumn, without food, and a fourth with the same number of men with a meal provided by the lord.

When, however, it was not at farm he used to work for five days a week from Michaelmas to Martinmas; and for four days a week from Martinmas to the feast of St John the Baptist; and perform carrying service as far as Eynsham on Sundays should it be necessary. He also rendered pannage, aid, and toll if he brewed for resale. He could not sell an ox or a male foal, or give his daughter in marriage without the lord's licence. A day's work was defined as follows: when threshing, he threshed one measure of wheat (four measures making one bushel), two measures of barley, three of oats or one of beans and peas; when ditching he dug one perch, two armslength deep; when hedging he did two perches.[17]

If it was at farm without labour services, he collected nuts for one day in the lord's wood, and took two loads of wood or four faggots to court for Christmas.

At the time of the mortality or pestilence, which occured in 1349, scarcely two tenants remained in the manor, and they expressed their intention of leaving unless Brother Nicholas de Upton, then abbot and lord of the manor, made a new agreement with them and other incoming tenants. And he made an agreement with them as follows:

16 A bede is a prayer and a bedereap (or bedrip) is a day's reaping nominally performed at the special request of the lord rather than as an obligatory service. In practice, as this reference implies, the requirement had become fixed. An alternative name for such services was boon works, because they were performed as a favour to the lord.

17 As a linear measure a perch (also called a rod or pole) varied from about 4½ yards to over 6 yards; in modern times it was standardised at 5½ yards.

that Walter and other tenants of the same standing would pay an entry fine to the lord whenever they took possession of a tenement; they would attend every court; they would give their best animal as heriot; they would not sell an ox or male foal, or give their daughters in marriage without the lord's licence. They would perform three boon-works or ploughings at the two sowings, with a meal provided by the lord for those using their own ploughs; perform three bedereaps with two men without a meal, and a fourth with the same number of men with a meal provided by the lord; reap the lord's hay or corn for 12 days without a meal; and render 13s 4d rent each year as long as it pleases the lord – and would that it might please the lord for ever, since the aforesaid services were not worth so much. However, lords in future must do as seems best to them.

97. A reduction in labour services

This agreement was recorded in the court roll of the manor of Aldham (Suffolk), under the entry for the court held on Wednesday 22 June 1351.

Suffolk Record Office (Ipswich branch), HA68:484:135.

As the result of a plea from various unfree tenants on various manors of the lord John de Vere, Earl of Oxford, concerning the waiving of part of the labour services and customs which they used to perform before the pestilence, and which now (as everyone knows) they lack the power to perform in their entirety, the said earl wrote to me, Thomas de Chabham (steward of all his estates) about the complaint of all the unfree tenants, authorising me, in my capacity as steward, to use my discretion in coming to an agreement with all the unfree tenants wherever it seemed to me that the lord's interests made it necessary, and, as a special favour on the part of the said earl, to release part of the works and customs which they used to perform before the pestilence. And since I have been given to understand by the earl's unfree tenants on his manor of Aldham that they cannot hold their land by performing all the works and customs which they used to perform before the pestilence, as has been very clearly demonstrated to the earl and his council, be it known to the steward, the auditors of the account, the tenants holding land there, the bailiffs, reeves and all the lord's officials that I, the said Thomas de Chabham, by virtue of the authority vested in me by the said letters, have, as a special favour, come to an agreement with the unfree tenants of the earl's manor of Aldham concerning part of their labour service and customs from the feast of the Purification last past [2 February] for the following three years.

At this court I have granted to all the unfree tenants who hold 15-acreware tenements in the said manor that a third part of their customary ploughing works and all their carrying services shall be waived annually during the said term.[18] Item, I have granted to all the tenants of 8-acreware tenements in the said manor that a third part of their ploughing service and all their carrying services be waived during the same period. Item, I have granted to Nicholas Aylwyne, Nicholas Skelman and John Crembel, cottars, who each owes 80 works a year, that 20 of the works and all the carrying services shall be waived annually during the same period. Item, I have granted to John Aylwyne who holds a two-acreware tenement and owes 40 works and carrying service, that 10 works and all his carrying service shall be waived during the same period. I have released the works and carrying services for the specified period because, according to the terms of the authority vested in me by the earl, it seems to me that the concession is necessary.

98. The ordinance of labourers, 18 June 1349

A. Luders *et al.* (ed), *Statutes of the Realm 1101-1713*, 11 vols, London, 1810-28, I pp. 307-8.

Since a great part of the population, and especially workers and employees,[19] has now died in this pestilence many people, observing the needs of masters and the shortage of employees, are refusing to work unless they are paid an excessive salary. Others prefer to beg in idleness rather than work for their living. Mindful of the serious inconvenience likely to arise from this shortage, especially of agricultural labourers, we have discussed and considered the matter with our prelates and nobles and other learned men and, with their unanimous

---

18 Peasant holdings on many East Anglian estates were expressed in *acreware*. *Ware* means defence, which implies that some feudal obligation was once attached to the land, although if so the obligation was obsolete by the fourteenth century. *Acreware* were not necessarily the same size as standard (or statute) acres and an eight *acreware* tenement might cover anything from six to ten acres. I owe this definition to Dr Mark Bailey.

19 The word translated here and elsewhere as employee is *serviens*, usually translated as servant. As this word now has rather narrowly domestic connotations I have preferred a more neutral term. The important point is that such people were contracted to work for one employer rather than freelancing.

advice, we have ordained that every man or woman in our realm of England, whether free or unfree, who is physically fit and below the age of sixty, not living by trade or by exercising a particular craft, and not having private means or land of their own upon which they need to work, and not working for someone else, shall, if offered employment consonant with their status, be obliged to accept the employment offered, and they should be paid only the fees, liveries, payments or salaries which were usually paid in the part of the country where they are working in the twentieth year of our reign [1346] or in some other appropriate year five or six years ago. Lords should have first claim on the services of their villeins or tenants, although they should retain only as many as they need and no more.

And if any man or women, being required to enter employment in this manner, refuses, and the fact has been proved by two men of legal standing before the sheriff, bailiff or constable of the vill where the incident took place, then let the person be immediately arrested by them or one of them and sent to the nearest gaol, there to remain in close captivity until they offer security that they will accept employment under these conditions.

And no reaper, mower, or other worker or employee of whatever standing who is in the employment of another person shall leave before the end of the agreed period of employment without reasonable cause or permission, under pain of imprisonment, and no one else is to receive or employ him under the same pain of imprisonment.

Moreover, no one should pay or promise wages, liveries, payments or salaries greater than those defined above under pain of paying twice whatever he paid or promised to anyone who feels himself harmed by it. And if no such person is willing to bring a prosecution, then the same to be paid to any member of the public who does so, and let the prosecution be brought in the court of the lord of the place where it happened. And if the lords of vills or manors presume to go against the present ordinance either in person or through their officials, then let them be prosecuted in our county, wapentake or trithing court, or in another of our courts, under penalty of triple the amount paid or promised by them or their officials.

And if it happens that someone, before the present ordinance was made, agreed to enter employment for a larger salary, the employer who made the agreement is not for that reason bound to pay any more than in the past, and should by no means presume to pay more under the abovesaid penalty.

Item, saddlers, skinners, tawyers, cobblers, tailors, smiths, carpenters, masons, tilers, shipwrights, carters and all other artisans and labourers ought not to receive for their labour and craft more money than they could have expected to receive in the said twentieth year or other appropriate year, in the place where they happen to be working; and if anyone takes more, let him be committed to gaol in the manner set out above.

Item, butchers, fishmongers, innkeepers, brewers, bakers, poulterers and all other dealers in foodstuffs should be bound to sell the food for a reasonable price, having regard to the price at which such food is sold in the neighbourhood. The price should allow the seller a moderate, but not excessive, profit, taking reasonable account of the distance he has transported the goods. And if a victualler should make a sale contrary to the ordinance, and be convicted for it, then let him pay twice what he has received to the injured party, or, failing him, to the person who has been willing to bring the prosecution. And the mayor and bailiffs of cities, boroughs, market towns and other towns shall have the power to question everyone to discover who has offended against the ordinance, and impose the penalty – which is to be paid to whoever brought the case against the guilty party. And if the mayor and bailiffs neglect to prosecute, and are found guilty before the justices appointed by us, then they should be compelled by the justices to pay damages of triple the value of the goods sold to the injured party or to the other person bringing the prosecution, and also to pay a heavy penalty to us.

And since many sturdy beggars – finding that they can make a living by begging for alms – are refusing to work, and are spending their time instead in idleness and depravity, and sometimes in robberies and other crimes; let no one presume, on pain of imprisonment, to give anything by way of charity or alms to those who are perfectly able to work, or to support them in their idleness, so that they will be forced to work for a living.

We firmly order you that every one of these requirements be proclaimed publicly in the cities, boroughs, market towns, ports and wherever else within your bailliwick you think appropriate, inside franchises as well as outside them.

99. An episcopal response to the ordinance

The ordinance of labourers was widely disseminated. Among the recipients
were bishops, who were requested to see that it was read out in parish
churches. They were also told to compel stipendiary priests to work for their
accustomed salary, and it is in response to this requirement that Hamo Hethe,
Bishop of Rochester, sent the following letter to his archdeacon on 1 July
1349.

C. Johnson (ed), *Registrum Hamonis Hethe diocesis Roffensis,* Canterbury and
York Society XLVIII, 1948, II pp. 884-5.

Recently, the most excellent prince, our illustrious lord the King of
England, took action to check the presumptuous excesses of certain
artisans and employees. Before the general pestilence of men arose in
the kingdom of England and destroyed a great part of the people, such
men used to earn their living through various crafts and the work of
their hands in a manner very useful to the state, but now that the
pestilence has (by God's grace) ceased, although there remain strong
and healthy men who are well able to work, yet they obstinately refuse
to enter employment or to work unless they receive intolerably high
payment for their work or their skill, to the great detriment of the
state. With the considered counsel of experienced men and with the
benefit of advice from all the other leading men, the king, with their
unanimous support, wholesomely ordained appropriate remedies for
those matters insofar as they concern lay people, and by his royal writ
ordered and caused them to be publicised and their due execution
ordered throughout the whole realm of England.

Moreover concerning the stipendiary chaplains and clerks in our said
city and diocese who likewise refuse to work without excessive
payment, our lord king ordered us that (insofar as it is our responsibility) we should restrain them from such excess, and compel them to
work for an appropriate salary, as is expedient, under pain of
suspension and interdict. We have accepted the royal commands, not
only because they are supported by reason but also because our office
constrains us to exercise our ministry for the public weal, and we
therefore order and command you that in every chapter held by you
before Michaelmas and in every parish church in our city and diocese
you warn each and every stipendiary chaplain and clerk in holy orders
celebrating or ministering within our jurisdiction, or ensure that
warnings are given to them on your behalf. This is to be done publicly,
generally and canonically, so that the admonitions are too forceful to

escape notice and nobody can plead ignorance as an excuse. Each one of them is henceforward to be content with the amount of salary or stipend which used to paid before the pestilence for the same type of work in the places where they happen to be employed, and should not dare to demand more. Nor should he presume to withdraw or remove himself from a lord whom he has been serving for an accustomed and appropriate salary, in the hope of obtaining a bigger salary elsewhere, unless he has the special and explicit permission of his lord. These things are to be obeyed under pain of suspension at least, which we will impose on any stipendiary chaplain or clerk contravening or doing anything against the commands set out here.

We order the sentence thus sent by us to be published solemnly and generally by you or by others in your name in the chapters held after Michaelmas, and the names and surnames of those offending or contravening these things are to be diligently sought out and, when they have been properly established, they are to be passed on to us. In addition we forbid you, on the obedience you owe to this letter (and we order you to forbid your official and all the deans in our diocese on our behalf and with our authority) to make or grant for love or money letters of good conduct or recommendation for any stipendiary chaplain or clerk in holy orders who wishes to leave the service of a lord who is paying him the accustomed salary, unless he has first lawfully demonstrated to you or to the dean making out the letters that he has free and explicit permission to leave from the lord in whose employment he has been. Where that is the case we want it to be stated explicitly in the letters of good conduct. Inform us in writing by the Feast of All Saints what you have done or caused to be done in this matter.

VII: Repercussions

100. Land values before and after the plague

During the Hundred Years War, alien priories (English religious houses which were the daughter houses of French foundations) were penalised in various ways by the crown. In 1350 the Cluniac house of Lewes (Sussex) offered Edward III eight advowsons[1] in return for the right to be treated as denizens – a right granted them in 1351. Lewes valued the advowsons at 200m, and Edward ordered an inquiry (carried out early in 1351) into whether their value had fallen since the plague. What is being valued is the income of the rector of the parish, consisting usually of his own land (the glebe); the tithes paid by his parishioners on agrarian products; and the altar dues, or offerings by lay people. The figures therefore give some idea of the plague's effect on the number of parishioners, as well as providing a direct comparison of land values before and after the plague.

Public Record Office, Chancery inquisitions miscellaneous, C 145/164/8.

Sandal (Yorkshire): the jurors say that the easement[2] of the houses belonging to Sandal rectory is worth nothing yearly after outgoings. They say moreover that there is 14s 8d in rents of assize there from various tenements at Easter and Michaelmas. Item, that there are 32 acres and 3 roods of land there, with adjoining meadow, and that each acre was worth, in an average year before the pestilence, 8d and is now worth 6d. Item, that there are 4½ acres of meadow there, of which each acre was worth, in an average year before the pestilence, 3s 4d and is now worth 2s 6d. Item, they say that the tithe of wool and lambs there was worth, in an average year before the pestilence, £6 p.a. and is now worth £4. Item, that the tithe of sheaves was worth, in an average year before the pestilence, £56 p.a. and is now worth £35 13s 4d. Item, that the altar dues and the small tithes of hay there were worth, in an average year before the pestilence, £20 p.a. and are now worth £12 13s 4d. Item, they say that the aforesaid church is charged with a pension of 6s 8d to the prior and convent of Lewes and to no one else.

Fishlake (Yorkshire): the jurors say that the easement of the houses of the rectory of Fishlake is worth nothing yearly after outgoings and

---

1 An advowson was the right to present a rector to a living.

2 An easement (in this context) is the enjoyment of a right or privilege in property not one's own. The jurors are saying that the rectory house has no cash value once its expenses have been met each year.

that there are 20 acres of land in the glebe there, of which each acre was worth 8*d* p.a. before the pestilence and is now worth the same amount. Item, there are 3 acres and 1 rood of meadow there, which were worth 8*s* 3*d* p.a. before the pestilence and are now worth 5*s* 5*d*. Item, the tithe of corn there was worth £40 before the pestilence and is now worth £33. Item, the tithe of hay with the profits of the garden there were worth £8 p.a. before the pestilence and are now worth £4 15*d*. Item, the tithe of wool and lambs there was worth £4 before the pestilence and is now worth 40*s* p.a. Item, the altar dues there were worth £20 before the pestilence and are now worth £13 6*s* 8*d*. Item, they say that the aforesaid church is charged with a pension of 20*s* to the prior and convent of Lewes and to no one else.

Kirkburton (Yorkshire): the jurors say that the easement of the houses of the rectory of the said church is worth nothing beyond outgoings. Item, they say that before the pestilence there were rents of assize of 15*s* 6*d*, payable at Martinmas and Pentecost, and that there is now 10*s*. Item, there are 21 acres of arable land there with adjoining meadow, of which each acre was worth, in an average year before the pestilence, 6*d* and is now worth the same amount. Item, the tithe of sheaves with the tithe from the mill were worth, in an average year before the pestilence, £12 p.a. and are now worth £10 17*s* 8*d*. Item, the tithe of wool and lambs there was worth, in an average year before the pestilence, £4 p.a. and is now worth 53*s* 4*d*. Item, the altar dues with the tithe of hay there were worth, in an average year before the pestilence, 108*s* and are now worth 66*s* 8*d*. Item, they say that the aforesaid church is charged with a pension of 3*s* to the prior and convent of Lewes and to no one else.

Harthill (Yorkshire): the jurors say that the easement of the houses of the rectory of the said church is worth nothing beyond outgoings. Item, they say that there are rents of assize there of 6*s* 9*d* payable at Pentecost and Martinmas, with 1 cock and 2 hens at Christmas and 1 boon work in autumn each year. Item, there are 65 acres of arable land there, of which each acre was worth, in an average year before the pestilence, 12*d* and is now worth 8*d*. Item, there are 3 acres of meadow there, each of which was worth 2*s* before the pestilence and is now worth the same amount. Item, the tithe of wool and lambs there was worth £6 13*s* 4*d* in an average year before the pestilence and is now worth 100*s*. Item, the altar dues there were worth £8 p.a. before the pestilence and are now worth 106*s* 8*d*. Item, the tithe of sheaves and hay was worth, in an average year before the pestilence, £41 6*s* 8*d* and is now worth £40. Item, there is a dovecote there which was worth 6s 8d p.a. before the pestilence and is now worth the same amount. Item, they say that the aforesaid church is charged with a pension of 26s 8d to the prior and convent of Lewes and to no one else.

Caxton (Cambridgeshire): the jurors say that the easement of the houses of the rectory of the vill of Caxton is worth nothing beyond outgoings. Item, they say that there are 80 acres of arable land in the glebe there, of which each acre was worth, in an average year before the pestilence, 10d p.a. and is now worth 6d. Item, that the tithe of hay was worth, in an average year before the pestilence, 13s 4d and is now worth the same amount. Item, that the tithe of sheaves was worth, in an average year before the pestilence, £20 and is now worth £13 6s 8d p.a. Item, that altar dues there, with the tithe of wool and lambs, were worth in an average year before the pestilence 106s 8d and are now worth 66s 8d p.a. Item, they say that the aforesaid church is charged with a pension of 40s to the prior and convent of Lewes and to no one else.

Whaddon (Cambridgeshire): the jurors say that the easement of the houses of the rectory of the vill of Whaddon is worth nothing beyond outgoings. Item, they say that there are 80 acres of arable land in the glebe there, of which each acre was worth, in an average year before the pestilence, 20d and is now worth 18d. Item, the hay there, both the tithe and the part of the meadow that belongs to the church, was worth, in an average year before the pestilence, 30s and is now worth the same amount. Item, there were rents of assize there of 21s 6d before the pestilence, payable at Easter and Michaelmas, and there is now 18s 6d. Item, that the tithe of sheaves there was worth, in an average year before the pestilence, £18 13s 4d, and it is now worth the same amount. Item, they say that the aforesaid church is charged with a pension of 50s to the prior and convent of Lewes and to no one else. Nothing is received from altar dues or from the tithe of wool and lambs because the vicar there receives it each year.

Gimingham (Norfolk): the jurors say that the easement of the houses of the rectory of the vill of Gimingham is worth nothing beyond outgoings. Item, that there are rents of assize of 23s 7¼d there from various tenants payable at Candlemas and St Peter *ad vincula*. Item, that the said tenants render 13 hens, price 2d each, and 2 cocks, price 1½d each, at Christmas. Item, that there are 13 autumn works, price of each work 2d. Item, that there are 30 acres of land there, of which each acre was worth, in an average year before the pestilence, 3s and is now worth the same amount. Item, that there are two pieces of meadow which were worth 10s p.a. before the pestilence and are now worth the same amount. Item, that the tithe of sheaves there was worth, in an average year before the pestilence, £52 6s 8d and is now worth £50. Item, they say that the altar dues of the said church with the tithe of wool and lambs were worth, in an average year before the plague, £7 6s 8d and are now worth £6 13s 4d. Item, they say that the aforesaid church is charged with a pension of 66s 8d to the prior and convent of Lewes and to no one else.

Ryston (Norfolk): the jurors say that the easement of the houses of the rectory of the vill of Ryston is worth nothing beyond outgoings. Item, they say that there was each year before the pestilence 25s in rents of assize payable at Easter and Michaelmas, and that there is now 16s 1d. Item, that there are 13 autumn works there, the price of each work 2d. Item, that there are 62 acres of arable land there, of which each acre was worth, in an average year before the pestilence, 4s and is now worth 2s. Item, that there are 2 acres of meadow which were worth 6s 8d before the pestilence and are now worth the same amount. Item, they say that the tithe of sheaves was worth, in an average year before the pestilence, 80m and is now worth 50m. Item, they say that altar dues with the tithe of lambs and wool were worth, in an average year before the pestilence, 20m and are now worth 10m p.a. Item, they say that the aforesaid church is charged with a pension of 40s to the prior and convent of Lewes and to no one else.

101. An increase in value

In 1356 Edward III ordered an inquiry into the value of the rectory of Bonby (Lincs) since the plague. The revenues of the church had been going to a French religious house and had therefore been seized by the crown.

Public Record Office, Chancery inquisitions miscellaneous, C 145/173/13.

An inquisition held at Glanford Brigg on 6 September 1356 before Hugh de Appelby and John de Elsham who have been appointed by royal letters patent to enquire into the value of the church of Bonby, currently in the king's hands, which was appropriated[3] to the alien priory of Saint-Fromond, and how much the rectory has been worth each year since the pestilence and the sources of its income. The jurors say on oath that the value of the church of Bonby each year derives from the tithe of sheaves and 11s 6d of rent from various lands and

3 For some examples of appropriations see 104.

tenements in Bonby and Saxby. And they say that the rectory of the church at the time of the pestilence, viz in 1349, was 8*m* including the said rent, and that it has been worth each year since then 10*m* p.a. and no more.

102. Diminished vills

Many settlements experienced a dramatic drop in the number of their inhabitants as a result of the plague. One indication of the decline comes from the records of the lay subsidy of 1354. In the East Riding of Yorkshire the proceeds of the Statute of Labourers were used to give relief to the vills most badly affected. The following extract lists the vills in Harthill wapentake[4] with the sum they were expected to pay and (in the second column) the amount of relief granted. Those marked with an asterisk [*] had ceased to exist as settlements by the late sixteenth century.[5] I have modernised all the place names.

Public Record Office, Subsidy rolls, E 179/202/53.

South Burton	£7 10s	£1 13s 6d
Scorborough	£1 2s	
Bubwith	£2 10s	10s
Kilnwick on the Wolds	£3 10s 15s	
Spaldington	£2 16s 8d	6s 8d
Willerby	£3	
North Ferriby	£2 16s 8d	13s 4d
Bentley	£3 2s 10s	
Houghton	£1 12s	
Skerne	£1 14s	
Braken	£4 17s 10s	
Hotham	£1 1s	£1[6]
Sancton	£1 14s 10s	
Wolfreton	£1 5s 4d	
Southburn	£3 7s	

4 A wapentake is the northern equivalent of a hundred: an administrative sub-division of a county.

5 The names of lost villages have been taken from the list in M. W. Beresford, 'The lost villages of Yorkshire, part II', *Yorkshire Archaeological Journal*, XXXVIII, 1952–5, pp. 56–70. I have noted only those villages whose disappearance can be firmly dated to the 150 years after the Black Death; several others vanished at some point before the eighteenth century.

6 Hotham (and Brantingham, below) were granted special exemption and the figures do not, therefore, reflect communities on the verge of disappearance.

Brantingham	£1 14s	£1 13s
Tibthorpe	£6	
North Cliffe	£1 4s	4s
Middleton	£4 13s 4d	£1
Anlaby	£3 16s	£1
Willitoft	14s	
Skidby	£6 10s	£1 10s
Riplingham	£1 18s	
Hessle	£8 13s 4d	£1 16s 8d
Shipton	£3 11s 2d	12s
Foggathorpe	18s	8s
Wauldby	£2	
South Cliffe	£1 7s	
*Arras	£1 8s	13s
Hunsley	£1 13s	
Neswick	£4 8s	10s
Elloughton	£6 9s	£1
Swanland	£5 10s	16s
Breighton	£2	
Harlthorpe	£1	
Beswick	£2 10s	5s
Hutton Cranswick	£5	£1 6s 8d
Sutton on Derwent	£1 15s	
North Cave	£4	£1 4s
Sculcoates	£1 14s	
*Kilnwick Percy	£1 10s	6s 8d
Lockington	£4 14s	
Easthorpe	£2 10s	13s 4d
Wilberfoss	£1 6s 8d	
Ellerton	£2 10s	
South Cave	£4	£1 13s
Gribthorpe	£1 4s	
Market Weighton	£8	£1
Laytham	£1	
Loftsome	15s	
Melbourne	£2 2s	
Burnby	£3	10s
Goodmanham	£1 10s	16s
Ousethorpe	6s 8d	3s 4d
Hayton	£4 13s 4d	£1 4s
Londesborough	£3 17s 11d	

Allerthorpe	£2 13s 4d	
Waplington	£1 8s 4d	11s 7d
Everthorpe	£2 10s	£1 10s
Sunderlandwick	12s	
Yapham	£1 16s	3s 4d
Aughton	£1 10s	
Full Sutton	£1 13s	
Bielby	£2 13s 4d	
Warter	£4 13s 4d	13s 4d
Seaton	£2 3s	12s
Catton	£1 11s	
Bolton	£1 13s 4d	
Thornton	£2 10s	
Fangfoss	£3	10s
Hundeburton & Stamford Bridge	£1 13s 4d	
Bishop Wilton	£3 18s	
Etton	£2 13s	
Huggate	£3 10s	
*Eastburn	£3 10s	
Rotsea	£1 8s 10d	
Wyton	£3 10s	£1 3s 4d
Ella	£5	
Holme on Spalding Moor	£5	15s
Bainton	£7 13s 4d	15s
Everingham	£3	
Newton on Derwent	£1 6s 8d	
Lund	£4 10s	£1 5s
Youlthorpe	17s	6s 8d
Meltonby	12s	3s 4d
Nunburnholme	£1 15s 2d	10s
Newsham & Arram	£3 3s	
Givendale	18s	
Kirkburn	£3	
Thorpe le Street	£1 6s 8d	
Gowthorpe	9s	4s
Wressle	£1 8s	
Molescroft	£1	
North Dalton	£4 10s	£1 6s 8d
Leconfield	£1 3s	
Faxfleet	£1 1s	

*Drewton	£1	10s
Watton	18s	
Cottingham	£22	

103. An early enclosure

A royal writ of 22 November 1357 ordering an inquiry into a planned enclosure of land in Oxfordshire. The jurors' verdict (not printed here) was that the plans were not to the king's damage and could go ahead.

Public Record Office, Chancery inquisitions miscellaneous, C 145/175/7.

Edward, by the grace of God King of England and of France and Lord of Ireland, to our beloved John de Estbury, our escheator[7] in Oxfordshire, greeting.

We have been approached by our beloved and faithful subject Roger of Cottisford concerning a certain royal highway which goes from Cot-tisford to Souldern and which passes through the middle of the hamlet of Tusmore which belongs to the said Roger and was, before the pestilence, entirely inhabited by Roger's serfs. Because of the death of those serfs it has been, from that time to this, empty of inhabitants, and so remains, and is intended to remain so in the future. Roger plans to enclose the hamlet and the said highway, but to do that he first requires our licence and he has asked that we should deign to grant him permission to enclose the said hamlet and highway and then hold them to him and his heirs for ever. It is agreed that Roger will have a replacement road built to an adequate standard on his own ground outside the enclosed hamlet.[8] We are prepared to grant this, if it can be done without damage or prejudice to us and, in order to receive full assurance of this, we order you to inquire carefully into the matter and send your findings to us, along with this writ, without delay.

7 The escheator was the royal official responsible for the king's land within a particular county. He is involved in this inquiry because the enclosure would absorb a length of highway, and highways were the king's.

8 The jury's verdict adds the detail that Roger had decided to build his road on the north side of the enclosed hamlet. The hamlet is one of those discussed in K. J. Allison, M. W. Beresford and J. G. Hurst, *The Deserted Villages of Oxfordshire*, Leicester, Department of Local History occasional papers 17, 1965, p. 45.

104. Appropriations of parishes

Appropriation entailed the granting of a parish church and its revenues to a religious house. After the plague several houses saw it as a way of recouping their reduced income. In the following examples only the explanations of why appropriation was thought necessary have been printed. The usual preamble setting out the bishop's obligation to nurture religion, and the details of how the appropriation should be effected have been omitted.

(a) Appropriation of Cotham near Newark (Notts) to the Augustinian Priory of Thurgarton by William Zouche, Archbishop of York; 1 December 1350.

York, Borthwick Institute of Historical Research, Reg. 10 fo. 145.

Your wholesome petition lately shown to us sets out that your priory, together with the lands, meadows and possessions which supply most of its income, are, as is well known, situated in low lying and watery country. Because of their infertility and the unusually large number of floods, these lands now yield virtually nothing and have not done so for many years past. Nor is it to be expected that they will yield profit and income in the future. You have frequently incurred various damages and losses, especially last year with the floods, the plague and the loss of tenants – which, as you point out, is through no fault of your own. You have lost goods and rents worth at least £200 and because of this, and for other essential and pressing reasons, have been obliged to borrow and are now so weighed down with onerous exactions, various unusual charges and other insupportable burdens that unless help is provided very quickly in the form of generous financial support, divine worship will be lessened in the priory and the exercise of hospitality and other pious works cease altogether because the priory will lack the resources to provide them.

(b) Appropriation of Whitchurch (Devon) to the monastery of Tavistock, by John Grandisson, Bishop of Exeter; 1 September 1351.

F. C. Hingeston-Randolph (ed), *The Register of John de Grandisson, bishop of Exeter*, II pp. 1107-8.

The wholesome petition presented to us by our beloved sons in Christ, Abbot Richard de Esse and the convent of the Benedictine monastery of Tavistock in our diocese, sets out that before the unprecedented pestilence which by the secret and just judgement of God recently laid waste not only England but almost the whole world, they had (thanks to the pious generosity of their founders and other faithful Christians) adequate means, in possessions and rents, for their running expenses, and also for supporting the poor, receiving pilgrims and strangers, and for performing other works of piety and meeting their parochial obligations. Now, however, the monastery has been so oppressed and so gravely damaged by various misfortunes which have affected it, and particularly because pirates have done enormous damage to the Isles of Scilly, which used to produce no small part of the monastery's income, that it is hardly to be hoped that the monastery will recover in our times. In the light of this, and because parental affection moves us to sympathise with them, we are prepared to grant them the parish church of St Andrew of Whitchurch for their own use, to be joined and annexed to them for ever. The church is in our diocese, situated near the monastery and within its patronage, will be profitable to them and was moreover granted to them by our predecessors.

(c) Appropriation of Kinver (Staffs) to the monastery of Bordesley by Robert de Stretton, Bishop of Coventry and Lichfield; 6 July 1380.

Lichfield Record Office, Reg. Stretton, B/A/1/5ii fo. 70-v.

The petition of the abbot and convent of the Cistercian monastery of Bordesley in our diocese relates that although their said monastery has been from the outset securely founded on land and its cultivation, those lands have been so badly affected by the scarcity of tenants caused by the various outbreaks of pestilence that they are next to useless and might as well be barren, so that the abbot and convent now receive little or nothing from them. The resources of their monastery are so slender and meagre as a result of the various exactions, tallages and levies imposed on the monastery (as on other churches in England) by the lord king to finance his wars, and because of the unusually large influx of travellers, both rich and poor, and the murrain of their cattle, that the said monastery – for these reasons and others which seem to be befalling them daily – has been so weakened and encumbered by an insupportable burden of debt that they now need to alienate their possessions to satisfy their creditors and will so lose them for ever. The monastery's resources are not adequate to maintain the requisite hospitality within the said monastery, or for the exercise of almsgiving and other works of charity and piety, or for the fitting support of those worshipping God within the monastery, the payment of their servants or the discharge of their parochial obligations.

105. An amalgamation of parishes

John de Trilleck, Bishop of Hereford, amalgamates the parishes of Great and Little Collington (Herefs); Sugwas, 24 April 1351.

J. H. Parry (ed), *Registrum Johannis de Trillek*, Canterbury and York Society, VIII, 1912, pp. 174–6.

As it is the responsibility of the pope to divide and unite bishoprics, so the uniting and dividing of parishes within his diocese is recognised to be the responsibility of a bishop. The wholesome suggestion and petition of our beloved children in Christ: Ralph of Yeddefen, patron of the parish churches of Great and Little Collington in our diocese; Sir John Hector, chaplain; Richard Carbonel, clerk; William and Robert Coly, parishioners of Little Collington; Sir John atte Broke, priest and rector of Great Collington; William Balle, sometime patron of the church of Great Collington and Alice Alisaundre, parishioners of that church, sets out that the most grave calamity – the plague of men, now ended, which overran the whole world – reduced the population of these churches so much that a great scarcity of residents and other inhabitants, a barrenness of land and notorious poverty has befallen these parishes and still persists, with the result that the parishioners and rents of both churches are scarcely enough to support one priest. Therefore the supplication humbly put before us on behalf of the said patrons and parishioners urges that we, for the reasons adequately expounded before us (and the truth of which was sworn to before us), should deign, at the prompting of charity and in our right as diocesan, to unite and annex the parish church of Great Collington to the parish church of All Saints of Little Collington.[9]

We, John, the bishop aforesaid, are inclined to the petitions and prayers of the said patrons and parishioners, due process having been observed in the proceedings, and moreover we find the whole suggestion and petition of the patrons and parishioners, as presented, to be true and to have been demonstrated clearly and lucidly before us, and we consider the suggestion and petition to have been and to be consonant with reason and the requirements of canon law. Bearing in mind also that the church of Little Collington is the better built, and is more convenient and nearer to the parishioners, we (first invoking the help of Almighty God) declare that the reasons set out above for the uniting and annexing of the church of Great Collington to the

9 These two parishes are now represented by the single settlement of Collington, north of Bromyard. The present church is nineteenth-century.

parish church of Little Collington are valid, just, true and have general support, and have also been demonstrated adequately and properly before us, and we accordingly annex and unite the church of Great Collington with all its rights and appurtenances to the parish church of Little Collington, and since everything necessary in the matter has been done we declare in this document that from now onwards it is united and annexed, and that the said church of Little Collington should enjoy the rights, liberties and privileges appropriate to a parish church on behalf of both churches, and that from this day forward all the sacraments and other divine offices should be celebrated and performed in the church of Little Collington and received by the parishioners there, and we have decreed in this document that the cure and rule of the souls of the parishioners of both churches is to remain with the rector of Little Collington for the time being and pertain to him for ever.

We also ordain and establish, by the present writing and with the agreement of the said Ralph, the patron of both churches, that one parson shall be presented to the said church of Little Collington by the said patron and his heirs, who shall have the patronage of the church in the future, and shall be admitted and instituted by us and our successors as Bishop of Hereford. Moreover we enact and ordain that the parishioners shall fully have, hold and recognise the church of Little Collington as their parish church with immediate effect, and shall hear vespers, matins, mass and all other divine offices there, and offer up prayers to God in it, and receive the sacraments of the church there, and faithfully offer and pay the real and personal tithes due to God to the said church of Little Collington and to its rectors for the time being.

All of these things – the annexation and union, our statutes and ordinances, and everything else ordained above with the consent of the patrons and parishioners of Little and Great Collington – we will, establish and ordain should be inviolably observed in all ages for ever.

106. Amendments to a chantry foundation, 1351

An agreement between Thomas de Cheddeworth, clerk, and Anglesey Abbey (Cambs) concerning his chantry in the abbey church.

The Register of Thomas de Lisle, Bishop of Ely: Cambridge University Library, Records of the Dean and Chapter of Ely: EDR G1/1 fo. 36v.

The prior and convent of St Mary of Anglesey in the county of Cambridge, according to a document sealed with their common seal, have been bound and obliged to provide, at their own expense, two suitable secular priests to celebrate mass for ever in the aforesaid church of Anglesey for my soul, the souls of my father and mother and of my ancestors, and for the souls of all those whom I am bound to benefit and pray for, in return for my giving and granting the prior and convent, and their successors for ever, all the lands, tenements, rents and services which I had in the town of Braughing (Herts). I have been considering that, following the great and various miseries which have arisen in these days because of the huge mortality of men – namely that lands everywhere are lying uncultivated, and that numerous tenements have been unexpectedly and suddenly demolished and thrown down – it is not possible to collect rents and services, nor to receive the accustomed yield but only very much less than the former value; and I do not wish that the aforesaid prior and convent or their successors should henceforth have to find the cost of the said chantry of two priests out of the said lands, tenements, rents and services. Know therefore that I have granted and released to the prior and convent of Anglesey and their successors for ever the cost and maintenance of one of those two priests, so that henceforward they shall only be obliged to find one suitable secular priest at their expense to celebrate mass as formerly. In other words, the priest in office should receive a salary of five marks each year from the prior and convent, payable quarterly at Christmas, Easter, Midsummer and Michaelmas, unless they come to some other suitable arangement which meets with the priest's approval.

107. Amendment of statutes governing a chantry, 1365

Robert de Stretton, Bishop of Coventry and Lichfield, revises the statutes of a chantry in Chesterfield at the request of the founder, to make the post less onerous and hence more attractive.

The explanatory preamble is given in full, but I have paraphrased the changes to the statutes.

Lichfield Record Office, Reg. Stretton, B/A/1/5ii fo. 47-v.

Our dear mother the church often ordains things reasonably and advisedly which she subsequently, persuaded by practical considerations, more advisedly and reasonably revokes or changes for the better. Our beloved son Sir Roger of Chesterfield, rector of the parish church of Wigginton in the diocese of Lincoln, prompted by piety and wishing to bring together heavenly with earthly things, by the authority and with the assent of Roger of blessed memory, our immediate predecessor as Bishop of Coventry and Lichfield, and of others who had an interest in the matter, founded a perpetual chantry of one chaplain in the parish church of Chesterfield in our diocese to celebrate divine service for ever. He endowed it adequately with his own possessions and set down and established statutes and ordinances which he wished and ordered should be observed by the chaplain henceforward. And although the ordinances and statutes so instituted prospered and were laudably efficacious, the mortality of pestilence which recently befell the realm of England and is now threatening again and will surely threaten many times in the future, has meant a scarcity of chaplains – with the result that it is not easy to find an honest, circumspect and literate person in priest's orders to whom the cure and rule of the aforesaid chantry might be committed. Because of this the aforesaid Sir Roger, the founder of the chantry, has asked us to rescind the statutes abovesaid and to make statutes and ordinances which the chaplain celebrating there should observe in the future, and to take pains to make, enact, ordain and determine this matter in accordance with justice and reason.

1. Where it was ordained that the chaplain, wearing a surplice, should say matins and the other canonical hours daily in the choir of the church with the vicar or the parish chaplains – an obligation which demanded continual residence – we now ordain that the chaplain should observe this requirement on Sundays and double feasts,[10] and that on all other days it shall be permissible for him to say the hours by himself or with others in the said church or in some other honest place. When absent he must find an honest chaplain to celebrate in his place.

2. It was ordained that the rents and goods of the chantry, after the necessary costs had been deducted, should be used entirely for chantry purposes and not spent on anything else; we now ordain that since the chaplain holds the chantry as a benefice it is lawful for him to receive

10 Double feasts were those of particular significance.

the profits and dispose of them freely, provided that the chaplain should answer each year for 6s 8d which is to be locked away in a box with two locks and put towards the cost of maintaining and repairing the houses belonging to the chantry.

3. It was ordained that the chaplain should bind himself to take on no other office or observance; this is to be taken as meaning no other office or observance incompatible with the requirements of the chantry.

4. Where the ordinances say that the chaplain shall totally abstain from visiting taverns, this is to be understand as meaning that he should not visit them habitually.

5. It was ordained that the chaplain should say every day after matins and before mass the 7 and 15 psalms, with the litany and all the usual prayers, and that after dinner he should say the office of the dead with the 9 psalms and 9 readings, and that every day at the tomb of the founder's parents he should say audibly, for bystanders to hear, the *De Profundis* with the accompanying prayers.[11] We now ordain that the chaplain shall say the 7 psalms daily, before celebrating mass, and the litany and the usual prayers when he conveniently can; and that he should say the office of the dead according to the Use of Sarum[12] every day, unless there is a genuine reason why he cannot; and the *De Profundis* with the prayers *Inclina* and *Fidelium* immediately after celebrating mass, before the altar, and should not be obliged to say them at the tomb in the presence of bystanders.

108. Effrenata

On 28 May 1350 the Archbishop of Canterbury, Simon Islip, issued the provincial constitution *Effrenata* (its title comes from its opening word: unbridled) which aimed to fix the salaries of unbeneficed clergy at pre-plague levels. It was reissued verbatim in 1362 because it had failed to take effect, and it is this reissue (sent to the Bishop of London on 16 July) which is printed here.

R. C. Fowler (ed), *Registrum Simonis de Sudbiria, diocesis Londoniensis AD 1362-1375*, Canterbury and York Society, XXXIV & XXXVIII, 1927-38, I pp. 190-3.

11 The 7 psalms were the seven penitential psalms, and the 15 psalms the psalms of degrees (for both of which see the notes to **33**). The 9 psalms associated with the office of the dead were 51, 65, 63, 67, Isaiah 38 (*Ego dixi*), 148, 149, 150 and Luke 1 (*Benedictus*). The *De Profundis* is psalm 130.

12 Each major church developed its own liturgical traditions. The liturgical usage of Salisbury (Sarum) was widely adopted in central and southern England.

Simon by divine permission Archbishop of Canterbury, primate of all England and legate of the apostolic see, to our venerable brother lord Simon, by the grace of God Bishop of London, greeting and fraternal love in the lord. A short time ago, after the first epidemic, we sent our letters to lord Ralph of happy memory, then Bishop of London, the tenor of which follows:

Simon, by divine permission Archbishop of Canterbury, primate of all England and legate of the apostolic see, to our venerable brother lord Ralph by the grace of God Bishop of London, greeting and fraternal love in the lord. The unbridled greed of the human race, out of its innate malice, would grow to such a point that charity would be driven off the earth, unless the strength of justice restrained its effects. The commons have properly brought their complaints to us, and experience, that effective teacher, also shows us that the priests of the present day, not realising that divine intervention spared them from danger in the past pestilence not for their own merits but so that they could perform the ministry committed to them for God's people and the public benefit, and not ashamed that their insatiable avarice is despicably and perniciously taken as an example by other workers among the laity, now take no heed to the cure of souls, which of all responsibilities should most properly be preferred by ministers of the church, and which bestows even greater lustre upon the man who takes up the burden in humble obedience against his own inclinations.

But priests now refuse to take on the cure of souls, or to support the burdens of their cures in mutual charity, but rather leave them completely abandoned and apply themselves instead to the celebration of commemorative masses and other private offices; and for these too they are not content with the payment of adequate wages but demand excessive salaries for their services so that they can revive old extravagances, and thus for the bare priestly name and precious little work they claim greater profits for themselves than those who have the cure of souls. Unless their unreasonable appetites are reined in, the multiplication of commemorative masses and the size of their salaries (moderated by no sense of balance) will mean that many, indeed most, of the churches, prebends and chapels, not only in your diocese but in ours and throughout the whole province, will be left completely destitute of the services of priests. For what distresses us particularly is that beneficed clergy, driven by the same idea, are eagerly turning to these private services and leaving their cures completely abandoned.

Wishing, therefore, to bridle this insatiable desire on the part of priests (because of the dangers mentioned above and the other grievous problems which would arise if we failed to provide some remedy) we order and urge you, Father, in the bowels of Jesus Christ, that, giving heed to the dangers posed to souls and to the causes mentioned above, you make healthy provision before all else for the care of each parish church, prebend or chapel where the cure of souls is at stake, appointing curates from the best and most suitable chaplains, in whoever's service they may be found, and that you use whatever ecclesiastical censures seem appropriate, canonically applied, to ensure that their relatives or supporters, or those retaining them in their service against our ordinance, do not rashly violate our ordinance, and that every chaplain or other person performing any kind of religious office anywhere in your diocese accepts a moderate salary.

And if anyone who rebels against you in this respect takes themselves into our diocese, or into that of one of our fellow bishops, we will and order that his name and surname be made known to us, or to the bishop into whose diocese he has passed, and that you should follow up the process you started, or they should do so on the authority of your letters; for we wish the process against those who have come into our diocese to continue along the lines initiated by you or another of our brethren, and to pursue the charges brought against them in due form. We also require and order that each of our fellow bishops should follow exactly the same policy within his own diocese.

And we have ordained that you should publicise what we have enacted concerning the level of salaries for our said diocese: that chaplains of a parish church, prebend or chapel with the cure of souls should be paid one mark more than was usual for ministers in the same cure in the past, but that the salary of a stipendiary priest should be limited to the going rate accepted in the past. We wish our present command to be made known by you to each of your fellow bishops and suffragans immediately after its receipt and that you order them to inform us in writing what they have done in the matter before the feast of the Nativity of the Blessed Virgin Mary next. Moreover we firmly order and enjoin you to tell us precisely and clearly in writing before the said feast what you have done about all the aforesaid articles; for you should know that once the feast has passed we intend (as our office requires) to take all necessary and legal steps in respect of any complaint which comes to our ears concerning your negligence or that of any of our brothers or suffragans.

But since this, and especially from the time of the ensuing epidemic, we have received, with much bitterness of heart, many more complaints, which demand a strict and speedy reformation of the excesses described above and of the even graver problems now added to them. For in these days the stipends which men used to pay to support priests of great probity and honest conversation are considered as nothing, and simple priests can scarcely be satisfied with salaries twice as big. They cite the evils of the present day as an excuse for their abuses, either forgetting or not knowing that it is not places and times which sanctify or pollute a man. On the contrary, it is their exaction of immoderate profit which leads them to overstep the bounds of proper behaviour. Their excessive affluence sucks them down into the whirlpool of voluptuousness: with the trimmings of their garments, their fancy hair styles, their haunting of taverns and gambling dens, and their disgusting pursuit of carnal lust. Having been unbridled by the *mores* of secular society, contrary to their priestly order and apostolic teaching, they impudently and publicly reject ecclesiatical benefices, and particularly the chantries founded with an adequate and honest endowment for the salvation of the dead. In their craftiness they aim to undermine any agreement which entails a modest remuneration and a traditionally plain standard of living.

It seems to us that our aforesaid letters have not hitherto been properly enforced, and we therefore require and urge you, brother, to put them into effect and so eradicate the excesses and abuses described above. For it seems to us and to several of your fellow bishops and to the other great men of the realm, that priests ought to be paid at the following rates: those looking after a lesser cure of souls, 5 marks; those entrusted with cures of middling size, 6 marks; and those constrained to look after major cures, 7 marks; except that responsibility for a very large parish should demand a larger sum, to be fixed at the discretion of the diocesan. And if you can think of anything which will allow these excesses and abuses to be more promptly and perfectly remedied, then you should do that as well, to the praise of God and his holy church.

109. Unwillingness to take on parochial responsibilities

John Thoresby, Archbishop of York, to the Dean of Harthill; Cawood, 20 January 1362.

York, Borthwick Institute of Historical Research, Reg. 11 fos. 204v-205.

A very serious complaint has been made to us on behalf of our beloved son Sir John, the rector of the parish of Hotham in our diocese. The pestilence in the said parish has grown and is now growing so strong that it is said to have carried off almost all the chaplains celebrating there. The rector accordingly asked a certain Sir Adam de Brantingham, a chaplain employed in the said parish to say mass for various souls, to serve as the parish chaplain of the said parish church of Hotham in return for an adequate salary, according to an ordinance made by our immediate predecessor.[13] But Adam did not choose to obey the ordinance of our predecessor and flatly refused to take on the job of parish chaplain, to the inconvenience of the rector and the manifest peril of the parishioners' souls; whereupon the rector has asked that a suitable remedy may be provided for him in the matter.

We, inclining to his supplications, order you to take lawful and effective steps to compel the aforesaid chaplain Sir Adam to be instituted as parish chaplain by the aforesaid rector Sir John within eight days of your command to him, in return for an adequate salary, according to our predecessor's laudable ordinance.

110. William Langland on gadding clergy

This passage come from the opening of *Piers Plowman*, where the Dreamer sees the field full of folk and enumerates all the vices of the age. It is part of a wide-ranging attack on clerical behaviour.

William Langland, *Piers the Plowman*, Prologue, lines 81-99.

Parsons and parish priests complained to the bishop
That their parishes were poor since the pestilence time,
And asked for permission in London to dwell
And sing masses for money, for silver is sweet.
   Bishops and bachelors, both masters and doctors,
That have charge under Christ, and are tonsured in token

---

13 This refers to an order by Archbishop Zouche which set 6 marks as the salary of a parish chaplain: A. Hamilton Thompson, 'Pestilences of the 14th century in the diocese of York', *Archaeological Journal*, LXXI, 1914, p. 118.

And sign that they should shrive their parishioners,
Preach and pray for them, and the poor feed,
Lodge in London, not only at Lent.
Some serve the king and tot up his silver
In exchequer or chancery; chase up his debts
From wards and wardmotes, waifs and strays.
    And some serve as servants to lords and ladies
And in place of stewards sit in judgement.
Their mass and matins, and liturgical hours
Are done undevoutly. I fear that at Judgement
Christ in consistory will find many guilty.

111. Simon Sudbury increases priests' wages

Simon Sudbury, Archbishop of Canterbury, to William, Bishop of London, 26 November 1378. The letter borrows the opening of *Effrenata*. I have omitted the closing section, ordering the bishops to publicise the constitution.

W. Lyndewood, *Provinciale seu constitutiones Angliae*, Oxford, 1679, appendix, pp. 58-9.

Simon, by divine permission Archbishop of Canterbury, primate of all England and legate of the apostolic see, to our venerable brother in the Lord, William, by the grace of God Bishop of London, greeting and fraternal love in the Lord. The unbridled greed of the human race, out of its innate malice, would grow to such a point that charity would be driven off the earth, unless the strength of justice restrained its effects. The commons have properly brought their complaints to us, and experience, that effective teacher, also shows us that the priests of today within the city, diocese and province of Canterbury, have been so infected with the sin of greed that, not satisfied with reasonable wages, they hire themselves out for vastly inflated salaries. And these same greedy and pleasure-seeking priests vomit out the enormous salaries with which they are stuffed. They are so mad with desire, so depraved, that there is no holding them; many gorge their bellies and afterwards work themselves up into a lather of lechery over various fleshly delights, until at last they are dragged down into the very vortex of the whirlpool of evil – a detestable scandal to the clergy and the worst possible example to the laity.

And although our predecessor lord Simon Islip, a former Archbishop of Canterbury, when he was alive decreed and ordained with the advice and agreement of his brethren that those chaplains celebrating anniversary masses and others whose responsibilities did not include the cure of souls should be content with an annual stipend of 5 marks, but those exercising the cure of souls in parish churches or chapels should have 6 marks, under pain of suspension from their office if they failed to observe the statute; yet we, mindful of the current state of affairs, with the advice and agreement of our fellow bishops and suffragans assembled on the 16 November 1378 in a chamber within the monastery of SS Peter and Paul of Gloucester, within the diocese of Worcester, ordain and appoint as follows concerning the salaries of parish priests and chantry priests within our city, diocese and province of Canterbury.

In the name of God, amen. We, Simon, by divine permission Archbishop of Canterbury, primate of all England and legate of the apostolic see, with the advice of our fellow bishops and suffragans, have ordained that each priest in our city, diocese or province celebrating masses for the souls of the dead shall receive 7 marks, or 3 marks and their keep; but those with a cure of souls shall receive 8 marks, or 4 marks and their keep; and in no way shall anyone receive more than this, unless the diocesan of the place has first given his permission, in consultation with those who have the cure of souls there. If any cleric presumes to go against this constitution, either in the giving or receiving of a stipend, he shall incur the penalty of excommunication by so doing, and that penalty can only be absolved by the diocesan of the place in which the offence was committed.

112. The statute of labourers, 1351

A. Luders *et al.* (ed), *Statutes of the Realm 1101-1713*, 11 vols, London, 1810-28, I pp. 311-3.

It was lately ordained by our lord the king, with the assent of the prelates, nobles and others of his council against the malice of employees, who were idle and were not willing to take employment after the pestilence unless for outrageous wages, that such employees, both men and women, should be obliged to take employment for the salary and wages accustomed to be paid in the place where they were working in the 20th year of the king's reign [1346], or five or six years earlier; and that if the same employees refused to accept employment in such a manner they should be punished by imprisonment, as is more clearly contained in the said ordinance.[14] Whereupon

14 For the ordinance of labourers see **98**.

commissions were issued to various people in each county to make inquiry and punish all those offending against the ordinance. And now the king has been given to understand by a petition of the Commons in the present parliament that the said employees – having no regard to the said ordinance but rather to their own ease and exceptional greed – withdraw themselves to work for great men and others, unless they are paid livery and wages double or treble what they were accustomed to receive in the said 20th year and earlier, to the great damage of the great men and the impoverishing of all the Commons, for which the said Commons pray for remedy. Wherefore, to restrain the malice of the said employees, the things below written have been ordained and established in the said parliament by the assent of the said prelates, earls, barons and other great men.

First, that each carter, ploughman, plough-driver, shepherd, swine-herd, dairy maid and other employees shall take the liveries and wages accustomed in the said 20th year and four years previously. In places where wheat was accustomed to be given, they shall take 10d for the bushel, or wheat at the will of the giver, until it shall be otherwise ordained. And that they be hired to serve for a whole year, or for the other usual terms, and not by the day. And no one shall take more than 1d the day for weeding the fields or hay making; and mowers 5d an acre or 5d a day; and reapers of corn 2d [the day] in the first week of August, and 3d in the second week and so until the end of the month, and less in places where less used to be given; without food or other bonus being asked, given or taken. And that such workers bring the tools of their trade openly to market and there shall be hired in full view and not secretly.

Item, that no one take more than 2½d for threshing a quarter of wheat or rye, and 1½d for a quarter of barley, beans, peas and oats, if so much used to be given. And in places where men were accustomed to reap by the sheaf and thresh by the bushel, they shall take no more, and in no other manner, than was usual in the said 20th year and before. And that the same employees shall be sworn twice a year before the lords, stewards, bailiffs and constables of every town that they shall uphold and observe these things. And that no one shall leave the town where he lives in the winter to work elsewhere in the summer if there is work for him in the same town, taking the wages abovesaid. Except that the people of Staffordshire, Lancashire, Derbyshire, Craven and the Marches of Wales and Scotland, and other places, may come and work in other counties in August, and return safely, as they were accustomed to do before this time. And those who refuse to take such an oath, or to perform what they have sworn or bound themselves to do, shall be put in the stocks for three days or more by the said lords, stewards, bailiffs and constables of the towns, or sent to the nearest gaol, there to remain until they submit themselves. And that stocks be made in each town for this purpose between now and Pentecost.

Item that carpenters, masons, tilers and other roofers shall not take more by the day for their work than in the usual manner, that is to say: a master carpenter 3d, and other carpenters 2d; a master mason working in freestone 4d, other masons 3d, and their assistants 1½d; a tiler 3d, and his lad 1½d; other roofers working in reed and straw, 3d and their lads 1½d. Item, plasterers and other workers on clay walls, and their lads, the same, without food or drink, that is to say from Easter to Michaelmas, and from that time less, at the discretion of the justices who are to be appointed. And those who transport goods by land or water are not to take more for each load than was usual in the said 20th year and four years before.

Item that cordwainers and shoemakers shall not sell boots or shoes or anything else touching their craft in any other manner than in the said 20th year. And that goldsmiths, saddlers, bit and bridle makers, spurriers, tanners, tawyers, and all other workers, craftsmen and labourers, and all other employees not otherwise specified, shall be sworn before the said justices to perform and carry out their crafts and jobs in the same manner as in the said 20th year and before, without any refusal on the grounds of this ordinance. And if any of the said employees, labourers, workers and craftsmen, after taking this oath, break this ordinance, let him be punished with a fine and imprisonment, at the discretion of the justices.

Item that the said stewards, bailiffs and constables of the said towns be sworn before the same justices that they will inquire diligently, by all the good ways they may, about all those who act contrary to the ordinance, and that they will certify their names to the justices whenever they come into the area to hold their sessions, so that the said justices, having received the names of such rebels from the stewards, bailiffs and constables, may have them arrested to appear before the justices and answer for their offences, so that they may make a fine and ransom to the king if they are convicted, and over that let them be sent to prison, there to remain until they find surety that they will take employment and wages, and carry out their work, and sell goods, in the manner specified above. And if anyone is convicted of breaking his oath he shall be imprisoned for 40 days, and if he is convicted a second time, he shall be imprisoned for a quarter of a year, and thus each time he offends and is convicted the penalty is doubled. And whenever the justices come into the area they shall inquire whether the said stewards, bailiffs and constables have made a good and loyal presentation, or have concealed anything in return for a gift or out of favour, and punish them by fine and ransom if they are found to have offended. And that the same justices shall have power to inquire into and impose due punishment on the said officials, workers, labourers and other employees; and also on hostelers, inn keepers and those who retail foodstuffs and other things not here specified, at the suit of the party as well as by presentment; and to hear and determine and to put the matter into execution by *exigent* after the first *capias*,[15] if need be; and to appoint as many deputies as they think necessary for upholding the ordinance. And those who choose to sue against such employees, workers and labourers for an excess charge shall recover that excess if the men are convicted at their suit. And in the event that no one sues for recovery of the excess, it shall be levied on the said employees, workers, labourers and craftsmen and paid over to the collectors of the fifteenth, to be credited to the vills where the excess was levied.[16]

Item that no sheriffs, constables, bailiffs, gaolers, clerks to the justices or to the sheriffs, or any other officials whatsoever shall by virtue of their office take from the said employees any fees, suit of prison or other payment; and if they have taken anything they shall pay it over to the collectors of the tenth and fifteenth, to help the Commons, during the time that the tenth and fifteenth are in force, both for time past and time to come. And that the said justices enquire in their sessions whether the said officials have received anything from the said

15 The writ *capias ad respondendum* (you shall seize [N] to answer) ordered the sheriff of the relevant county to arrest an individual to answer to a charge. If the sheriff could not find the individual, he would return an answer to that effect, and when this had been done three times the proceedings would move to the next stage, that of summoning the defendant by a writ of *exigent* and outlawing him if he did not appear. This clause of the statute is designed to speed up the process by requiring only one writ of *capias*.

16 The fifteenth was a tax on moveables levied on rural areas (cities paid at the higher rate of a tenth). By this date the tax had ceased to be calculated on the possessions of individuals and had fossilised as lump sums levied on towns and villages. Setting the income from the statute against the tenth and fifteenth thus meant that local people could reduce their tax bill by enforcing the legislation. In 1352 about half of the tax bill of Essex (c.£600 out of c.£1200) was met in this way. For an example of the income being used to help the poorest vills, see above 102.

employees, and if these enquiries reveal that the officials have received anything, then the justices are to levy it from each of the said officials and pay it to the said collectors, along with the excess charges, fines and ransoms, and also the amercements from all those amerced before the justices, and the amount credited to the vill, as abovesaid. And in the event that the excess collected in one vill exceeds the amount of the fifteenth due from the vill, the remainder of the excess shall be paid by the collectors to the poorest of the neighbouring vills, to help with their fifteenth, by the advice of the justices. And that the fines and ransoms, excess charges and amercements from the said employees and labourers for the time to come, during the life of the said fifteenth, shall be paid over to the said collectors by indentures made between them and the justices, so that the collectors may be charged with the amount in their accounts on the evidence of the indentures, in case the said fines, ransoms, amercements and excess charges are not paid to help with the fifteenth. And when the fifteenth ceases, the money shall be levied to the king's use and the sheriff of the county be answerable for it to him.

Item, that the said justices hold their sessions in every county of England at least four times a year, that is to say at the feasts of the Annunciation [25 March], St Margaret [8 or 20 July], St Michael [29 September] and St Nicholas [6 December], and also at all times when it seems necessary, at the discretion of the justices. And that those who speak in the justices' presence or do anything in their presence or outside it to encourage or maintain the said employees and labourers against this ordinance shall be heavily punished at the discretion of the said justices. And if any of the said labourers, craftsmen or employees flee from one county to another because of this ordinance, the sheriffs of the counties where these fugitives shall be found shall cause them to be arrested, on the order of the justices of the counties whence they fled, and bring them to the county gaol, there to stay until the next session of the same justices; and that the said sheriffs return these commands to the justices at their next session. And that this ordinance be upheld and kept within the city of London as well as within other cities and boroughs and elsewhere, within franchises as well as without.

113. A case under the ordinance of labourers

A plea before the justices of labourers for Surrey, held at Guildford, 1 June 1350.

B. H. Putnam, *The Enforcement of the Statutes of Labourers 1349-1359*, Columbia, 1908 pp. 248*-250*.

William atte Merre of Merrow has been arrested to answer Peter de Semere. It has been ordained that every man and woman in the kingdom, being sound of body and under the age of 60, not supporting themselves by trade or by the exercise of a craft and not engaged in the cultivation of their own land or in the employment of someone else, is, if offered employment appropriate to their status, obliged to accept it and to take such fees, allowances, payments or salary as were accustomed to be paid in that place in the 20th year of the present reign or five or six years earlier. And Peter said that on 8 February 1350 at Merrow in the presence of John atte Dene and William Hereward he offered the said William appropriate employment in the vill of Merrow, and the said William flatly refused to work for the said Peter, and still refuses, in contempt of the lord king and contrary to statute, and to the damage of Peter of 100s.

And the said William denied the charge and said that he was unable to work for the said Peter because he was a serf of the prior and convent of St Mary at Boxgrove on the priory's manor of Merrow, and that the present prior was seised of him and his services, and the prior and his predecessors had been so seised of him and his ancestors time out of mind. And he said that the prior and convent had leased the manor and its appurtenances to John Chene of Tortington for life; and the said John Chene had him, William, in employment which was necessary to the manor. And he asked judgement on whether he ought to accept employment from the said Peter.

And because the justices had doubts about William's claim, they had a book placed before him on which he could swear the truth of these matters, and after taking the oath he repeated what he had said earlier. And therefore it was decided that Peter should not have brought the complaint and that William should work for John Chene as his lord. And therefore he was handed over to Walter de Wernham, John Chene's bailiff, to work for him according to the statute and the custom of the said manor.

114. Cases brought under the statute of labourers

This is a sample of the cases from Kingsbridge hundred (Wiltshire) presented to the justices of labourers sitting at Devizes, 11 June 1352. The paraphrase of the entries is my own.

E. M. Thompson, 'Offenders against the statute of labourers in Wiltshire, AD 1349', *The Wiltshire Archaeological and Natural History Magazine*, XXXIII, 1903–4, pp. 403–6.

Philip Heryng of Chisledon, carpenter, took an excess of 6*d* from various men contrary to statute. He came before the deputy justices at Chisledon and put himself in the king's grace. John Tyburn and Robert Westroup stand surety that he will satisfy the king for the excess at the next session of the justices; fine 12*d*.

John Laurok came at Chisledon, a vagabond out of employment, and acknowledged that he had left the employment of William de Stratton of Oxfordshire. Therefore he is committed to the custody of the bailiff of the hundred until details of the withdrawal are known. Afterwards Thomas Whytsyde and John Goddard stood surety that he will come before the justices at their next session and stand to judgement if he cannot prove that he withdrew with the permission of the said William.

It was presented that William le Coupere of Elcombe, who had sworn before the justices to exercise his craft according to statute, took an excess of 6*d* from various men. He came before the deputy justices at Nether Wroughton and said that he was not guilty and put himself on his country.[17] Therefore the bailiff of the hundred is ordered to bring 12 lawful men from his bailiwick to Swindon on 1 May. Walter Gylemyn and John le Smyth stand surety that he will be there on the said day. And the jury say on their oath that he is not guilty and he is acquitted.

John Boltash, carter of the parson of Elingdon, acknowledged that he received a livery of one quarter of corn for 10 weeks, of which 2 bushels were of wheat, although he used to be given a quarter for 11 weeks of which one bushel was of wheat.[18] Therefore he remains in custody of the bailiff. Afterwards Thomas de Lyl and Philip Shayl stand surety that he will come before the justices at their next session

17 In other words, elected that his claim be tested by a jury of local people.

18 Wheat was the most valuable grain grown by medieval farmers. Medieval weights and measures tended to vary somewhat from region to region, but in modern terms a bushel is eight gallons; a quarter is eight bushels.

and answer to the king for the excess.

[Similar cases involving two other servants of the parson]

Edward le Taillour of Wootton, employee of the prior and convent of Bradenstoke under an agreement made between them to run from Michaelmas 1351 for one year, receiving his diet and accustomed salary, left his employment before the feast of St Nicholas [6 December] without permission or reasonable cause, contrary to statute. Therefore the bailiff of the hundred is ordered to make him come before the justices in their next session.

John Deth of Wroughton acknowledges that he took an excess of 6s 8d from John Lovel for reaping his corn. John Shayl and Walter Whyte stand surety that he will come before the justices at their next session.

Richard the cobbler of Clack, who had sworn before the justices that he would exercise his craft according to statute, took an excess of 40d from various men for shoes sold to them, contrary to the statute and his oath. Richard has not appeared before the deputy judges because the bailiff of the hundred presents that he cannot be found. Therefore the bailiff is ordered to take him and bring him before the justices at their next session in Devizes. Richard does not come at Devizes, taking flight when he saw the bailiff coming. Afterwards he was taken and came before the justices, accused of contempt as well as the excess charge. Richard seeks to acquit himself of this and puts himself on the king's grace. Fine 2 marks.

115. A selection of cases from Lincolnshire

(a) A plea of the crown heard at Lincoln, 30 September 1353.

B. Putnam, *Enforcement of the Statute of Labourers*, pp. 195*-196*.

The jury present that last summer one John Skit was in the employment of Sir John Dargentene as a ploughman, and one Roger Swynflete, keeper of the manor of the Abbot of Selby at Stallingborough, hired the said John outside his existing employment, for this winter, for 6s and wheat (no other grain), and for as much land as could be sown with two bushels of corn for one suit of clothes, and also an acre sown with peas for another suit of clothes; and for such a large payment he left the employment of the said Sir John at the feast of St Martin last [4 July]. And afterwards the said John Skit was afraid that he would be indicted before the justices and therefore did not dare to stay, but took himself off to distant parts, and thus Sir John lost his service, by the default and malice of the said Roger and contrary to the statute of the lord king.

(b) Inquisition in the soke of Bolingbroke (Lincs), 16 November 1360. Rosamund Sillem (ed), *Some Sessions of the Peace in Lincolnshire, 1360-1375*, Lincolnshire Record Society, XXX, 1937, p. 1.

The jurors say that Alan Bishop of Freiston, living in Sibsey, and others wished to leave the employment of Lady Roos before the end of their contract. On 5 October this year William son of Petronilla and Hugh de Orby, the constables of the vill of Sibsey, came with the intention of arresting them, and the said Alan refused to submit to the constables and resisted them, in contempt of the king's statute, and is self-evidently a breaker of the statute. When charged, Alan sought to acquit himself of the offence and placed himself on the grace of the lord king and made a fine of 40*d*.

(c) A presentment before the justices in Lindsey, 1374. *Ibid*, p. 70.

The jurors of the wapentake of Wraggoe present that John Fisshere, William Theker, William Furnes, John Dyker, Gilbert Chyld, Alan Tasker, Stephen Lang, John Hardlad, Cecilia Ka, Joan daughter of Henry Couper, Matillis de Ely, Alice wife of Simon Souter, all of Bardney, labourers, were on 3 August 1374 required by the constables of Bardney, Simon Tele and Richard Gladwyn, to work in Bardney during the following autumn for the Abbot of Bardney and others, receiving the wages specified by statute. John Fisshere and the others refused to work there, and on the same day they left the town to get higher wages elsewhere, in contempt of the king and contrary to statute.

(d) A presentment before the justices in Holland. *Ibid*, p. 241.

The jurors present that, because he refused to work by the year according to the statute of the lord king, one Richard Rote, a vagabond, was placed in the stocks by Stephen de Redynges and John Lyne, constables of the vill of Wyberton, until he submitted. On 29 December 1373 there came Stephen the chaplain, rector of Wyberton, John Candeler, chaplain, Robert Chaumberleyn and John, a servant of the said rector, with force and arms, viz with swords and bows and arrows, and assaulted the said constables and beat and wounded them so that their life is despaired of, and tried to take the said Richard Rote from the stocks, in contempt of the lord king and contrary to his peace.

116. Cases before the justices in Kesteven, 1371

These are taken from a roll of 192 indictments made before the justices of the peace for Kesteven (one of the three administrative divisions of Lincolnshire – the others, represented in 115 above, are Holland and Lindsey). All the cases of excess wages are printed here, and a sample of those concerning over-charging for victuals.

Sillem, *Some Sessions of the Peace*, pp. 154–182.

Walter, chaplain of the parish of Barrowby and John Sire of the same, proctors of the said church, accuse Robert Tasker of Londonthorpe in a plea of breach of covenant, in that the said Robert was hired by Walter and John at the feast of St Martin in winter [11 November] 1370 to thresh all their grain, of whatever kind, receiving for his wages the amount specified by statute; and Robert left his employment in return for the offer of a higher salary, contrary to statute, and to the loss of Walter and John of 15s.

John Tawerner of Sleaford is a freelance[19] fisherman and he sold fish and herrings to William Croftes of Sleaford on the first Monday in Lent 1371, at 6 herrings for 1d instead of 8 for 1d as he ought, and he sold at the same rate to everyone else during Lent to their grave damage; excess 2s.

Simon Olyer of Old Sleaford sold a gallon of oil at Sleaford to Alice Skynner of Sleaford on 25 February 1370 for 16d when he ought to have sold a gallon for 10d. The excess is 2s since he sold at the same price to all who bought oil of him.

William Kote of Evedon is a freelance weaver of woollen cloth and on 9 May 1370 he took from Henry Stork, chaplain, living in Evedon 3d per yard, when he ought to have taken only 2d; excess 12d.

Thomas Tygow of Hale is a freelance roofer and he took at Hale from Hugh Skynner of Little Hale on various occasions in 1370 a daily wage of 4d and his dinner, contrary to statute; excess 3s 4d.

Richard [lost] took from John de Burton at Hale on 12 August 1370 4d and his dinner, and did this on various days throughout autumn, when he ought to have taken only 2d and food; excess 12d.

William Deye of Ingoldsby is a freelance ploughman and took from Gilbert Deye at Ingoldsby on 2 December 1370 3d and food, and did

---

19 Literally a 'common' [*communis*] fisherman, which is how this and similar phrases are normally translated. The point is that such 'common' workers were not contracted to a single master but were available to work for anyone.

this for the rest of the week, and received the same from others in the following year; excess 12*d.*

William de Breton of Ingoldsby is a freelance roofer and refused to work in the said vill, but worked outside the vill to earn excessive money, and he took from Thomas Smyth at Bitchfield on 18 November 1370 4*d* and food, contrary to statute, and thus for the whole week the excess was 6*d.*

Thomas de Stafford sold wine from Gascony in Grantham for 14*d* the gallon, when other people were selling it for 12*d* in the same town.

William Sudde of Catthorpe carpenter took from Thomas son of Matilda of Sudbrooke for 3 days work 40*d* and his dinner, contrary to statute; excess 2*s* 4*d.*

John Couper, carpenter, refused to work by the day in order to earn excessive money, and he took a lump sum from William Burton of Sudbrooke; excess estimated to be 2*s.*

Thomas Havenyld of Normanton and Adam Attonesende of Catthorpe, masons, took 40*d* for 2 days work from Walter at Boure of Sudbrooke and refused to work by the day; excess estimated at 18*d.*

Hugh Beaumares, employee of Richard Thorald of Marston, took for his allowance rye and wheat, where he ought, according to local practice, have taken rye and peas, and he took 4*s* 4*d* for his year's wages; excess 40*d.*

John Nethird and Richard de Colyngham, employees of Richard Thorold of Marston, took their allowance in rye, refusing to take peas, contrary to statute and local custom; the excess from Michaelmas to now [January] estimated at 18*d.*

John de Wyluby of Marston and Robert Scephird, employees of John Trippolow, rector of Haugham, take rye and wheat for their allowance, refusing peas, contrary to statute and local custom; the excess of both of them estimated at a quarter of rye, price 6*s.*

[2 similar cases follow]

Richard, employee of Nicholas de Merston, has an allowance this year of 20*s,* where he ought to take only 10*s;* excess 10*s.*

117. Additions to the statute of labourers, 1388

The six chapters of the statute printed here are concerned not only with the wage levels of those in employment, but their freedom of movement and how they should spend their leisure time. I have also included the chapters concerned with able-bodied beggars: a group who were beginning to trouble the authorities.

Statutes of the Realm, II pp. 56-8.

It is ordained and agreed that all the statutes of artificers, labourers, employees and victuallers made in the time of the present king as well as in the time of his noble grandfather, whom God assoil, which have not been repealed shall be firmly held and kept and duly executed; and that the said artificers, labourers, employees and victuallers shall be subject to the jurisdiction of the justices of the peace at the suit of the king as well as at the suit of the party, as the said statutes require; and that the mayors, bailiffs and constables of towns and seigneurial stewards duly perform their offices concerning such artificers, labourers, employees and victuallers; and that there shall be a pair of stocks in every town for the same employees and labourers until they submit to judgement, as is ordained in the said statutes.

Moreover it is ordained and agreed that no employee or labourer, whether male or female, shall depart at the end of his term of employment from the hundred, rape or wapentake where he is living to work or live elsewhere, or go from thence on a claimed pilgrimage, unless he carry a letter patent[20] containing the reason for his going and the time of his return (if he is to return) under the king's seal, which shall be assigned and delivered for this purpose to some worthy man of the hundred or hundreds, rape or wapentake, city or borough at the discretion of the justices of the peace; and it shall be kept to make such letters as necessary and not for any other purpose, and he shall take an oath to that effect; and the name of the county shall be written around the seal, and the name of the hundred, rape, wapentake, city or borough diagonally across the seal. And if any employee or labourer be found in any city or borough or elsewhere *en route* from another place and wandering about without such letters he shall be immediately taken by the said mayors, bailiffs, stewards or constables and put in the stocks and kept there until he has found surety to return to his employment, or to work or labour in the town from which he came, or

20 Letters patent were sealed open – that is, with the seal hanging from a tongue of parchment cut from the bottom of the sheet – so that they could be read without destroying the seal which validated them.

until he secures a letter permitting his departure for a reasonable cause. And it should be remembered that an employee or labourer at the end of his term may freely leave his employment and work somewhere else, provided that he has a certain offer of employment and has a letter as described above. But it is not the intention that employees who ride or go on their lords' or masters' business should be brought within the terms of this ordinance during the time of that business.

And if anyone carries a letter which is found to be forged or false he shall be imprisoned for forty days for the deception, and then until he finds surety to return to his former work or employment. And that no one shall harbour an employee or labourer who has left their hundred, rape or wapentake, city or borough without a testimonial letter; or harbour them for more than one night if they have such a letter, unless it is because of sickness or some other reasonable cause, or because the letter allows them to work or labour there, under a penalty to be established by the justices of the peace.

And employees and apprentices, and also artificers and master craftsmen of no great standing, active in trades and crafts which are not in much demand during harvest time, shall be compelled to work during the harvest, to reap, stack and carry in the corn. And these statutes shall be duly executed by the mayors, bailiffs, stewards and constables, under a penalty to be established and decided by the justices of the peace during their sessions. And no one shall take more than a penny for making, sealing and delivering such a letter.

Because employees and workers refuse, and for a long time have refused, to work and labour except for an outrageous and excessive sum (much more than has been given to such employees and labourers at any time in the past), so that because of the lack of such employees and labourers husbandmen and tenants[21] cannot pay their rents and can scarcely make a living from their land, to the great damage and loss of the lords as well as of all the Commons; and because the rate for the said employees and labourers has not previously been established, it is accorded and agreed that a bailiff in husbandry shall receive 13s 4d p.a. and a suit of clothing once a year at most; the master

---

21 This clause is distinguishing between the small tenant farmers, who could not afford the high wages, and the great landowners who (by implication) could, but who were losing out because their tenants could no longer afford to pay their rent. The 1351 statute had drawn a similar distinction.

hind[22] 10s; the carter 10s; the shepherd 10s; the oxherd 10s; the cowherd 6s 8d; the swineherd 6s; a female labourer 6s; the dairymaid 6s; the plough driver 7s at most; and each other labourer or employee according to his status; and less in those regions where less used to be paid; without clothing, presents or other kinds of rewards by contract.[23] And no one employed by artificers or victuallers in cities, boroughs or other towns shall take more than the labourers and employees listed above, according to their status; without clothing, presents or other rewards by agreement as abovesaid. And if anyone gives or takes by contract more than is specified, then for the first offence both giver and recipient shall pay the value of the excess payment; for the second offence double its value, and for the third offence triple its value; and if the recipient has no money with which to pay the excess he shall go to prison for forty days.

It is ordained and agreed that any male or female who works as a carter or ploughman, or in any other agricultural occupation until they reach the age of 12, shall from then on remain in the same employment, without being put to learn any trade or craft; and if any agreement or indenture of apprenticeship shall later be made to the contrary it shall be void.

It is decided and agreed that no employee in husbandry, or labourer or employee of an artificer or victualler shall in future carry any baselard, dagger or sword upon pain of forfeiture, except in war time for the defence of the realm (and then only under the supervision of the arrayers for the time being) or when travelling through the countryside with their masters or on their masters' business. But such employees and labourers shall have bows and arrows and use them on Sundays and holy days, and entirely leave off playing handball and football, and the other games called quoits, dice, stone throwing[24] and skittles, and other such unsuitable games. And the sheriffs, mayors, bailiffs and constables shall have the power to arrest all those contravening the statute, and to seize the said baselards, daggers and swords and keep them until the session of the justices of the peace and

22 A hind is a skilled agricultural worker. The master hind was the man who ran the practical farming side of things, as distinct from the bailiff who had a more general executive responsibility.

23 In other words workers could be given *ad hoc* gifts but these were not to become an invariable supplement to their wages.

24 To judge from the context, the reference is probably to shying stones at a target, but the phrase could cover a range of games, from knuckle-bones to ducks and drakes.

then present the weapons and the names of their owners to the justices. But it is not the king's intention that this should be to the prejudice of the franchises of lords as far as their right to forfeitures is concerned.

It is decided and agreed that everyone who goes begging and is able to work or labour shall be treated like the people who leave a hundred or other place without a testimonial letter, as abovesaid; except for members of religious orders and hermits with supporting testimonial letters from their ordinaries. And that beggars unfit to work shall remain in the city or town where they are living at the time this statute is proclaimed; and if the people of the said city or town will not or cannot support them, the said beggars shall take themselves off to other towns within the hundred, rape or wapentake, or to the town where they were born, within forty days of the proclamation, and shall remain there for the rest of their lives. And everyone who goes on pilgrimage as a beggar, and is fit to work, shall be treated like the said employees and labourers without testimonial letters, unless they have testimonial letters concerning their pilgrimage sealed under the said seals. And that the scholars of the universities who go begging shall have testimonial letters from their chancellor under the same penalty.

It is ordained and agreed that men who claim to have travelled beyond the realm and there to have been imprisoned shall carry testimonial letters from the captain of the place where they were living, or from the mayor and bailiffs of the place where they arrived in this country; and the same mayor and bailiffs shall inquire of such people where and with whom they have lived, and where they live in England; and the mayor and bailiffs shall make them letters patent under their official seal, testifying what day they arrived and where they have been, according to their account; and the mayor and bailiffs shall make them swear that they shall go straight back to their home area, unless they have letters patent under the king's great seal allowing them to do otherwise. And if any traveller is found without such letters he shall be treated like the said employees and labourers; and this ordinance shall apply to travellers who go begging through the countryside after their arrival.

118. Difficulties in finding tenants

These extracts from the Durham hallmoot book covering the period 1350-55 show the continuing difficulties which lords experienced in finding tenants – and in keeping them. The entries are printed in chronological order, except that later developments are printed (indented) after the first mention of a case. For earlier material from the same source see 95 above.

[summer 1350]
William de Kirkeby, coroner of the ward of Chester le Street, testifies that Thomas Short, John son of Patrick, William Chir, John son of Richard, Robert Jenkynson, Thomas Colman, Richard Robertson, Thomas son of Adam, John son of Matilda, the lord's serfs, said openly in the hearing of the coroner that they wanted to run away from the lord's land and take holdings elsewhere; and they paid nothing for the term of St Cuthbert in March last in the 5th year of Bishop Thomas [1350]. And in addition they maliciously and with malice afore-thought surrendered their plough shares to the lord at Auckland on the Thursday before Pentecost [13 May]. And for these reasons they have been arrested and were imprisoned at Durham until the Saturday before Trinity Sunday [29 May], when they were released by Sir Thomas Gray the steward, with the advice of William de Westle the receiver, on condition that they and their neighbours pay all the debts from the term of St Martin and other sums arising from the great hallmoots up to the term of St Cuthbert in March last, and as much for the terms of St Cuthbert last and St John the Baptist and fines from the great hallmoots as Sir William the receiver shall decide, on the basis of what seems to him best for the lord bishop, under the supervision of Sir Thomas Gray the steward. And the aforesaid Thomas and his fellows named above found sureties, namely Reginald de Wermouth of Whitburn and William Tymprum of Whitburn, and also bound themselves and each other to remain within the estates of the lord bishop.

[Boldon, 7 June 1350]
The jurors claim that the whole vill is so weakened that they can pay nothing, nor can any tenant be found to make a fine for any of the land in the lord's hand; two of the existing tenants have offered money to render up their land, but no one has taken it.

[Benfieldside, 17 June]
Walter Walker takes an acre of land and a fulling mill, which William de Brandon held and which fell into the lord's hands, and no one of William's blood kin came after proclamation was made. And Walter will maintain the mill and its pond at his own expense, except that the bishop will supply him with great timbers.[25] And he gives half a mark of new increment on top of the one mark formerly paid. And he will hold it on these terms until another tenant comes who is prepared to

25 In other words, the bishop would supply the massive tree trunks necessary to form the drive shaft of the mill.

pay an entry fine or to give the lord a larger sum. And it is agreed that he
will begin to pay the whole farm at the feast of St John the Baptist next.

[Sedgefield, 8 November]
Thomas de Carleton, the lord's serf, who ought to have held a bondage
tenement, has fled. And the tenement is committed to Richard Stere on
the surety of Adam Kirkman and Vynt his brother, to answer to the
lord for all charges until they bring back the said Thomas.

[Killerby, 4 April 1351]
The villages[26] of Heighington, Ricknall, Middridge and Killerby refuse
to hold their lands at pennyfarm[27] unless they pay 12d. The steward
does not agree.

[Tunstall, 15 July]
Land lying waste which belonged to John de Duresme is committed to
the village, who are to satisfy the lord for the farm until a tenant can
be found.

[Sedgefield, 23 February 1352]
Nothing from William de Hedlem who has refused to hold a bovate of
land imposed on him by his neighbours.

[Killerby, 27 February]
An agreement is struck with the village of Killerby by Sir Thomas
Gray the steward that they should work all the land lying in the lord's
hands in the vill on condition that this shall be at pennyfarm for all
works and carrying services, except that they will pay the tender of
malt, wheat and oats at the rate in force when the payment falls due;
and that they will perform the usual carrying services for the bishop
in his comings and goings. And this agreement shall last for three
years from the feast of St Cuthbert in March, 1352.

[Killerby, 9 March 1355]
The tenants of Killerby make complaint that there is no way they
can hold their land by paying a farm, malt and labour services.
Therefore they discuss with the steward whether, as a favour from
the lord, he would be willing to allow them to pay cash for the malt
and labour services. And let it be done in secret, because of the bad
example it sets to the other villages, for two or three years.

26 *Villata* – the men who make up the community of the vill. I have deliberately not
used the modern word 'villagers' which would now imply all the residents; *villata*
is more selective.

27 'Pennyfarm' is the local term for a cash rent paid instead of labour services for a
bondage (villein) holding. Here and elsewhere to 'farm' land is to pay rent for it, not
(as now) to cultivate it.

[Byers, 27 February]
12*d* has now been waived from each acre which used to pay 2*s* until the world improves or other tenants can be found who are prepared to pay the whole farm; and this is to come into force at the feast of St Cuthbert next [20 March].

[Lanchester, 31 October]
15 acres lying waste in the lord's hands because of the departure of Alan de Falderby are committed to the village to answer for the farm.

[Ryton, 18 February 1353]
It is presented that William Bacon, the lord's serf, is living in Winlaton, and the jurors say that he is able to hold a bondage tenement in Ryton. Therefore it is ordered that he be fetched back.

[Ryton, 13 November 1356]
Be it noted that William Bacon, the lord's serf, is living in Winlaton on the land of Lord Neville. Therefore the coroner is ordered to bring him home to hold land, since he is wealthy.[28]

[Ryton, 6 February 1357]
Be it still noted that William Bacon, the lord's serf, is living in Winlaton. The coroner is ordered to bring him back to the lord's land.

[Wearmouth, 19 February]
The jury present that most of the lord's houses in Wearmouth are falling down for want of tenants. Therefore the coroner is ordered to go and look at the houses and report the names of those whose default has led to the dereliction of the houses to the steward before the next hallmoot.

[Easington, 20 February]
All the neighbours of Easington are ordered to put waste cottages upon employees or others who can be charged with the farm before the next hallmoot, or otherwise the said cottages will lie upon the said village.[29]

[Whickham, 21 October]
The jury present that Agnes Dowe, the lord's serf, has abandoned the land of the lord and fled to Newcastle, where she has married a cobbler without the lord's licence, but they do not know his name.

28 In other words, he has the resources to pay the rent for the land.

29 A 'cottage' was not (as now) simply a small domestic dwelling, but the land which went with it – hence the references among these entries to a derelict cottage (the building) and a cottage (the land) not being worked.

[Cassop, 23 October]
The jury present that John de Byrden, who took a cottage, has
abandoned it and is now living on the prior's land at Pittington.
Therefore be it noted that the coroner is to have his goods and chattels
seized until the cottage is rebuilt, because it has been ruinous for a long
time.

[Middleham, 24 October]
It is found by the coroner, Richard Stere, and the other jurors that
William Meggison and Thomas Saynyng are capable of holding a
waste land called the land of John Batell. And it has been committed
to them. And they are to begin to pay at the feast of St Cuthbert in
September next [4 Sept].

[Middridge, 28 October]
The villages of Heighington, Killerby, Ricknall and Redworth present
that Wiliam Woderose has the capacity to hold half a waste land.
Therefore the said land has been committed to him. And he is to begin
to pay at the feast of St Cuthbert in September next.

[Sedgefield, 3 July, 1354]
The jury present that John Cose is not capable of holding the waste
cottage committed to him to work. Therefore it has been taken into the
lord's hands until Walter Dynaund and the four jurors can find
another tenant.

[Middridge, 7 July]
One land out of three in the lord's hand is committed to William
Woderof in his absence because it is presented by Roger de Tykhill
that he is capable of holding the said land. And he is to begin to pay
at the feast of St John next.

[Hartburn, 27 October]
The jury present that William de Elleton who lives in Long Newton
is a serf, as do the jurors of Carlton who present that he was a serf in
the same vill. Therefore the coroner is ordered to take him to
Hartburn, to the land which Adam Dobbe held, who is now incapable
of holding the land, and it is ordered that the tenants should answer
for the farm until William arrives.

[Hartburn, 3 July 1355]
The coroner is ordered to bring home William de Elton, the lord's
serf who is living in Long Newton, to hold the land or to perform
service for the same.

[Ricknall, 9 March 1355]
The coroner testifies that William Standupryght is so quarrelsome and
rancorous that none of the lord's tenants can bear to live in the vill
because of him, and he has caused the vill to be deserted. Therefore the
coroner is ordered to have his goods and chattels seized.

Peter de Hessewell is charged with the farm of the said vill because the
tenants have voluntarily withdrawn from their land.

[Killerby, 2 November 1355]
Peter de Hessewell is ordered to distrain all the tenants of Ricknall
and Killerby who have fled from their lands except those who are
infirm, wherever they can be found between Tyne and Tees.

[Ricknall, 14 March 1356]
Richard del Graunge, Gilbert de Rikenall, William Standupryght
and the rest of the husbandmen have fled from the vill of Ricknall.
Therefore the coroner Peter de Hessewell is ordered to distrain
them wherever they can be found in his bailliwick, to make them
answer for the farm due to the bishop and for the damage to the
houses.

[Cassop, 1 July 1355]
Be it noted that there are people among them capable of holding land
but they refuse.

[Cornforth, 2 July]
Because it was ordered at the last hallmoot that Hugh Carter and Alice
his wife should come today to hold land for which they have made a
fine, and they have not come, it is ordered that the neighbours should
work the land and answer for the farm.

[Escomb, 6 July]
John Arowsmyth, whom the lord's council says is a serf, claims to be a
free man, and it is thought likely that he will try to flee. Therefore he
finds sureties: Roger Malson, John Baret, Thomas Mareshall and
Roger de Tikhill.

119. Rebellious serfs at Wawne

The legal expedients pursued by a group of disaffected serfs on the East
Riding estates of Meaux Abbey recorded by the monastic chronicler.

E. A. Bond (ed), *Chronica Monasterii de Melsa*, 3 vols, Rolls Series, 1866-68, III
pp. 127-42.

It should not be passed over in silence, since it deserves to be remembered, how our serfs at Wawne turned stubborn and refused their service which they owed to us. Those serfs, who were serfs by birth, being descended from certain unfree tenants of ours at Dimlington, sought to lighten the yoke of servitude, under which they and their ancestors were subjugated. In order to turn them from their evil ways, we felt obliged to use the force at our disposal against the ringleaders, and we imprisoned three or four of them. But one of them, called Richard Cellerer, escaped away secretly and contrived to avoid that punishment. He then announced that he and all his ancestors were free from servitude, or (when he felt like making a less extreme claim) that he and all his family could trace their descent from serfs on the royal manor of Easington, and they admitted themselves to be the king's serfs, invoking the protection of royal power against us.[30] They apparently considered it more glorious to be considered – indeed, to *be* – royal serfs than to offer the meritorious due of service to the church of God and to our monastery.

Therefore the said Richard Cellerer went to William Fyllylott, then the king's escheator in Holderness, and filled his ears with his made-up stories: that he and the rest of those imprisoned by us, and their ancestors, were from of old royal serfs of the manor of Easington. Whereupon the escheator made an official inquiry among the serfs of Easington, and on their evidence accepted that John the son of Robert Cellerer, Thomas Cellerer and the others held in chains in our abbey, and Richard Cellerer, were serfs belonging to the king and his progenitors as of his manor of Easington, and that they had removed themselves and their belongings from the manor twenty years ago and had gone to Wawne. By virtue of that finding William the escheator seized the persons and possessions of the serfs into the king's hands, with the result that they remained in the king's service for some little while.

We realised what a threat this loss of our rights posed to us and our monastery, for – as long as it looked as though we had been worsted by our serfs – it would serve as a model for the unbridled malice of the

---

30 The Cellerers are unlikely to have been motivated only by the desire for a powerful protector – although this is the angle the Meaux chronicler chooses to emphasise. It was widely believed that the king's villeins enjoyed privileges not shared by ordinary villeins, and the Cellerers in the 1350s were pursuing a strategy which was to be taken up by whole communities in the late 1370s, when villeins turned to Domesday Book in an attempt to prove that their manor had once been part of the royal demesne: R. Faith, 'The 'great rumour' of 1377 and peasant ideology', in R. H. Hilton and T. H. Aston (eds), *The English Rising of 1381*, Cambridge, 1987, pp. 43-73.

others and bestow even greater audacity on the troublemakers who wanted to withhold their service. We duly addressed a petition against Wiliam the escheator to the king's council. In it we explained how the escheator, by virtue of his official finding, had seized our serfs as royal serfs and asked that a commission, made up of men of some standing, should be appointed to inquire into the truth of the matter, and bring the case to a conclusion, as law and justice require. Whereupon the king sent a writ to William the escheator, ordering him to give an account of the matter and of the taking of the serfs. His answer was that he had seized the serfs with their belongings and dependents for no other reason than the finding of the inquiry, and so, because we were claiming that the serfs were men and serfs of our manor of Dimlington, the king ordered letters patent to be sent to William the escheator and to others, authorising them to inquire by the oath of men of standing whether the serfs were royal serfs, from the king's manor of Easington, or our serfs by right of our manor of Dimlington; and, if the serfs were the king's, then by what title, how, and in what way, and if they were ours, then from what time, by what title, how, and in what way; and they were then to notify the king accordingly.

The inquisition was held at Hedon in December 1358 and the jurors said that serfs, viz John, Richard and Thomas, were not serfs of the king and never had been, but were at the time serfs of our Abbey of Meaux, and that time out of mind their ancestors had been serfs of the present abbot and his predecessors, in right of their church. When asked by what title, the jurors replied that one Geoffrey Gybwyne had owned a serf called Robert Hurt, the ancestor of the said John, Richard and Thomas; and that Robert fathered Adam, who fathered Robert, who fathered Robert Cellerer, John Cellerer and William Cellerer, and that Robert fathered the above written John and others, And Robert's brother John fathered the aforesaid Richard Cellerer; and William their brother fathered Thomas Cellerer. Geoffrey Gybwyne gave the aforesaid Robert Hurt with all his dependants to the Abbot of Meaux and his successors, and by virtue of that grant the present abbot and his predecessors, time out of mind, had owned Robert Hurt and his dependants as their serfs, until John, Richard and Thomas took themselves off less than ten years ago. In witness of the truth of their findings the jurors set their seals to the inquisition, which was sent to the king's chancery.

The king then sent a writ to the Sheriff of York ordering him to render up to us immediately our fugitive serfs with all their belongings and dependants wherever they might be found, unless they were in the king's demesne, and the sheriff duly arranged for us to have John and Thomas with their dependants and belongings. But Richard Cellerer (who was still pursuing the matter against us, regardless of the findings of the inquisition) could not be found and so the sheriff could not hand him over; but he arranged for us to have his belongings, according to his instructions from the king. A short time afterwards, John Cellerer and his son William made a complaint against our abbot to the king, alleging that the abbot, before the taking of the inquisition described above, had used force to seize and detain a number of men employed by them as ploughmen, in contempt of the king and in contravention of the statute and ordinance of labourers. The damage to each of them was assessed at £5. One day when our lord abbot was at Hedon to discuss the matter with the auditors of the lord king and of his daughter Isabel, then lord of Holderness for life, his horses were seized to make him answer the king and the aforesaid John, William, Thomas and William concerning the said accusation. The horses were taken away and impounded at Burstwick, and the abbot had to borrow others in order to get back to the monastery.

On the appointed day the abbot returned to Hedon to answer the charges before William de Belkethorp and his colleagues, justices of labourers. In making his reply he denied that there was any case to answer, because John, William, Thomas and William were his serfs, and the serfs of our church of Meaux, and that the abbot and his predecessors had owned them time out of mind, and asked the judges to rule whether he was obliged to answer the charge. The said John, William, Thomas and William were then examined individually, without warning, and they (as God willed) frankly admitted that they and their ancestors were serfs of the abbot and monastery, and that the abbot and monastery owned them, as described above. But they claimed that this did not mean that the abbot need not answer them, because it did not alter the fact that he had committed an offence in taking away their employees contrary to statute; and they sought a judgement, with compensation of £5 each. But it seemed to the judges and the court that there was no case to answer, since John, William, Thomas and William had individually confessed themselves to be serfs of the abbot and monastery, and the ruling was that the serfs should get nothing for their claim, but should be in the king's mercy, and that the abbot should withdraw quit, *sine die.*

But the serfs, undeterred by the fact that they had admitted their servile status and that judgement had been given against them accordingly, still pursued the matter. Richard Cellerer put it to the king that William de Belkethorpe and his colleagues had given an unjust judgement against them, and the king accordingly ordered William to send a record of the proceedings into chancery for examination. In pursuing the case the serfs, in the person of Richard Cellerer, continued to make false accusations against the abbot, claiming (in spite of the findings of the inquisition described above) that Richard, and the aforesaid John and Thomas (fathers of the two Williams) were the king's serfs from his manor of Easington, and backed up their claims with this genealogy. Hugh Hert, a serf of the Count of Aumale, held a toft within Easington and fathered Robert Hert within wedlock. And Robert Hert held the toft after the death of his father Hugh and fathered Adam Hert; and Adam held the toft after his father's death until he granted it and his service to a monk of Meaux, who had been cellarer there for a long time, and it was because of this that he became known as Adam Cellerer. Afterwards the Abbot of Meaux granted him land in Wawne and there he fathered three sons: Robert, John and William. And Robert fathered John Cellerer, against whom false charges were brought by the Abbot of Meaux.

As a result of all this a new suit was begun against us by the king concerning the ownership of these serfs. The king, who had been badly advised by some members of his council who were hostile towards us, acted on Richard's claim and dispatched writs to our abbot and to the Sheriff of York. That to the abbot told us to hand over to William Fyllylott, the escheator in Holderness, the persons of the said John, Richard and Thomas, along with all their belongings and dependants at Wawne, whom we had just taken into our hands as our serfs. So we handed over the persons of John and Thomas with their dependants and belongings to the escheator by indenture. We could hardly hand over Richard, because we had never managed to get our hands on him, but we handed over his belongings to the escheator.

Another writ to our abbot instructed him (under pain of total forfeiture) to be at London on a certain day to answer the king in person concerning the injury done to these men – whom the king described as his serfs. The abbot came down to London early and by means of various hefty gifts presented to the king's chancellor, the Bishop of Winchester, was able (in the teeth of opposition from other members of the royal council) to secure the right to present his case by attorneys rather than in person. That achieved, he appointed two attorneys to act for him and headed back home. The attorneys presented a bill to the king asking him to send letters to the chancellor to the effect that, if it could be shown by the original commission and inquiry that the said John, Richard and Thomas were serfs of our abbot and monastery, he should arrange for them and their belongings to be handed over to our abbot. The attorneys guaranteed on the abbot's behalf that he would be answerable to the king or to the lady Isabel his daughter for the said serfs with their dependants and belongings, or for the value of their belongings as set out in an indenture drawn up between the lady Isabel and our abbot. So we got back our serfs, with their dependants and belongings, just as we had held them before their seizure into the king's hands, while discussion continued about whether they properly belonged to the king and his daughter or to us and our monastery.

When we had got possession of the serfs in this manner, considering the extreme gravity of their offence, we imprisoned them within the abbey, in a room in the bursary below the monks' dormitory. One night John Cellerer, who was one of the men imprisoned there, managed to escape by climbing down the latrine shaft into a ditch called Dog Dyke and then made his way to the king, again with the intention of proving his freedom. To that end he procured a writ, on behalf of himself and his son William, addressed to the Sheriff of York and ordering that, if John and William found surety to prove their freedom, then he should put the matter before the judges at the next assize at York, and in the meantime he should have John and William under his protection. And our said abbot would have to attend the assize if he wanted to prove the servile status of John and William.

When John and William had made proof of their freedom at the assize Nicholas Damery, one of the king's knights, William de Skypwith, justice, and others were appointed by the king to investigate, by the oath of worthy and respectable men from Holderness, whether John, Richard and Thomas had been, or by rights ought to be, serfs of the king and his daughter, or of our abbot; and, if serfs of our abbot, from what time, by what title, how and in what way; and to get more fully at the truth of all the attendant circumstances; and to do full and speedy justice both for the king and his daughter and for our abbot; and to hear and determine the whole matter according to the law and custom of England; and to deliver possession of the said John, Richard and Thomas and their dependants and belongings to whichever of the parties they were adjudged to belong to.

This was nearly frustrated, for Nicholas Damery, who favoured the serfs, demonstrated his hostility against us. A day had been assigned for the case to be heard at Hedon, but Nicholas Damery concealed his arrival, in the hope that we, by failing to pursue the case, would lose all the ground we had gained earlier. But we were afraid that he might turn up at short notice and so we summoned worthy men to be in readiness for the occasion, so that our right should not be lost through any lack of support engineered by the malice of our ill-wishers. So when Nicholas turned up at the very last minute (as if he had only just arrived) he found to his surprise our abbot, his countrymen, the worthy men who had been summoned and others, all ready to hear the case. He thereupon claimed that the crowd of people had been gathered to uphold the abbot against the king, and because (according to him) this had the appearance of a conspiracy against the king's right and would be deeply damaging to his prerogative, he announced that he was not going to be party to holding an inquiry or reaching a decision. And he accordingly withdrew, and made no attempt to proceed any further in the matter, so that the business was held up for almost a year.

Finally the king sent letters patent to the justice William de Skypwyth and to others, repeating what had been said in the original commission and ordering them to inquire into the matter. On the appointed day four knights and eight other worthy men came before William at Hedon and stated, on their oath, that John Cellerer, Richard Cellerer and Thomas Cellerer had been and by right ought to be the serfs of our Abbot of Meaux, of his manor of Dimlington; and that the abbot and all his predecessors time out of mind had owned the said serfs and their ancestors and all their dependants, in right of the church of St Mary of Meaux and his manor of Dimlington. Asked who the predecessors of Abbot Robert were, who had owned the ancestors of the said John, Richard and Thomas as their serfs, they replied that Thomas and Alexander, who had been abbots of Meaux in the time of king John, the great-great-grandfather of the present king, had in turn owned one Hugh Hurt, the great-great-grandfather of John, Richard and Thomas, and all his dependants, as his serf of his manor of Dimlington, in right of the church of Meaux. Hugh Hurt had fathered Robert Hurt, his son, who was born within wedlock, and Hugh, Geoffrey and Michael, formerly abbots of Meaux and the successors of Thomas and Alexander, had in turn owned Robert Hurt, Hugh Hurt's son, and all his dependants during the reign of King Henry, great-grandfather of the present king, as his serf of his manor of Dimlington. Robert Hurt fathered Adam Hurt, who was born within wedlock, and William, Richard, Robert and Richard, formerly abbots of Meaux and the predecessors of the said Abbot Robert, had in turn owned Adam Hurt during the reign of King Edward, grandfather of the present king; and, because Adam Hurt lived for a long time with the cellarer of Meaux he took the name Adam Cellerer. They said further that Adam fathered three sons: Robert, John and William. The present John Cellerer is the son of Robert son of Adam, and Richard Cellerer the son of John son of Adam, and Thomas Cellerer the son of William son of Adam. And Roger and Adam, predecessors of Robert as abbots of Meaux during the reign of Edward II, owned Robert, John and William, the sons of Adam, and all their dependants as their serfs of their manor of Dimlington. And concerning John, Richard and Thomas, who made the false accusations, the jury said that Hugh, William and John, predecessors of Abbot Robert, and Robert himself, owned them and their dependants as their serfs of their manor of Dimlington during the reign of King Edward the present king, in right of their church of St Mary of Meaux, until John, Richard and Thomas withdrew themselves from the abbot's jurisdiction.

But since this business partly concerned the king the justice William de Skypwyth and the others were afraid to make a judgement or proceed further in the matter without special authorisation from the king. Therefore the business was deferred until an agreed date so that in the interim a royal writ could be obtained which would authorise them to proceed to execution. On that day, both our abbot and the said John, Richard and Thomas presented themselves in person before the justices. The justices, citing the king's writ, urged our abbot not to seek vengeance on the serfs for what they had done, but to treat them with moderation. And then judgement was given by the judges to the effect that our abbot should recover the serfs and own them, along with their belongings and dependants, as serfs of his manor of Dimlington. And accordingly, there in the court, the serfs were handed over to the abbot, to hold as his serfs, according to the force and effect of the judgement in the case. For greater security the abbot secured an exemplification of the proceedings and judgement in the form of royal letters patent.

During the proceedings all the royal officers in the court tried to put obstacles in the abbot's way – all, that is, except for the chancellor, who, because of the gifts he had received, could hardly do other than favour the abbot. But the escheator, William Fyllylott, gave us a great deal of help (as far as it was proper for him to do so) in pursuing our right. Without him the business could not have been brought to such a speedy conclusion.

120. The sin of pride

This brief extract comes from an anonymous fourteenth-century sermon. The preacher has structured his sermon around the seven beatitudes [Matthew 5] which he sees as seven rungs on the ladder of salvation. The extract is taken from his discussion of the first rung: 'Blessed are the poor in spirit, for theirs is the kingdom of heaven' [Matt. 5.3].

Cambridge University Library, Ii.iii.8 fo. 145v.

The first virtue is poverty of spirit, that is to say, humility of heart, and this is the foundation of all virtues and the first rung of this ladder.... Christ instructed us in this, saying, 'Learn of me, because I am meek, and humble of heart' and he continued, which is significant, 'and you shall find rest to your souls' [Matt. 11.29], which is as much as to say that the proud man does not have rest in his soul. Indeed, how can he, when he does not know what new fashion to follow;[31] when he worries about precedence, not knowing whether to ride before or behind or when he can carry a weapon; always terrified that someone will gain more admiration than he; and never having a moment's peace while he can see a neighbour who exceeds him in status or respect. But the humble and meek of heart do not fret about such things, and therefore have rest in their souls, as Christ said, 'Learn of me etc. And you shall find rest to your souls'.

It is much to be regretted how few now follow this precept. Instead men prefer to learn the lesson of Lucifer – and then put it into practice.[32] There is scarcely a villein today who is satisfied with his lot. Little men are always bustling about to make themselves the equals of their betters – or even, if they can wangle it somehow, to make themselves greater than them. This plague – by which I mean the plague of pride – is the mother and principal of all sin. It is capable of intoxicating a man's intelligence, so that he barely recognises himself. For if he gave serious thought to who he is, where he came from and where he is heading for, he would find precious little to glory in. For our proud man comes from nothing; he inhabits a body which will be

31 The preacher here uses the English word *disgyse*. A literal translation of the phrase is 'He does not know how he will be able to *disgyse* himself'. The word did not yet have its modern meaning of concealing one's identity, but had the sense of changing from what was normal and proper to something strange and outrageous.

32 Lucifer rebelled against God and was cast out of heaven with his followers to become devils in hell. It was a medieval commonplace that his fall was due to pride, which was accordingly often seen as the first of the deadly sins. There are brief references to the story in 2 Peter 2.4 and Jude 6.

nothing but dust and ashes, and food for worms; and his soul, in a state of mortal sin, will go to the devil. Look hard. This is hardly the stuff of glory!

121. Sumptuary legislation, 1363

This was the first attempt to regulate clothing according to social status. The attempt was repeated regularly thereafter, with the reissues usually prefaced by expressions of dismay that past attempts had been ineffective.

Statutes of the Realm, I pp. 380-82.

Item, for the outrageous and excessive apparel of many people, contrary to their estate and degree, to the great destruction and impoverishment of the whole land, it is ordained that lads[33] (including the servants of lords as well as those employed in crafts and manufacturing) shall have meat or fish to eat once a day, and at other times other food appropriate to their estate, such as milk, butter and cheese. And those given cloth for their clothing or stockings shall have cloth worth less than 2 marks a cloth[34] and use no cloth of a higher value, whether purchased by them or otherwise, and shall use nothing of gold or silver, embroidered, decorated, or of silk. And their wives, daughters and children shall do likewise and shall wear no veils worth more than 12*d.*

Item, that craftsmen and those of the status of yeoman shall not receive or wear cloth worth more than 40 shillings for a whole cloth for their garments or stockings, whether purchased or otherwise. Nor wear bejewelled cloth or cloth of silk or silver; any belt, knife, clasp, ring, garter, brooch, ribbon, chain, knot,[35] seal or anything else of gold or silver; or any sort of embroidered, decorated or silk clothing. And their wives, daughters and children shall do likewise and shall wear no veil of silk, but only of yarn made within the realm, and shall wear no

33 *Garçons.* The word, as in modern French, is used of the humblest level of servant or employee, and does not necessarily imply a child or even an adolescent. It is analogous to the colonial English term 'houseboy' which could be used of an adult domestic servant. In a seigneurial household the English equivalent would be groom (the translation used in *Statutes of the Realm*).

34 Medieval cloth came in standard sizes and pricing was therefore 'by the cloth' rather than, as today, 'by the yard' or metre. The standard English broadcloth was about 24 yards long by 1½ or 2 yards wide. Thus the amount used to make a garment would cost very much less than the 2 marks (£1 6*s* 8*d*) of the whole cloth.

35 Knots of rich ribbon or cord were attached to clothing as decoration or as a livery badge.

fur or budge,[36] but only lamb, rabbit, cat and fox.

Item, that esquires and all gentlemen below the rank of knight, who do not have land or rent worth more than £100 p.a. shall not receive or wear cloth for their garments or stockings worth more than 4½ marks for a whole cloth, whether purchased or otherwise. Nor wear any cloth of gold, silver or silk; any embroidered garment; any ring, clasp, brooch, ribbon, belt, or any other garment or harness[37] of gold or silver; jewels or any kind of fur. And that their wives, daughters and children shall do likewise, and have no turned-back facings or fur linings in their garments; and have no slashings, jagged edges or fripperies; and wear no cloth of gold or silver or bejewelled cloth. But esquires who have land or rents worth more than £200 p.a. may receive and wear cloth worth 5 marks for a whole cloth, and cloth of silk and silver, with ribbons, girdles and other things reasonably trimmed with silver. And their wives, daughters and children may wear fur facings of miniver, but not ermine or lettice;[38] and may not wear any jewelled item of clothing other than a head-dress.

Item, merchants, citizens, burgesses, manufacturers and craft masters of London and elsewhere who have goods and chattels worth more than £100 net per annum, and their wives and children, may dress in the same way as esquires and gentlemen with land or rent worth £100 p.a. And merchants, citizens and burgesses with goods and chattels worth more than £1000 net, and their wives and children, may dress in the same manner as esquires and gentlemen with land or rent worth more than £200. And no groom, yeoman or employee of merchants, manufacturers or craft masters shall dress otherwise than as specified for the grooms and yeomen of lords, above.

Item, that knights who have land or rent to the value of 200 marks p.a. shall receive and wear cloth worth 6 marks for the whole cloth and not more. And they shall not wear cloth of gold; or a cloak, mantle or gown furred with pure miniver[39] or ermine; or clothing embroidered

36 Budge or bogey was fine black lamb fleece, originally from North Africa. In other words the lamb worn by the wives of craftsmen was not to include exotic foreign varieties.

37 Harness can mean armour, but here refers to non-fabric items of attire, such as belts, buckles and straps.

38 Lettice was the fur of the snow-weasel, used as a less expensive substitute for ermine. Miniver was less expensive again and was the white belly-fur of the Baltic squirrel.

39 Pure miniver was miniver with the surrounding grey fur trimmed away to give a pure white pelt. Untrimmed (or gross) miniver was cheaper.

with jewels or in any other way. And their wives, daughters and children shall do likewise and shall wear no facings of ermine or miniver, or slashed clothes, or any jewelled item of clothing other than a head-dress. But all knights and their ladies who have land or rent worth more than 400 marks but less than 1000 marks p.a. shall wear what they like, except ermine and lettice, and items of clothing hung with jewels or pearls other than a head-dress.

Item, that clerks who hold office in a cathedral, collegiate church or university, and royal clerks whose status requires the wearing of fur, shall wear the designated fur. All other clerks who have more than 200 marks of rent p.a. shall wear the same as knights who have the same rent; and other clerks with 200 marks shall wear the same as esquires with £100 of rent. And all the clerks entitled by this ordinance to wear fur in winter shall wear lawn in the summer.

Item, that carters, ploughmen, drivers of the plough, oxherds, cow-herds, shepherds, swineherds, dairymen and all other keepers of livestock, threshers and all other agricultural workers, and everyone involved in husbandry of the status of a groom, and everyone with goods and chattels worth less than 40s shall receive and wear no sort of cloth other than blanket or russet[40] price 12d, and shall wear belts of fabric appropriate to their standing. And living-in servants shall receive appropriate, not excessive, food and drink. And it is ordained that if anyone dresses or behaves contrary to this ordinance, he shall forfeit to the king all the clothing which breaches the ordinance.

122. The unprepared death

This extract comes from the best known English literary treatment of the Black Death, the Pardoner's Tale in Chaucer's *Canterbury Tales*. The tale is a powerful sermon on the sin of greed, structured around an *exemplum* of three young men who kill each other for possession of a cache of gold. The story is set against the backdrop of a plague epidemic, and within the context of a moral laxity which many moralists thought characteristic of the plague. I have printed the original text, followed by a free prose 'translation'.

Geoffrey Chaucer, 'The Pardoner's Tale', lines 1-20, 199-222.

In Flaundres whilom was a compaignye
Of yonge folk that haunteden folye,
As riot, hasard, stywes, and tavernes,

---

40 Russet was originally a type of coarse, homespun woollen cloth rather than, as now, a colour.

Where as with harpes, lutes and gyternes,
They daunce and pleyen at dees bothe day and nyght,
And eten also and drynken over hir myght,
Thurghe which they doon the devel sacrifise
Withinne that develes temple in cursed wise
By superfluytee abhomynable.
Hir othes been so grete and so dampnable
That it is grisly for to heere hem swere.
Our blissed Lordes body they totere –
Hem thoughte that Jewes rente hym noght ynough –
And ech of hem at otheres synne lough.
And right anon thanne comen tombesteres[41]
Fetys and smale, and young frutesteres,
Syngeres with harpes, baudes, wafereres,[42]
Whiche been the verray develes officeres
To kyndle and blowe the fyr of lecherye,
That is annexed unto glotonye.

***

Thise riotoures thre of whiche I telle,
Longe erst er prime rong of any belle,
Were set hem in a taverne to drynke,
And as they sat, they herde a belle clynke
Biforn a cors was caried to his grave.
That oon of hem gan callen to his knave:
'Go bet', quod he, 'and axe redily
What cors is this that passeth heer forby;
And looke that thou reporte his name weel.'
'Sire', quod this boy, 'it nedeth never-a-deel;
It was me toold er ye cam heer two houres.
He was, pardee, an old felawe of youres,
And sodeynly he was yslayn to-nyght;
Fordronke, as he sat on his bench upright.
Ther cam a privee theef men clepeth Deeth,
That in this contree al the peple sleeth,
And with his spere he smoot his herte atwo,
And wente his wey withouten wordes mo.

---

41 Tombesters were tumblers or acrobats. They were regarded with great disapproval
   by moralists, who considered their contortions indecent. Salome, who danced
   seductively before her step-father King Herod [Mark 6] is often shown in medieval
   art as an acrobat.

42 Wafereres sold wafers – or, in modern terms, waffles.

He hath a thousand slayn this pestilence.
And, maister, er ye come in his presence,
Me thynketh that it were necessarie
For to be war of swich an adversarie.
Beth redy for to meete hym everemoore;
Thus taughte me my dame; I sey namoore.'

[Once upon a time in Flanders there was a band of young people who lived for pleasure: running wild, gambling, frequenting brothels and taverns, where they dance to the accompaniment of harps, lutes and citterns; play dice day and night; and eat and drink much more than they can hold. Their loathsome excesses constitute a sinful sacrifice at the devil's altar. Their blasphemous swearing by parts of God's body (appalling to hear), dismembers him again, as if the Jews had not torn him enough already. They each laugh at the sins of the rest. Slinky acrobats soon come along, young fruit-sellers, singers with harps, pimps, sweet-sellers – officers of the devil, who kindle and blow the fire of lechery, which always follows closely after gluttony.... Long before prime, these three roisterers were already drinking in a tavern, and as they sat there they heard a bell being rung before a corpse that was being carried to its grave. One of them called his page and said, 'Go quickly, and ask around to find out who the corpse is; and be sure you get the name right'. 'Sir', said the boy, 'there's no need for all this fuss; I heard who he was two hours before you arrived. He was an old friend of yours, by God. He was killed suddenly last night, blind drunk, while he was still sitting at table. A secret thief passed by – men call him Death – who is killing all the people in this country, and he split his heart in two with a spear thrust and went on his way without a word. He's already killed a thousand in this pestilence. And, master, before you find yourself in his presence, I think it would be a good idea to prepare yourself so that you are ready to meet him at any time, for he's a dangerous enemy. That's what my mother taught me. I've no more to say'.]

123. The prepared death

The *Ars moriendi* (the art of dying) was a popular late-medieval handbook on how to make a good death. The first chapter explains how the living should prepare for death. Subsequent chapters (not printed here) detail the individual's proper conduct during the process of dying.

The English original includes numerous Latin quotations, which the author always renders immediately into English. For reasons of space I have omitted the Latin and printed only the translations. As well as modernising the spelling I have amended the wording and syntax where the original might cause problems for the modern reader, but I have made no attempt to rewrite it completely in modern idiom.

C. Horstmann (ed), *Yorkshire Writers*, II, London, 1896, pp. 407-8.

[Chapter 1]

Though bodily death be the most dreadful of all fearful things, as the philosopher says in the third book of Ethics, yet the spiritual death of the soul is as much more horrible and detestable as the soul is more worthy and precious than the body, as the prophet David says: 'The death of a sinful man is the worst of all deaths' [Ps 33.22], but as the same prophet witnesses: 'The death of a good man is ever precious in the sight of God' [Ps 115.15], whatever manner of bodily death they die. And you shall understand also that not only the death of holy martyrs is so precious, but also the death of all other righteous and good Christian men; and furthermore doubtless the death of all sinful men, however long, cursed and wicked they may have been all their life before their last end, if they die in the state of true repentance and contrition and in the true faith and unity and charity of holy church, is acceptable and precious in the sight of God; as St John says in the Apocalypse: 'Blessed be all dead men that die in God' [Apoc 14.13].

And therefore God says in the fourth book of Wisdom: 'A rightful man though he be hastily or suddenly dead, he shall be had to a place of refreshment' [Wisdom 4.7]. And so shall every man that dies, if it so be that he keeps himself stably and governs himself wisely in the temptations which he shall have in the agony or strife of his death, as shall be declared afterwards. And therefore of the commendation of the death of good men a wise man says thus: 'Death is nothing else but a going out of prison, an ending of exile, a discharge of a heavy burden (that is the body), a finishing of all infirmities, an escaping of all perils, a destroying of all evil things, a breaking of all bonds, a paying of the debt of natural duty, a turning again into his country, and an entering into bliss and joy'. And therefore it is said in the seventh chapter of Ecclesiastes: 'The day of a man's death is better than the day of his birth' [Eccl 7.2], and this is to be understood only of good men and the chosen people of God, for to evil men and the reprobate neither the day of their birth nor the day of their death may be called good.

And therefore every good Christian man, and also every other man, although he be but imperfectly and lately converted from sin, if he is truly contrite and believes in God, should not be sorry or troubled, nor dread the death of his body, in whatever manner or for whatever cause he is put thereto; but should take his death gladly and willingly, with the reason of his mind that rules sensuality, and suffer it patiently, conforming and committing his will fully unto God's will and disposition alone if he will go hence and die well and surely.[43] Witness the wise man saying: 'To die well is to die gladly and willingly', and therefore he adds: 'Neither many days nor many years cause me to say and feel that I have lived long enough, but only the reasonable will of my heart and of my soul'.... Since we may neither flee or escape nor change the inevitable necessity and passage of death, therefore we ought to take our death when God wills, willingly and gladly, without any grudging or contradiction, through the might and boldness of our soul, virtuously disposed and governed by reason and true discretion, though the lewd sensuality and frailty of our flesh naturally grudge or strive against it. Whereof Seneca says thus: 'Suffer easily, and blame not what you may not change or avoid', and the same clerk adds: 'If you would escape what you are straitly trapped in, it is not enough that you should be in another place but that you should be another man'.

Furthermore, for a Christian man to die well and surely it is necessary that he knows how to die; as a wise man says: 'To know how to die is to have a heart and soul ever ready to go Godwards', so that whenever death comes he may be found ready, and without any retraction or withdrawing receive him as a man would receive his welbeloved and trusty friend and fellow whom he had long awaited and looked for. This knowledge is the most profitable of all knowledge; in the which knowledge religious men in particular, more than other men, should every day study more diligently than other men so that they might grasp it, for the religious state asks and requires it more of them than of others; notwithstanding that every secular man, both clerk and layman, whether he is disposed to die or not, must nevertheless die when God wills. Therefore every man, not only religious but also every good and devout Christian man that desires to die well and surely, ought to live in such wise and so behave himself always that he may safely die at whatever hour God wills, and so he should have his life in patience and his death in desire, as St Paul had when he said: 'I desire and covet to be dead and with Christ' [Phil 1.23].

124. 'It is good to think on death'

---

43 To die 'surely' is to die safely; in other words, in such a way as to achieve ultimate salvation.

These ten lines preface a late-medieval debate poem: 'A disputation betwixt the body and worms', in which the corpse of a beautiful woman takes issue with the worms which are devouring it.[44] The poem is set 'In the season of huge mortality, of sundry diseases, with the pestilence heavily reigning', and begins with the poet visiting a church, where he reads the epitaph on a tomb. The first four lines below are to be understood as the epitaph he reads, the rest is an exhortation to the reader to make good use of the disputation which follows. I have printed the original, followed by a prose paraphrase.

British Library, Additional MS 37049 fo. 32v.

Take hede un to my fygure here abowne
And se how sumtyme I was fresche and gay
Now turned to wormes mete and corrupcion
Bot fowle erth and stynkyng slyme and clay.
Attende therfore to this disputaccion written here
And writte it wysely in thi hert fre
[Th]at ther at sum wisdom thou may lere
To se what thou art and here aftyr sal be
When thou leste wenes. venit mors te superare
When thi grafe grenes. bonum est mortis meditari.

[Look at my image and see how I was once fresh and gay, who am now turned to worms' meat and corruption; just foul earth, stinking slime and clay. Pay attention to the disputation written here and inscribe it upon your heart so you may learn some wisdom from studying it, and realise what you are and what you shall become. When you least expect it death comes to conquer you. While your grave is still undug[45] it is good to think on death.]

125. The fate of the sinful

This is an extract from John Gower's poem, *Vox Clamantis*. 'The Voice of one Crying' – a reference to Mark 1.3, where John the Baptist urges men to prepare for the coming of Christ. Gower's poem, completed in the last decade of the fourteenth century, is a bitter attack on the sins of the times. This section comes towards the end of the poem, where the poet meditates on the bodily corruption which awaits the sinner after death. Each chapter is prefaced by a brief statement of its contents, but I have printed the preface only to chapter 9, which adds a dimension not made explicit in the poem itself.

44 For the poem itself see John W. Conlee, *Middle English Debate Poetry*, East Lansing, Michigan, 1991, pp. 51-62.

45 This phrase could be interpreted as 'when your grave grins [i.e. gapes]', but this seems to go against the sense of the prologue, which urges the reader to think of death before it is too late.

John Gower, *Vox Clamantis*, Book VII, chapters 9-15.

9. Here he speaks of how man, who is a lesser world,[46] will go the way of all flesh and pass from the world into death. And just as man, while he was alive, caused the world's corruption through the sins of his body, so in death he will be forced to endure the corruption of his body. And first he talks of the corruption of the dead body appropriate to pride.

What will you have to say for yourself when the breeze no longer stirs your hair, when your throat is dry and can utter no words and your bloodless face is colourless, when your eyes are set in their gloomy sockets, when your mouth cannot be moistened and inside it your tongue stiffens against the roof of your mouth, when blood no longer throbs in your veins, when your neck cannot bend or your arms embrace, when your foot cannot take a step?

What does that proud dead man reply now? Let him say what vain glory has to offer him now; now that all the honour enjoyed by that lifeless corpse, which so lately despised others, has died. And, because the body bore itself so haughtily just a little while ago, now its flesh is degraded to food for worms. His eyebrow is not raised now as if in disdain, nor does his hand lingeringly smooth his flanks. The power of death has overcome his manly strength and, look, the backbone of a fly is stronger now than his. If he was in the bloom of elegance or beauty a little while ago, grace is now driven away by his foulness. If he was wise, he is now far otherwise – he has reached a conclusion about which he knows nothing: death has in a moment dissolved the subtleties he pursued in long study. He may have been learned in many fields, but now the man of experience finds himself contracted to a narrow span;[47] his reasoning now unreasonably stops as death abruptly blanks out reason. He now knows less of the learning he taught than an ass, and not a jot or tittle remains in his understanding. He no longer passes intellectual judgement on others, his own lifelessness prevents his bragging. The man who used to bask in the honour of a pretended virtue is now openly shown for what he was.

46 Man (the microcosm) and the universe (the macrocosm) formed an integrated system. Just as the universe, through the configuration of the heavens, could influence man; so man could influence the macrocosm – not the universe, which was perfect and unchanging, but the world. Gower is making the same point as many of the commentators on the plague: that it is man's sins which have corrupted nature.

47 This rather free translation is an attempt to capture Gower's play on *artes* (skills or accomplishments) and *artus* (confined or narrow).

The fact that he once knew lots of languages helps him not at all, now that death has stopped his mouth. No music, either the sound of an organ or the plucking of a harp, can please a dead listener. Efforts to beautify the body with artificial means are proved worthless now that it has lost all its natural good looks. No finery, no mounting on horses, can exalt a body once it's stiff. A beautiful house or the obedience of servants means nothing to him now. No one greets him among the crowds in the market place. Now a serpent shall be his servant, a pit his hall, and a stinking hole his bedchamber. Because vain glory lately deluded him, nothing is now left to him in which he can take pride.

10. Behold the man who, through envy, gnawed like a dog;[48] now a dog or worm must gnaw him. He once jeered at the fame of others, because it cut him to the quick, now his deceitful tongue is silent – rotten. He laughed at the difficulties of others and wept at their prosperity, now he cannot laugh because his mouth has no lips. His heart, once full of grudges, is now rotted away and a pathway lies open to its very centre. Now that he lies unpraised his ambition cannot deflect the praise due to a colleague or assert his own superiority. The bile which then hid under honeyed words is now hidden indeed, for without a mind there can no longer be any pretence. That mind, once on fire with envy, can no longer prick everyone with the poisonous goad of spite.

11. The man whom fierce wrath recently inflamed can no longer toss his head impatiently. He who, not so long ago. troubled his neighbours with his quarrelling cannot make a sound, ruin leaves him dumb. Once so voluble, he can no longer even whisper; death calls and he is silent, unable to answer back. He who used to terrorise the helpless with terrible threats is powerless against maggots. Rage no longer drives him to war; he cannot make a truce with the worm. No one can fear the sword of a man who allows a worm to pierce his heart. He who now lacks all power of reason can no longer distort his reason by physical hatred.

12. What good does avarice do the miser now? He is left with no more than a narrow wooden box. Of the land which he worked so hard to

48 Dogs generally carry negative connotations in medieval literature, largely due to their bad press in the Old Testament. A dog gnawing a bone (which is the reference intended here) symbolised a jealous refusal to share, which was held to be a form of envy. Canine greed and jealousy were thought to extend to denying others the enjoyment of something the dog did not want itself – as in the still-proverbial image of the dog in the manger. The only exception to this negative canine image was the hound (an aristocratic hunting dog) which was a symbol of loyalty.

secure, he now holds just seven feet. The man who, not so long ago, was a predator preying on others is now the prey of the predator death. He who lately spread his nets to catch wealth (vain wealth!) is now caught in a net from which there is no escape. He gathered together great riches, and guarded them obsessively, but now someone else is squandering his treasure. His assets, which seemed almost boundless, have changed hands, and suddenly he has nothing left. His wife is enjoying a new husband and keeps no place in her heart for the old one. His son and heir is having a wonderful time, never thinking of his father. Not one friend remains to the dead man. He who amassed possession after possession, field after field, now gets nothing for his efforts; what he gathered in a year has been lost in one day, and his long labours are all in vain. He who shut his purse to the poor is now a beggar himself, all his money worthless. Neither guile nor cunning, deviousness nor perjured greed avails his body now.

13. **Sloth** refuses to allow the slothful man to pamper his body as he wishes. The man who gave himself over to sleep now has more sleep than he wants, in that long sleep from which there is no waking. He who not so long ago sought out soft straw for his bed now lies under the cold ground, his covering infested with snakes. He who recently shirked tasks in pursuit of idleness now finds that there is nothing he can do to better his situation. He once had the opportunity to learn what is good, but now it is too late and there is no school which can teach him to be wise. He can only lament the waste of so much time. Once he hardly ever came to church to pray – now he cannot be carried from church, but he still does not pray. The man who sowed thinly reaps thinly; he now wishes that he had done what he failed to do when he had the chance.

14. **Gluttony** which, a little time ago, he practised every day, now gives no pleasure to belly or mouth. His bowels, which used to be stuffed tight with food, are now emptied and can hold nothing. He gourmandised on dainties and drank sweet wines, and now in their place there is nothing but shit and soil. Around his middle, where his blubber was stored, there now lurks a serpent gorging itself on his fat. His pot-belly, as big as a pregnant woman's with boozing, has burst open, and a toad occupies his gaping throat. The odours of cooking which he enjoyed recently are gone, and in their place the stink of corruption fills his nostrils. Excessive drinking, which he never gave up even on fasting days, has no effect on him now that his stomach has burst.

15. Who used to think the vice of **lechery** so sweet! A serpent now sucks his private parts. He no longer does the rounds of the brothels, and his hand can get no satisfaction in groping women. He cannot feign a wanton glance to entice some silly woman to give him what he wants. No deceitful songs, couched in the language of love, can help him with their feigned promises; singing is nothing to him now, and nor is dancing, for he no longer has a throat, or a foot to stand on. Dead, he can no longer commit incest or violate a virgin. All his previous lasciviousness is now turned to corruption, and the heat of sexual intercourse has chilled to icy coldness. What was a body just a short time ago is now a corpse, and what was ashes returns to ashes.

Suggestions for further reading

This is only a selection from a large number of general and specialist studies available. Fuller bibliographies can be found in several of the works cited here, including the books by Biraben, Campbell and Poos.

Bean, J. M. W. 'Plague, population and decline in England in the later middle ages', *Economic History Review* 2nd series XV, 1963, pp. 423-38.

Benedictow, O. *Plague in the late medieval Nordic Countries*, Middelalderforlaget, Oslo, 1992.

Beresford, M. & Hurst, J. G. *Deserted Medieval Villages*, Lutterworth Press, London, 1971.

Biraben, J-N. *Les hommes et la peste en France et dans les pays européens et méditerranéens*, 2 vols, École des Hautes Études en Sciences Sociales, Paris, 1975-6.

Bolton, J. L. *The Medieval English Economy 1150-1500*, Dent, London, 1980 (reprinted with supplement 1985).

Bowsky, W. M. (ed) *The Black Death: a turning point*, Holt, Rinehart & Winston, New York, 1978.

Bridbury, A. R. 'The Black Death', *Economic History Review*, 2nd series XXVI, 1973, pp. 393-410.

—'Before the Black Death', *ibid* XXX, 1977, pp. 393-410.

Britnell. R. H. 'Feudal reaction after the Black Death in the palatinate of Durham', *Past & Present* CXXVIII, 1990, pp. 28-47.

Campbell, A. *The Black Death and Men of Learning*, Columbia Univ. Press, New York, 1931.

Campbell, Bruce M. S. (ed) *Before the Black Death: studies in the 'crisis' of the early fourteenth century*, Manchester Univ. Press, Manchester, 1991.

Courtenay, W. J. 'The effect of the Black Death on English higher education', *Speculum* LV, 1980, pp. 696-714.

Coville, A. 'Écrits contemporains sur la peste de 1348 à 1350', *Histoire Littéraire de la France* XXXVII, 1938, pp. 325-390.

Crawfurd, R. *Plague and Pestilence in Literature and Art*, Oxford Univ. Press, Oxford, 1914.

Davies, R. A. 'The effect of the Black Death on the parish priests of the medieval diocese of Coventry and Lichfield', *Historical Research* LXII, 1989, pp. 85-90.

Dols, M. W. *The Black Death in the Middle East*, Princeton Univ. Press, Princeton, N.J.,1977.

Dyer, C. *Standards of Living in the Later Middle Ages: social change in England, c. 1200-1520*, Cambridge Univ. Press, Cambridge, 1989.

—'The social and economic background to the rural revolt of 1381' in R. H. Hilton and T. H. Astons (eds), *The English Rising of 1381*, Cambridge Univ. Press, Cambridge, 1984, pp. 9-42.

Gasquet, F. A. *The Great Pestilence*, Simpkin Marshall, Hamilton, Kent & Co, London,1893.

Goldberg, P. J. P. 'Mortality and economic change in the diocese of York, 1390-1514', *Northern History* XXIV, 1988, pp. 38-55.

Gottfried, R. S. *Epidemic Disease in fifteenth-century England: the medieval response and its demographic consequence*, Leicester Univ. Press, Leicester, 1978.

Harvey, B. F. 'The population trend in England between 1300 and 1348', *Transactions of the Royal Historical Society*, 5th series XVI, 1966, pp. 23-42.

Hatcher, John *Plague, Population and the English Economy 1348- 1530*, Macmillan, London & Basingstoke, 1977.

—'Mortality in the fifteenth century: some new evidence', *Economic History Review*, 2nd series XXXIX, 1986, pp. 19-38.

Levett, A. E. & Ballard, A. 'The Black Death on the estates of the see of Winchester' in P. Vinogradoff (ed), *Oxford Studies in Social and Legal History* V, 1916.

Lomas, R. A. 'The Black Death in County Durham', *Journal of Medieval History* XV, 1989, pp. 127-40.

Mate, M. 'Agrarian economy after the Black Death: the manors of Canterbury cathedral priory', *Economic History Review* 2nd series XXXVII, 1984, pp. 341-54.

Meiss, M. *Painting in Florence and Siena after the Black Death*, Princeton Univ. Press, Princeton, N.J., 1951.

Miller, E. & Hatcher, J. *Medieval England: rural society and economic change 1086-1348*, Longman, London, 1978.

Ormrod, W. M. 'The English government and the Black Death of 1348-9' in *idem* (ed), *England in the Fourteenth Century: proceedings of the 1985 Harlaxton Symposium*, Boydell and Brewer, Woodbridge, 1986, pp. 175-88.

Poos, L. R. *A Rural Society after the Black Death: Essex 1350-1525*, Cambridge Univ. Press, Cambridge, 1991

Putnam, Bertha *The Enforcement of the Statutes of Labourers during the first decade after the Black Death, 1349-1359*, Columbia Univ. Press, New York, 1908.

Razi, Z. *Life, Marriage & Death in a Medieval Parish: economy, society and demography in Halesowen 1270-1400*, Cambridge Univ. Press, Cambridge, 1980.

Rees, W. 'The Black Death in England and Wales, as exhibited in manorial documents', *Proceedings of the Royal Society of Medicine* XVI, 1923, Section of the History of Medicine pp. 27-45.

—'The Black Death in Wales', in R. W. Southern (ed), *Essays in Medieval History*, Macmillan, London, 1968, pp. 179-199.

Shrewsbury, J. F. D. *A History of the Bubonic Plague in the British Isles*, Cambridge Univ. Press, Cambridge, 1970.

Slack, Paul *The Impact of Plague in Tudor and Stuart England*, Oxford Univ. Press, Oxford, 1985 (reprinted with corrections, 1990).

Thompson, A. Hamilton 'The registers of John Gynewell, Bishop of Lincoln, for the years 1349-1350', *Archaeological Journal* LXVIII, 1911, pp. 301-360.

—'The pestilences of the fourteenth century in the diocese of York', *ibid* LXXI, 1914,
· pp. 97-154.

Tristram, P. *Figures of Life and Death in Medieval English Literature*, Paul Elek, London, 1976.

Twigg, Graham *The Black Death: a biological reappraisal*, Batsford, London, 1984.

[Wellcome Institute] *The Pest Anatomized: five centuries of the plague in Western Europe*, Wellcome Institute for the History of Medicine, London, 1985.

Williman, D. (ed) *The Black Death: the impact of the fourteenth-century plague*, Centre for Medieval and Early Renaissance Studies, Binghamton, 1982.

Ziegler, Philip *The Black Death*, Penguin, Harmondsworth, 1969 (reprinted with illustrations, Alan Sutton, Stroud, 1990).

Index

Abingdon, Oxon, abbey, 87
advowsons, 237, 292-6
agriculture, 33, 47, 60, 63, 70, 72, 73,
    78, 79, 80, 120, 133, 287, 313-14,
    324-5, 342
air, corrupted, 29, 40, 46, 49, 56-7,
    59, 100-1, 106-7, 118, 120, 159-
    61, 163, 172, 173-7, 177-82, 185,
    188, 194, 203-4, 205, 207
Albertus Magnus, 159, 160, 180
Aldham, Suff, 239, 286-7
Alfonso, king of Castile, 250
alien priories, 292
Alsace, 210, 224
Amounderness, Lancs, 262-6
Andrew, king of Hungary, 44
Anglesey, Cambs, abbey, 304
Anonimalle Chronicle, 62, 85, 88-9
anthrax, 7
Antichrist, 83, 99-100, 110, 154-5,
    210n; and see Last Days
appropriations, 295, 300-2
Aristotle, 158-9, 164, 168, 184, 345
Ars moriendi, 344-6
astrology, 16, 48-9, 50, 101-5, 159-
    60, 163-72, 185-6
Austria, 9, 59-61, 110, 178, 208-10
    duke of see Habsburg, Albrecht
Averroes, 186
Avesbury, Robert of, 64-5, 153-4
Avicenna, 174, 176, 180, 186, 188,
    192
Avignon, 4, 9, 20, 41-5, 46, 56, 62, 69,
    74, 76, 82, 86, 96, 207, 222, 252

Babylon, 20
Bacon, Roger, 168
Baker, Geoffrey le, 10, 80-2
Barnet, John, bishop of Worcester, 87

basilisks, 106, 178, 183-4, 214
Bath and Wells, bishop of,   see
    Shrewsbury, Ralph
bathing, 101, 163, 175, 176, 186
Bavaria, 9, 178
beggars, 70, 223, 242, 287, 289, 326
Bergen, 10
Bern, 211
Beverley, Yorks, 269
biblical exemplars, 35, 112, 113, 120;
    and see Noah's Flood; Sodom
Biel, Gabriel, 108-9
Bircheston, Simon, abbot of West-
    minster, 74
Black Sea, 9, 17
blood-letting, 25, 188-92, 194
Boccaccio, Giovanni, 26-34, 101, 107,
    108, 243, 245n, 246
Bologna, 87, 207
Bonby, Lincs, 295-6
Bordeaux, 9, 250
Bordesley, Warw, abbey, 301-2
Boxgrove, Suss, priory, 317
Brabant, 50
Bradwardine, Thomas, archbishop-
    elect of Canterbury, 71-2, 74, 78
Bransford, Wolstan de, bishop of
    Worcester, 268, 277
Braughing, Herts, 304
Bridgnorth, Salop, 274-5
Brinton, Thomas, bishop   of
    Rochester, 11, 98, 100, 137-48
Bristol, 10, 62, 63, 77, 81
Bruges, 10, 41, 77
Brussels, 218
Bryan, Reginald, bishop of Worces-
    ter, 85, 87
Burgundy, 87
Burgundy, John of, 106, 160n, 184-95

burial, 3, 21, 23, 31-3, 34, 36, 39, 44, 52, 53, 70, 74, 196-8, 201-2, 245, 267
Bury St Edmunds, Suff, abbey, 87
butchery, 100, 108, 198-9, 200, 203-5

Caffa, 9, 17, 18, 46
Calais, 77, 80, 81, 118, 130n
Cambridge, 91, 154, 205
Canterbury, archbishops of, see Bradwardine, Thomas; Islip, Simon; Langham, Simon; Offord, John; Stratford, John; Sudbury, Simon
monastery (Christ Church), 86, 96, 253
Carcassonne, 222-3
Carinthia, 129, 178, 181
Castile, king of, see Alfonso
Catania, 37-41
cats, 8, 36, 54, 201n
cauterisation, 189n
Caxton, Cambs, 294
Cellerer family, 331-8
cemeteries, 43, 61, 64, 65, 69, 81, 82, 245n, 266-71; and see burial
chancery, 88, 204, 205, 311
chantries, 241, 250-1, 274-5, 304-6, 309; and see mass for the dead
Charles IV, king of Bohemia, 128, 209
Charlton, Lewis, bishop of Hereford, 87
Chaucer, Geoffrey, 13, 102, 342-4
Chesterfield, Derbs, 304-6
children, 11, 12, 85, 86, 88, 98, 126, 134-5, 136, 146, 172
Chillon, 211-14
China, 9, 18, 25
Clement VI, pope, 26, 44-5, 46, 56, 66, 71-2, 74, 96, 110, 120, 122, 128, 221-2, 273
clergy, 15-16, 55, 69, 72, 78-9, 86, 127-30, 136-7, 143, 155, 235, 241, 273-4, 290-1, 306-12; and see friars; parish priests
Clynn, John, 3, 82-4, 96, 99
Cobham, Reginald, 85, 87

Cockerham, Lancs, 265
Collington, Herefs, 302-3
Cologne, 110, 208, 210, 219-20
comets, 55, 104, 162, 174
confession, 36, 40, 54, 56, 75, 77, 112, 138, 147-8, 149, 241, 271-3; and see last rites
Constable, John, 246
Constance, 209
Constantinople, 8, 9, 38n
Cotham, Notts, 300
Courtenay, William, bishop of London, 311-12
court rolls, 11, 230, 256-62, 276, 283-4, 286-7, 326-31
Coventry and Lichfield, bishop of, see Stretton, Robert de
Covino, Simon de, 163-7
Craven, Yorks, 313
Crich, Derbs, 250
Crimea, 9, 17
Cyprus, 76

Damascus, bishop of, see Hugh
death, 10, 19, 32, 40, 56, 244-6, 249, 250, 252, 342, 344-7; and see burial
death rate, 3, 11-12, 20, 33-4, 43, 44, 47, 49, 51, 53-4, 55-6, 58, 63, 64, 65, 66, 68, 71, 77, 82, 86, 92, 207, 223, 230-6, 252, 262-6, 267
de la Mare, Thomas, abbot of St Albans, 74, 252-3
de Lisle, Thomas, bishop of Ely, 71, 85, 87
de' Mussis, Gabriele, 9, 10, 14-26, 107, 246
Dene, William, 3, 11, 70-3, 99, 240
Derbyshire, 313
de Venette, Jean, 12, 54-7, 107, 110, 242
de Vere, John, earl of Oxford, 286
devils, 38, 99, 133, 339n
de Vinario, Raymond Chalin, 6
Devon, 10, 63, 81, 266, 275
Diessenhoven, Heinrich Truchess von, 208-10
digestive process, 105-6, 163, 175

di Tura, Agnolo, 246-7
doctors *see* physicians
dogs, 8, 33, 34, 38, 54, 349
Dorset, 10, 63, 64, 81, 112, 266
Drakelow, Ches, 280-3
Drogheda, 82, 84
drought, 87
Dublin, 82, 84
Durham, bishop of, *see* Hatfield, Thomas
    county, 237, 238, 239, 283-4, 326-31

earthquakes, 5, 25, 34, 59, 68, 76, 83, 99, 101, 129, 161, 162, 177-82
Easington, Yorks, 332, 335
eclipses, 25, 87, 105, 166, 169, 170-1
Edendon, William, bishop of Winchester, 115-17, 335
Edward III, king of England, 77, 95, 113, 114, 117-18, 128, 240, 241, 246, 266, 274
    daughters of, 87, 246, 250, 334, 336
    wife of *see* Philippa of Hainault
Effrenata, 72n, 241, 306-9, 311
elements, 103-4, 159, 168
Ely, bishops of, *see* de Lisle, Thomas; Langham, Simon
enclosure, 299
Enoch and Elias, 99, 210; *and see* Last Days
Essex, 92, 276
Euclid, 182-3
Eulogium, 12, 63-4, 131-2
exchequer, 88, 237, 274, 275, 277-80, 311
excommunication, 153, 312
Exeter, bishop of, *see* Grandisson, John
    city, 115
Eynsham, Oxon, abbey, 285-6

famine, 5, 12, 56, 83, 113, 160, 235
fashion, 23, 98, 131-4, 339
fear of the sick, 22-3, 28, 30-1, 36, 40, 43, 83-4, 84-5, 246-7, 271
feudal reaction, 239-40
fish, 45, 73, 172, 190

Fishlake, Yorks, 237, 292-3
Fitz Waryn, Aymer, 275
Fitzwaryn, William, 85, 87
flagellants, 44, 50, 60, 96-7, 110, 150-4
Flanders, 10, 48, 77, 97, 153, 342
fleas, 5, 6-7, 8, 195n, 233n
flight, 29-30, 37, 61, 108-9
floods, 5, 54, 61, 88, 133, 172, 179, 300
Florence, 20, 26-34, 35, 100, 101, 246
food and drink, 28-9, 101, 104, 160, 179-80, 183, 186-7, 190, 340, 342
football, 89, 325
Fordun, John of, 84, 88
France, 9, 20, 46, 50, 54-8, 70, 77, 80, 112, 128, 207, 223
fraternities, 31, 96, 197, 202, 245
Frederick II, Holy Roman Emperor, 100, 155-7
friars, 22, 36, 75, 76, 83, 91, 155, 202
Fulford, Yorks, 270
funerals *see* burial

Galen, 185, 192
gambling, 53, 128, 218, 242, 309
games, 242, 325
Garstang, Lancs, 263, 265
Gascony, 9, 46, 56, 63
Geneva, 216, 219
Genoa, 14, 18-19, 20, 36, 42, 46
Germany, 9, 50, 56, 80, 100, 108, 109, 128-9, 151-3, 177, 178, 181, 207-10
Gigas, Herman, 207
Gilling, Yorks, 271
Gimingham, Norf, 294-5
Gloucester, 10, 81, 108, 312
Gog and Magog, 73, 99; *and see* Last Days
Gower, John, 347-51
Grandisson, John, bishop of Exeter, 115, 300-1
Greece, 18, 42, 59, 70, 80
Gregory the Great, pope, 35, 95
Gregory IX, pope, 89
Guisborough, Yorks, priory, 271

Gynwell, John, bishop of Lincoln, 77

Habsburg, Albrecht, duke of Austria, 110, 209-10
Hatfield, Thomas, bishop of Durham, 239, 283, 327
Haerlebech, Jean, 48-9
Hainault, 131n, 218
Haly Abbas, 168
Harthill, Yorks, parish, 293-4
    wapentake, 296-9
Henry, earl (later duke) of Lancaster, 77, 85, 87
Hereford, bishops of, see Charlton, Lewis; Trilleck, John
    city, 79
Herford, Heinrich von, 127-30, 150-3
heriots, 230, 235, 256-62, 276, 286
Hethe, Hamo, bishop of Rochester, 11, 71, 73, 253-6, 290-1
Heyligen, Louis ('Socrates'), 4, 9, 10, 41-5, 248-9
Hillingdon, Midds, 278
Hippocrates, 161, 162, 185, 192
Holy Roman Empire, 9, 20, 59-61, 128-9, 178
Hotham, Yorks, 310
Hugh, bishop of Damascus, 269-71
humours, 57, 104-6, 163, 172, 185, 187
Hungary, 44, 50, 178

India, 9, 18, 25, 41-2, 49, 70, 76, 80
indulgences, 26, 44, 56, 66, 68-9, 74, 77, 89, 96, 112, 114, 115, 117, 272
Ireland, 3, 82-4, 207
Islip, Simon, archbishop of Canterbury, 11, 72, 95, 118-19, 241, 306-9, 311
Italy, 9, 10, 19-22, 26-41, 42, 46, 59, 97, 181, 194-203, 217

Jacmé, Jean, 173
Jerusalem, 46, 83, 99
Jews, 49, 50, 56, 99, 109-10, 207-22, 225, 343
John II, king of France, 128

John VI, Byzantine Emperor, 4n
Jubilee Year (1350), 26, 75, 96
justices of labourers, 314-22, 334
justices of the peace, 240, 323, 325-6

Kent, 11, 71
Kilkenny, 3, 84
Kingsbridge, Wilts, hundred, 318-19
Kinver, Staffs, 301-2
Kipchak Khanate, 9
Kirkburton, Yorks, 293
Kirkham, Lancs, 263, 264
Knighton, Henry, 10, 75-80, 85, 130, 239, 240
Knutsson, Bengt, 107, 162n, 173-7

labourers, ordinance of, 71, 79, 117n, 238, 240, 287-9, 290, 312-13, 317
    statute of, 237, 240-1, 242, 296-8, 312-16, 318-26
labour services, 80, 238-9, 278-80, 285-7, 293, 294, 295, 328
labour shortages, 64, 66, 70, 72, 78-9, 80, 242, 287
Lancashire, 262-6, 313
Lancaster, earl (later duke) of, see Henry
    parish, 264-5
land values, 57, 68, 237, 277-80, 292-6, 304
Langham, Simon, abbot of Westminster (later bishop of Ely, archbishop of Canterbury), 74, 87, 89
Langland, William, 98, 135-6, 241, 310-11
Last Days, 98-100, 110, 128n, 155n, 193n, 210n; and see Antichrist
last rites, 21, 22, 44, 54, 56, 58, 92, 149, 252, 271-2; and see confession; Sacrament
Lausanne, 210-11
Leatham, Yorks, 270
Leicester, 77, 85
leprosy, 81
Lewes, Suss, priory, 237, 292-5
Lewis IV, Holy Roman Emperor, 128-9

li Muisis, Gilles, 7, 10-11, 45-54, 125, 179, 242
Lincoln, bishop of, see Gynwell, John
Lincolnshire, 10, 66-7, 295-6, 319-22
livestock, 28, 33, 47, 60, 63, 64, 77-8, 90, 133, 180-1
London, bishops of, see Courtenay, William; Northburgh, Michael; Stratford, Ralph; Sudbury, Simon
city, 10, 11, 65, 81, 86, 88, 107, 108, 153, 203-4, 205, 266-8, 310-11
Louth Park, Lincs, abbey, 66-7, 85-6
Lucifer, 193, 339
Lydgate, John, 124-5
Lytham, Lancs, 263, 265-6
Lythe, Yorks, 269

Mainz, 129, 210
Malling, Kent, nunnery, 71, 253-6
Manney (Marney), Walter, 81, 266-7
Marseilles, 42, 43, 46, 76, 130, 178, 207
mass, 25-6, 69, 83, 95, 111, 117, 120-4, 140
for the dead, 52-3, 69, 241, 304, 306, 307, 309, 311-12; and see chantries
Meaux, Yorks, abbey, 10, 67-70, 240, 331-8
Meaux, Geoffrey de, 102-3, 104, 105, 167-72
medicine, 27, 106, 109, 163, 169, 172, 185-6, 187-8, 189-91
Mediterranean Sea, 9, 42
Melcombe, Dorset, 10, 63
Merevale, Warw, priory, 96, 148-9
merry-making, 29, 58, 61, 107-8, 243
Messina, 36-40, 130
Michael, abbot of St Albans, 74, 252
Montgomery, John, 81
Montpellier, 46, 76, 106-7, 167, 173, 177, 182, 207
Montreux, 212-13, 215
moral decline, 29, 31, 57, 61, 72, 75, 85, 117-18, 242-3, 309, 311, 342-3
Mowbray, John, 85, 87

murrain, 63, 66, 77, 301

Naples, 44n, 76
Narbonne, 222-3
Neuberg, 59-61, 107-8, 243
Newark, Notts, 269
Noah's Flood, 3, 35, 67, 145, 165, 193, 242
Norfolk, 91
Northburgh, Michael, bishop of London, 85, 87
Norwich, 154
Nostell, Yorks, priory, 273-4

Offord, John, archbishop-elect of Canterbury, 71-2, 74
ordinations, 273
Oxford, city, 10, 81, 167
earl of, see de Vere, John

Padua, 3, 34-5
Palaeologus, Andronikos, 8
Papal Curia see Avignon
Paris, 7, 9, 47, 55-8, 109, 158
parish priests, 22, 72, 78-9, 86, 136, 241, 271, 273, 274, 307-9, 310, 312
Parliament, 204, 205-6, 313
Pedro, Infante of Castile, 250
penance, 13, 95-8, 111-19, 145, 151, 176, 271; and see flagellants; indulgences
Persia, 9, 18
Petrarch, Francesco, 41, 246, 248-9
Philip VI, king of France, 158
Philippa of Hainault, wife of Edward III, 131n
physicians, 6, 22, 27, 35, 60, 105-8, 109, 163, 167, 175, 185-6, 192, 214
Piacenza, 14, 21-2
Piazza, Michele da, 35-41
pilgrimage, 26, 47, 54, 67, 82, 96, 97, 148-9, 242, 323
pirates, 301
Pisa, 20, 35
Pistoia, 108, 194-203

plague *see* death rate; fear of the sick; flight; regimen; remedies; spread; symptoms; transmission

planets, 16, 59, 60, 83, 89, 101-5, 133, 145-6, 150, 159-60, 163-72, 174-5, 183, 185, 223, 252; *and see* astrology

Pleshy, Essex, 276

Polychronicon, 62-3, 85

popes *see* Clement VI; Gregory the Great; Gregory XI

population movements, 12, 232-3; *and see* death rate

Poulton, Lancs, 263, 264

prayer, 111, 113, 114, 117, 118, 119, 120, 124-6

pregnancy, 22, 57, 64

Preston, Lancs, 263-4

prices, 57, 64, 73, 77-8, 79, 80, 88, 92, 232, 240

processions, 10, 27, 38, 44, 60, 69, 95, 111-13, 119-20

prodigies, 5, 25, 38-9, 41-2, 55, 59, 69-70, 87, 91, 129

prophecies, 83, 99-100, 150, 154-5

Ptolemy, 162, 168-72

Ravenna, 181

Reading, Berks, abbey, 87, 133

Reading, John of, 11, 74-5, 86-8, 133-4

Reggio, 203

regimen, 163, 171, 176-7, 181, 186-7

remedies, 25, 28-9, 45, 106, 176-7, 188-92, 194

rents, 11, 80, 235, 238, 239, 278-80, 280-3, 294, 295

Ribchester, Lancs, 265

Richmond, Yorks, archdeaconry, 262-6

Rochester, bishops of, *see* Brinton, Thomas; Hethe, Hamo monastery, 73

Rome, 26, 35, 46, 59, 75, 95, 96, 99, 154

royal demesne, 332

Rudby, Yorks, 270-1

Rudheath, Ches, 238, 281, 283

Russia, 9

Ryston, Norf, 295

Sacrament, 21, 51, 91, 272; *and see* last rites

St Agatha, 37-8

St Albans, Herts, abbey, 10, 252 abbots of, *see* de la Mare, Thomas; Michael

Saint-Denis, abbey, 11, 58

St Mary, 38-9, 47, 69, 97, 124-5, 138, 148

St Michael, 95, 252

St Roche, 97

St Sebastian, 26, 54, 97, 125-6

St Thomas Cantilupe, 79

Sandal, Yorks, 292

sanitary regulations, 27, 34-5, 52, 100, 108, 194-206

Saracens, 16-17, 18, 20, 46, 64, 66, 69, 76, 80, 82, 154

Savoy, 110, 211-19

scholars, 326

Scilly Isles, 301

Scotland, 11, 64, 78, 81, 84-5, 88, 89-91, 98, 108

sea, 100, 160, 172, 178, 193-4

serfs, 243, 284, 286-7, 299, 317, 327-31, 331-8

sermons, 11, 48, 98, 108-9, 115, 135-6, 137-48, 339-40

Seuse, Heinrich, 109, 223-6

sexual intercourse, 69, 85, 87-8, 101, 116, 130, 134, 141, 142, 163, 175, 176, 184, 343, 351

sheriffs, 274, 275, 288, 315, 316, 333, 335

Shrewsbury, Ralph, bishop of Bath and Wells, 112, 241, 271-3

Shropshire, 274-5

Sicily, 19, 20, 35-41, 42, 46, 246

Siena, 35

simony, 71, 126, 128-9

sin, 11, 14-16, 23-4, 75, 95-8, 100, 111, 113, 116, 120, 126-7, 133, 137-43, 165, 176, 193, 339, 347-51

Skelton, Yorks, 271

social mobility, 243-4
Sodom, 113, 141, 146, 180, 193
Somerset, 63, 81, 112, 266
Southampton, 10, 77
Spain, 9, 20, 42, 46, 56, 222-3, 250
spices, 29, 45, 100-1, 187
spread, 9-11, 18-19, 26-7, 34, 42, 46,
    49, 56, 59-60, 76, 80-1, 82, 266
Staffordshire, 313
Stokesley, Yorks, 271
Stow, John, 266-8
Strassburg, 209, 210-11, 219-20
Stratford, John, archbishop of Can-
    terbury, 71, 74, 113, 114
    Ralph, bishop of London, 81, 113-
    15, 118, 267-8, 307
Stratford upon Avon, Warw, 277-8
Stretton, Robert de, bishop of Coven-
    try and Lichfield, 148, 239, 301-2,
    304-6
Sudbury, Simon, bishop of London
    (later archbishop of Canterbury),
    87, 95, 120, 143, 307, 311-12
suicides, 268
sumptuary laws, 243, 340-2
Surrey, 317
sweating sickness, 13, 107
symptoms, 4, 5-6, 8, 17, 24-5, 27, 35,
    36, 40, 42-3, 55, 60, 74, 81, 84,
    106, 179, 183-4, 188-9, 194

Tana, 9, 17
tanning, 100, 199, 200
Tarsus, 76
Tartars, 16-17, 34, 46, 154
taverns, 241, 242, 306, 309, 342-4
Tavistock, Devon, abbey, 300-1
taxation, 79n, 237, 296-9, 301, 315,
    316
Tech-Moling, 82
teeth, 57, 75
Terribilis 113-14
Thoresby, John, chancellor (later
    bishop of St Davids, Worcester,
    archbishop of York), 74, 95, 119,
    277n, 310
Three Living and the Three Dead, 245

thunder and lightning, 14-15, 41,
    112, 130, 162, 174; and see weather
Thurgarton, Notts, priory, 300
Tickhill, Yorks, 274
tithe, 292-5
Toledo, 212, 214
tombs, 245, 347
Toulouse, 9, 47, 207, 217
Tournai, 10, 45-54
tournaments, 69, 97-8, 130
trade, 9-10, 21, 42, 59, 139, 195-6,
    216-17, 235
transmission, 5-6, 8, 17, 27-8, 34, 36,
    42, 55, 60, 83, 106-7, 108, 175-7,
    182-4, 214, 223
Trilleck, John, bishop of Hereford,
    87, 302-3
Tripoli, 83
Turks, 18, 34, 80, 129
Tusmore, Oxon, 299
twins, 57, 168

Venice, 18-19, 20, 34, 59, 178, 207,
    216-17
venomous animals, 25, 41, 59, 207;
    and see basilisks; vipers
Vienna, 4n, 9, 61
Villach, 59, 178
Villani, Matteo, 70, 98
Villeneuve, 212-16, 218, 219
vipers, 26, 129
Visconti, Bernabò, 108, 203
Vortigern, king of Britain, 78
Vox in Rama, 115-17

wages, 30, 57, 70, 72, 78-9, 232, 238,
    240-1, 242, 287-91, 306-9, 310,
    311-16
Wakebridge family, 250-1
Wales, 81, 313
Walsham le Willows, Suff, 237, 256-62
Walsingham, Thomas, 11, 65-6, 85,
    88-92, 98, 154
Waltham, Essex, 276
war, 48-9, 57, 61, 77, 78, 89-91, 98, 99,
    113-14, 118, 119, 120, 128, 130,
    141, 172, 292

Wawne, Yorks, 239-40, 331-8

weapons, 130, 134, 325-6, 339

weather, 7, 54, 62, 66, 74, 89, 133, 160, 161-2, 172, 173-4, 177, 179, 186-7

well-poisoning, 45, 49, 50, 56-7, 110, 207, 208, 210, 211-19, 220, 222-3, 224-5

Westminster, abbey, 74, 131, 268, 275
  abbots of, see Bircheston, Simon; Langham, Simon

Whaddon, Cambs, 294

Whitchurch, Devon, 300-1

wills, 230n, 244, 262-4

Winchester, bishop of, see Edendon, William
  estates, 231, 238n

wind, 42, 49, 86, 105, 130, 133, 136, 160, 161, 162, 174, 175, 176, 178; and see weather

Winterthur, Johann von, 155-7

wolves, 60, 87

women, 24, 30-1, 85, 87-8, 127, 130, 131, 136

Wood Eaton, Oxon, 285-6

Worcester, bishops of, see Barnet, John; Bransford, Wolstan de; Bryan, Reginald
  city, 268
  estates, 277-80

Yersinia pestis, bacillus, 5-6, 7-8

York, archbishops of, see Thoresby, John; Zouche, William
  city, 10, 65, 89, 92, 270

Yorkshire, 269-71, 296-9

Zouche, William, archbishop of York, 10, 95, 111-12, 119, 269-71, 273, 300